D0966819

Dissociation in Children and Adolescents

Dissociation in Children and Adolescents

A Developmental Perspective

FRANK W. PUTNAM, MD

The Guilford Press
New York   London

© 1997 The Guilford Press
A Division of Guilford Publications, Inc.
72 Spring Street, New York, NY 10012
www.guilford.com

Printed in the United States of America

This book is printed on acid-free paper.

Last digit is print number: 9 8 7 6 5 4 3 2 1

Library of Congress Cataloging-in-Publication Data
Putnam, Frank W. 1947–
    Dissociation in children and adolescents : a developmental
perspective / Frank W. Putnam
      p. cm.
    Includes bibliographical references and index.
    ISBN 1-57230-219-4 (hardcover)
    1. Dissociative disorders in children.   I. Title.
RJ506.D55P87 1997
618.92'8523—dc21   97-20444
                                            CIP

*To my mother and father,
for all of the love and support
that you have given me
all of my life*

Contents

✿ Chapter One

Introduction

In the fall of 1996, the U.S. Department of Health and Human Services (1996) released details of the Third National Incidence Study of Child Abuse and Neglect. This national study found that physical and sexual abuse of children doubled from 1.4 million to 2.8 million during the period 1986 to 1993. During the same period, the number of children seriously injured by maltreatment increased almost fourfold, from 143,000 to 570,000. By 1993, only about one in four child abuse cases (28%) were being investigated by state child protective service agencies—a significant decline from roughly half (44%) of such cases in 1986. Drug abuse, poverty, and the breakdown of family structure were implicated in the rise of cases. Children from single-parent homes were at an 80% higher risk for abuse and neglect. Children living in homes with annual incomes below $15,000 were 22 times more likely to be physically abused, 18 times more likely to be sexually abused, and 56 times more likely to be neglected than those whose family incomes exceeded $30,000. This study is only one among many indices of a shocking rise in the numbers of maltreated children in the United States.

During the same period, we have learned a great deal about the outcomes associated with child maltreatment. We now know that this flood of maltreated children will become, with time, a torrent of psychiatric and medical patients requiring enormous expenditures of health care dollars to treat lifelong disorders. A substantial percentage of these children will eventually commit suicide. A substantial number will assault others. Many will abuse drugs and alcohol their entire lives. A sizeable percentage will abuse their own children—continuing a generational pattern that is steadily propelling the United States toward uncontrollable crime, violence, substance abuse, and social breakdown.

There are many adverse outcomes associated with child abuse and neglect; these are discussed in this book. The larger focus, however, is on the dissociative disorders, particularly multiple personality disorder (MPD),* in children and adolescents. We now recognize that a percentage of child maltreatment victims go on to develop dissociative disorders. Among the dissociative disorders, the prevalence of MPD in particular appears to be closely related to the prevalence of child maltreatment. We are learning something about the ways in which child abuse and neglect produce MPD and other negative outcomes. We have also learned that if we wish to understand MPD, we must take a developmental perspective.

This book organizes current knowledge about childhood-onset dissociative disorders in a manner that permits the reader to grasp the fundamental nature of pathological dissociation as it arises from childhood traumatic experiences. Seemingly bizarre dissociative symptoms—for example, the existence of multiple, alternative senses of self as manifested in MPD—are understood as failures in basic developmental processes, such as the consolidation of identity and maturation of metacognitive integrative functions. Understanding pathological dissociation from a developmental perspective informs clinical interventions, particularly with children and adolescents, who are still traveling these developmental pathways toward adulthood.

It is a daunting task to introduce readers coherently to so many concepts and so many data in a single, clinically oriented book. In particular, when symptoms are being discussed many mental processes operating at different levels are simultaneously relevant. This depth and breadth of effects make it difficult to craft a smooth, linear progression of information and ideas. Thus, to aid readers, references to earlier or later discussions of the relevant ideas and data are embedded throughout the book.

HISTORICAL PERSPECTIVE ON THE DISSOCIATIVE DISORDERS

Dissociative phenomena are associated with trauma, healing, and religious experiences in virtually all cultures. Western medical tradition includes a strong tradition of trance and dissociation in the form not only of clinical syndromes, but of altered states of consciousness induced by certain healing practices. The emergence of distinct dissociative disorder

---

*With the publication of the *Diagnostic and Statistical Manual of Mental Disorders, Fourth Edition* (DSM-IV; American Psychiatric Association, 1994), the name of this diagnosis was officially changed to "dissociative identity disorder" (DID). However, for reasons I discuss in Chapter Five, I prefer "multiple personality disorder" (MPD) and use that term throughout this book except when referring directly to DSM-IV.

diagnoses is closely intertwined with the development of modern psychology and psychiatry (Ellenberger, 1970). Clinical descriptions of pathological dissociation can be traced to the 17th century and become relatively plentiful by the 19th century (Ellenberger, 1970; Crabtree, 1988). A comparison of late-19th-century and modern cases reveals a strong clinical consistency over the last 100 years (Putnam, 1989a). Stability of core features (e.g., amnesias, trance states, automatisms) across time and cultures is one of many indicators that pathological dissociation is a fundamental form of psychopathology.

The clinical investigation of dissociation during the late 19th century was especially rich. Ellenberger's (1970) informative and readable text provides the best introduction. Other interesting accounts include Hacking's (1995) book and Crabtree's (1988) annotated bibliography. This history, much of which centers around turn-of-the-century events at the Salpêtrière Hospital in Paris, has been subjected to different readings (e.g., Ellenberger, 1970; van der Hart and Friedman, 1989; Hacking, 1995; McHugh and Putnam, 1995). No one has a definitive view of what "really" happened back then, but whichever reading one subscribes to, all parties appreciate that events at the end of the 19th century still influence our thinking today.

Foremost among 19th-century clinicians was Pierre Janet, a French psychiatrist and psychologist, whose clinical research led to the dramatic rise of interest in dissociation. Largely forgotten or ignored after World War I, Janet has only recently received recognition for his many contributions and his steadfast pursuit of knowledge about dissociation (Putnam, 1989b; van der Hart and Friedman, 1989b). Our belated recognition of Janet's legacy occurs in the midst of a resurgence of interest in dissociation that began in the late 1970s.

Trained successively as a philosopher, psychologist, and psychiatrist, Janet is additionally credited with the first clinical description of bulimia nervosa (Pope, Hudson, and Mialet, 1985), the first discussion of obsessive–compulsive disorder (Pitman, 1987), and the first articulation of a transference theory of psychotherapy (Haule, 1986). Hacking (1995) and others maintain that Janet lost interest in dissociation, multiple personality, and hysteria by 1909. However, Janet's autobiographical essay, published in 1930 at age 71, makes clear that he always remained invested in his early work:

> These studies have been somewhat forgotten today because of the discredit thrown on observations relative to hysteria since the death of Charcot in 1895. Hysteria patients seemed to disappear because they were now designated by other names. It was said that their tendency toward dissimulation and suggestibility made an examination dangerous and interpretations doubtful. I believe these criticisms to be gross-

ly exaggerated and based on prejudice and misapprehension, and I still am under the illusion that my early works were not in vain and they have left some definite ideas. . . . From the medical viewpoint, I still believe that one will eventually be compelled to return to interpretations of neuropathic disorders similar to those which I have proposed in regard to hysteria. (p. 127)

Indeed, we have returned to many of Janet's formulations—and perhaps with time we will embrace yet others. It is true that in his later years Janet deemphasized the centrality of trauma in hysteria, although trauma always retained a prominent place in his thinking about dissociation.

Certainly there are interesting parallels between our present situation and the investigation of dissociation a century ago. Perhaps most importantly, the credibility of the dissociative disorders, particularly MPD, is again being aggressively questioned (e.g., Merskey, 1992; Piper, 1994; McHugh and Putnam, 1995). The arguments made against MPD today are remarkably similar to those offered in the past. The persistence of this dispute, and the emotional nature of the arguments made for and against the validity of MPD, reflect fundamental disagreements about the source and nature of the dissociative disorders. This difference of opinion becomes most sharply focused around the approach a therapist should take toward dissociated aspects of self, such as the alter personalities of MPD. (The question of the validity of MPD is be taken up in more detail in Chapter Five.)

Now, as in the 19th century, dissociative disorders as a clinical specialty seem disproportionately to attract people interested in the workings of the human mind and in "mind–body" questions. The result is a heterogeneous group of mental health professionals and others who speak different clinical languages and have little in common with regard to training or guiding theory. This diversity is both a strength and a weakness. On the one hand, it provides the field with a wealth of perspectives and models to draw upon; on the other, it acts to discourage critical evaluation of theories and data, because of the inherent difficulties of communication across disciplines and professions. As a consequence, outrageous claims by a few practitioners often go unchallenged and may even be passed along as "clinical lore." Of course, similar processes occur in all areas of human inquiry, but few fields attract as diverse a following as the dissociative disorders.

From our late-20th-century perspective, the disappearance of the dissociative disorders from mainstream psychology and psychiatry at the beginning of the century appears to have been driven by concerns about the credibility of MPD and fears that cases were being iatrogenically produced in suggestible patients. Other influences—such as the inclusion of MPD patients under the diagnosis of schizophrenia (Rosenbaum, 1980), the rise of psychoanalytic theory with its emphasis on repression (Hart, 1926), and experiments by Messerschmidt (Messerschmidt, 1927–1928; White and Shevach, 1942) "disproving" the independence of dissociated processes—also contributed to a loss of interest in dissociation after the 1920s. The decline in the use of dissociative diagnoses is evidence that aggressive challenges to credibility can lead to their disuse in mainstream psychiatry. In turn, the current interest shows that the unique disturbances of memory and identity seen in pathological dissociation demand a viable clinical formulation and an effective therapeutic response.

CHILD AND ADOLESCENT DISSOCIATIVE DISORDERS

The history of childhood dissociative disorders parallels that of adults in terms of the ebb and flow of professional interest. Early child cases, such as Despine's (1840) report of Estelle (well reviewed by Fine, 1988), demonstrate considerable clinical continuity with modern cases. Compared with case reports of adults, fewer 19th-century child and adolescent cases are known. But the number of rediscovered old cases is growing as historians revisit dusty journals with eyes newly sharpened for dissociative symptoms in children (e.g., Bowman, 1990; Hacking, 1991).

The beginnings of modern interest in childhood and adolescent dissociative disorders are subject to debate. Congdon, Hain, and Stevenson's (1961) case of an adolescent with dual personality is arguably the first modern case report, although the authors understood little about the origin and nature of MPD. Cornelia Wilbur and Richard Kluft each reported treating children and adolescents with MPD during the late 1970s. Certainly Richard Kluft made the most significant contributions during the 1980s. In a series of articles beginning in 1984, Kluft presented case vignettes with detailed clinical phenomenology, generated a list of childhood MPD predictors to increase clinical awareness, and sketched out a treatment course and strategy (Kluft, 1984a, 1984b, 1985a, 1985b, 1986). His articles and lectures provided the field with its first coherent conceptualization of childhood MPD. Taking a life span perspective, Kluft detailed the natural history of MPD and its many clinical presentations over the life course (Kluft, 1985c, 1991).

The paper by Fagan and McMahon (1984), in which the authors drew on four cases to develop a clinical predictor list, was also influential. Single case reports published in the respected *Journal of the Ameri-*

can *Academy of Child* (later *Child and Adolescent*) *Psychiatry* further increased the credibility of childhood dissociative disorders among child psychiatrists (e.g., Bowman, Blix, and Coons, 1985; Weiss, Sutton, and Utecht, 1985; Malenbaum and Russell, 1987).

Predictor lists circulated by Kluft (1984a, 1985a), Fagan and McMahon (1984), and myself (Putnam, Helmers, and Trickett, 1993) during the early 1980's played an important role in advancing the recognition of child and adolescent cases. Independently generated from each author's clinical experience, the predictor list items were strikingly similar in many areas (see discussions in Putnam, 1986b; Reagor, Kasten, and Morelli, 1992; Tyson, 1992; Putnam et al., 1993). These initial predictor lists helped to reframe a set of apparently unconnected symptoms and behaviors into a coherent syndromic picture that is more readily recognized.

As with the adult dissociative disorders, single-case reports initially dominated the child clinical literature. Subsequent reviews served to consolidate the clinical picture and to inform revisions of predictor lists (e.g., Vincent and Pickering, 1988; Peterson, 1990). By the early 1990s, single-case reports were giving way to collected case series ranging from 10 to 50 or more children (e.g., Dell and Eisenhower, 1990; Hornstein and Tyson, 1991; Hornstein and Putnam, 1992; Reagor et al., 1992; Coons, 1994a). In most respects, results from these support earlier observations drawn from single cases. In addition, the larger case series provide a look at some of the heterogeneity of dissociative children and adolescents.

Although our data base on child and adolescent dissociative disorders is small by comparison with the adult literature, sufficient information is available to enable us to begin formulating a clinical approach. Much remains to be learned. This book is designed to acquaint the reader with pathological dissociation in children and adolescents. The intention is to provide an understanding of the principles of pathological dissociation, and of its impact on the cognition and behavior of a developing child.

DEFINING DISSOCIATION

The challenge "Define your terms!" is often heard when two parties begin arguing about the existence of something or other. Unfortunately, once the definitional fray is joined, little further progress is usually made; definitions are easy to disagree about and very hard to agree on. This is particularly true in such fields as psychology and psychiatry. As a consequence, we have largely replaced simple definitional approaches to psychiatric diagnosis with multicriterion-based systems such as the *Diagnostic and Statistical Manual of Mental Disorders* (DSM) and the *International Classification of Diseases* (ICD). The "Chinese menu" approach of such classification systems generates a larger definitional space to encompass individuals with variations on a disorder.

Still, some believe that the DSM approach is insufficiently validated and that the diagnostic categories were created too arbitrarily to capture the crux of some pathological processes. Such critics advocate the use of dimensional rather than categorical measures to assess psychopathology. The problem of selecting the "best" approach to identifying psychopathology is particularly relevant in assessment of the mental health needs of children, who often do not fit well into the adult-oriented DSM categories. The tension among the basic approaches to psychiatric diagnosis, which I refer to as the "definitional," the "descriptive DSM," and the "dimensional" approaches, will become a familiar theme in subsequent chapters.

The term "dissociation" has been defined on many occasions from many different perspectives. The descriptive DSM approach identifies the essential feature of the dissociative disorders as "a disruption in the usually integrated functions of consciousness, memory, identity, or perception of the environment" (American Psychiatric Association, 1994, p. 477). Hypnosis researchers, such as Ernest Hilgard (1986), define dissociation as "a special form of consciousness such that events that would ordinarily be connected are divided from one another "(p. 80). Adopting an information-processing model, Louis Jolyon West (1967) defines dissociation as "a psychophysiological process whereby information—incoming, stored, or outgoing—is actively deflected from integration with its usual or expected associations" (p. 890).

Other examples can be cited, but the point is that definitional approaches converge around the concept that dissociation involves a failure to integrate or associate information and experience in a normally expectable fashion. Experts disagree on whether the process is "psychophysiological" or "active" or a "special form of consciousness," but they do agree that dissociation interferes with the associative integration of information. General agreement, however, does not readily translate into meaningful diagnostic criteria.

The descriptive DSM approach to psychiatric diagnosis is to delineate disorders by specifying a list of criteria for each disorder. Many DSM diagnoses contain mixable sets of major and minor criteria. For example, the diagnosis of posttraumatic stress disorder (PTSD) requires that in addition to a person's fulfilling criteria A, E, and F, one or more of five B criteria must be met; three or more of seven C criteria must be met; and two or more of five D criteria must be met (American Psychiatric Association,

(1994). These combinations provide a minimum of 36 symptom configurations that fit within the diagnosis of PTSD. However—with the exception of dissociative disorder not otherwise specified (DDNOS), which is defined by examples—the DSM dissociative disorders are defined by simple lists without mixable options (American Psychiatric Association, (1994). It does not have to be this way. Alternative criteria systems and other dissociative disorders have been suggested (e.g., Putnam, 1993b; Peterson and Putnam, 1994). (See Chapter Five for further discussion.)

Over the last decade, the dimensional approach has made significant contributions to our understanding of normal and pathological dissociation. Dimensional measures, such as the Dissociative Experiences Scale (DES; see Chapter Four) approach dissociation from the perspective of a continuum of experience ranging from normal to pathological (Bernstein and Putnam, 1986; Waller, Putnam, and Carlson, 1996). There are problems with this approach; however, it has facilitated scientific investigation of the correlates of dissociation in normal and clinical populations. It also provides an opportunity to empirically investigate categorical (e.g., DSM diagnoses) versus dimensional models of dissociation (Putnam et al., 1996a; Waller et al., 1996). The categorical and dimensional approaches to defining and describing dissociation are discussed in greater detail in Chapter Four and elsewhere.

A related issue is the question of whether dissociation should be viewed as a "state" or a "trait" process. The "state" model assumes that an individual periodically enters into a special type of consciousness, the dissociative state. The trait model assumes that dissociation is a characteristic quality or property of an individual—one that is often assumed to have a significant heritable component. Clinical models often combine (or perhaps conflate) dimensional and categorical, state and trait distinctions. If left to definitional resolution alone, these contradictions would forever hamper our understanding of dissociation. Fortunately, they are open to empirical investigation. For the moment I will speak of "normal dissociation," meaning dissociation that is not associated with maladaptive responses, and "pathological dissociation," which includes the DSM dissociative disorders and is defined as dissociation that contributes to maladaptation. This distinction should become clearer as the book progresses.

DEVELOPMENTAL PSYCHOPATHOLOGY: A CONCEPTUAL FRAMEWORK

To understand the long-term effects of child abuse and neglect, we must understand how these experiences interact with children's psychological and biological growth and development. This is a formidable task. It requires a guiding developmental theory with which to integrate diverse information and against which to formulate testable hypotheses. Various developmental theories exist and serve to underpin specific clinical models of psychopathology. Classic Freudian psychoanalysis is an example of a therapeutic approach closely wedded to a theoretical model of psychological development. For reasons that will become apparent, I believe that the conceptual framework provided by the field of developmental psychopathology offers the best vantage point from which to understand the long-term outcomes of child abuse and neglect.

Developmental psychopathology is a conceptual framework that defines a scientific approach to normal and abnormal development. The field of developmental psychopathology is made up of researchers and clinicians from many disciplines and backgrounds who have come to appreciate the power of this approach to understanding the interactions between individuals and their environments. As initially conceived by Sroufe and Rutter (1984), developmental psychopathology was defined as *"the study of the origins and course of individual patterns of behavioral maladaptation,* whatever the age of onset, whatever the causes, whatever the transformations in behavioral manifestation and however complex the course of the developmental pattern may be" (p. 18, original italics). In endorsing this approach, the Institute of Medicine's *National Plan for Research on Child and Adolescent Mental Disorders* expanded the definition to include investigation of "the emerging behavioral repertoire, cognitive and language functions, social and emotional processes, and changes occurring in anatomical structures and physiological processes of the brain" (National Advisory Mental Health Council, 1990, p. 14).

Developmental psychopathology concerns itself with the "ontogenetic, biochemical, genetic, biological, physiological, cognitive, social-cognitive, representational, socioemotional, environmental, cultural, and societal influences on behavior" (Cicchetti and Cohen, 1995b, p. 5). Obviously, it is a multidisciplinary field that examines multiple domains of behavior and function with multiple kinds of measurements. To some this may all seem too much to keep track of, but anything less does not do justice to the complexity of the questions that the field concerns itself with. Each of these domains makes independent and interactive contributions to an individual's development over the life span.

As yet, there remains a demonstrable gap between the lofty theoretical ideals and the collection and integration of actual experimental data (Cicchetti and Cohen, 1995b). This becomes apparent in the ensuing discussions of our understanding of the developmental progression of pathological dissociation. Despite these current shortcomings, a developmental-psychopathological perspective is the most informative and comprehensive one to adopt in examining the origin and course of normal and pathological dissociation.

Core Principles of Developmental Psychopathology

The Developmental Process

A central tenet of developmental psychopathology is that individuals move between pathological and nonpathological modes of functioning (Cicchetti, 1993). Thus investigations of normal and abnormal behavior are regarded as reciprocally informative. Research in developmental psychopathology also concerns itself with the boundary area between normal and abnormal functioning.

A related focus is an interest in the mechanisms and processes that determine the ultimate outcome of risk factors (e.g., poverty and maltreatment) and protective factors (e.g., high IQ, a nurturing adult). Both normal and abnormal behavior are viewed as resulting from a dynamic transaction among these mechanisms and factors, both within the individual and between the individual and the environment. These mechanisms are revealed in the context of a series of developmental tasks that span the life of the individual and have a special salience at certain developmental stages. (See the discussions of risk and protective factors for maltreatment outcomes in Chapter Three and for pathological dissociation in Chapter Nine.)

Individual development is conceptualized as a pathway traversing a series of qualitative reorganizations within and among the biological, emotional, cognitive, and social systems of the individual (Cicchetti and Cohen, 1995b). These reorganizations involve the incorporation of older reorganizations into the current organizational structure. Thus early experience and adaptations are carried forward in time and incorporated within current adaptations. Deficits, maladaptations, and developmental shortfalls from one period may lie dormant during a later developmental stage and may reappear as problems when the individual confronts new challenges at a much later life stage. Within a given domain (e.g., socialization or cognitive functioning), developmental lags may result from maladaptation to the challenges of the environment. During later developmental reorganizations, these delays have an impact on the organizational integration of abilities and functions within and across domains. Over time, problems in one domain increasingly influence adaptation and function in other domains.

Thus, abnormal development is viewed as the progressive incorporation of problematic or pathological component structures. In such cases, Cicchetti and Cohen (1995b) observe that "the organization of the individual may then appear to consist of an integration of poorly integrated component systems" (p. 6). This seems to be very much the case for many of the psychiatric outcomes associated with serious childhood maltreatment (see Chapter Two).

As I began to grapple with a developmental-psychopathological conceptualization of pathological dissociation, I found Kurt Fischer's (Bidell & Fischer, 1992) metaphor of a "developmental web" helpful. The concept of a developmental web stands in contrast to the common notion of a "developmental ladder." A developmental ladder conjures up an image of simple linear growth—that is, moving up a ladder in a stepwise fashion—whereas a developmental web implies interconnected growth radiating in many directions. A developmental web represents the periodic interconnection of developmental threads or dimensions at various nodes, and the progressive expansion and strengthening of a fundamental but complex behavioral structure.

Final Outcomes

In any consideration of the "final" outcomes of normal and abnormal development, a number of principles need to be articulated (Cicchetti and Cohen, 1995b). The first is the principle of "equifinality"—that is, the idea that the same outcome may be achieved through a diverse set of developmental pathways. This is well illustrated by research on alternative pathways to delinquent behavior in boys (e.g., Loeber, Stouthamer-Loeber, Van Kammen, and Farrington, 1991). The second principle is the notion of "multifinality"—that is, the observation that a given developmental dimension or domain may operate differently, depending on the organization of the systems that include it (Cicchetti and Cohen, 1995b). For example, insecure attachment may contribute differently to the individual's adaptation, depending on life circumstances.

Equifinality and multifinality are both frequently present in group outcomes. For example, Cicchetti and Cohen (1995b) point out that maltreated children exhibit many symptoms in common, despite the differences in their specific life experiences (equifinality). Yet maltreated children show a wide range in the severity of outcomes, with a few children even manifesting no discernible disruption in normal development (multifinality).

The third principle involves the existence of critical or sensitive periods during development, when an individual's susceptibility to chance or directed experiences is markedly increased. Critical periods exist for the shaping of psychological, social, and biological capacities. Biological critical periods are the best demonstrated in animal studies (e.g., the well-known failure of kittens to develop functional vision if their eyes are sewn closed during early development). The existence of similar psychological and social critical periods can be inferred from research on the development of the attachment response. At certain points in the life course, individuals may be more profoundly affected by the loss of their parents or more influenced—for better or for worse—by who their friends and teachers are. For empirical examples, see research by Loeber et al. (1991) on the different developmental pathways to antisocial behavior in teenagers.

The final principle is the existence of individual differences—for example, differences in the array of intelligences possessed by an individual (for a discussion of the multiple forms of intelligence, see Gardner, 1983), or the presence or absence of specific talents or handicaps. These are often mistakenly viewed as essentially genetic factors, but cumulative life experiences make substantial contributions to long-term individual differences. Life experiences may set biological thresholds and alter physiological regulation (see discussion in Chapter Seven). The empirical investigation of individual differences through "DF" analysis (a regression model using kinship pair data) and other techniques make it possible to assess the extent to which genetic and environmental contributions differ across the range of individual differences found in a general population (Plomin and Rende, 1991).

How Is Developmental Psychopathology Used in This Book?

Developmental psychopathology provides a powerful overall framework within which we can organize and understand the diverse array of outcomes associated with childhood trauma. A central tenet of this book is that childhood maltreatment affects various developmental domains and functions that are central to the modulation and integration of behavior. These domains and functions, which are extracted from reviews of clinical data in Chapters Two and Three, individually and interactively contribute to the various psychological, social, and biological problems associated with childhood maltreatment. In particular, I focus on one key process, the modulation of behavioral states, as a core mechanism through which traumatic experiences affect different domains in a developmentally cumulative fashion that contributes to abnormal dissociative developmental trajectories.

I do not claim to be a full-fledged developmental psychopathologist. I came to adopt this conceptual approach as a result of working with traumatized children and adults. My application of developmental-psychopathological theory is best exemplified by the longitudinal study of sexually abused girls that Penelope Trickett and myself (Putnam and Trickett, 1997). Since 1987, we have followed—with a multimethod, multidomain design—the psychological, social, and biological development of a group of sexually abused girls and a group of matched comparison girls. I have learned something about how to conduct this kind of research and how to analyze and interpret the results. Nonetheless, I regard myself as an apprentice in many areas of developmental psychopathology. I point the interested reader toward the excellent two-volume textbook edited by Dante Cicchetti and Donald Cohen as the definitive reference on this exciting multidisciplinary field (Cicchetti and Cohen, 1995a).

The "Discrete Behavioral States" Model of Dissociation

Embedded within the developmental-psychopathological framework is a mechanistic model of dissociation and dissociative psychopathology, the "discrete behavioral states" (DBS) model of pathological dissociation. The DBS model seeks to account for the symptoms, behaviors, physiology, and phenomenology associated with pathological dissociation and to provide insights into therapeutic interventions. The DBS model, as presented in this book, represents a synthesis and extension of ideas and observations by a number of researchers, most notably the work of Peter Wolff (1987) and Charles Tart (1972, 1975). Unlike many theoretical models of psychopathology, the DBS model is supported by a respectable body of physiological, behavioral, psychological, and developmental data.

The model is covered more extensively from Chapter Eight on. In brief, the DBS model proposes that the behavior of children, particularly young children, is organized as a series of discrete behavioral states that follow each other in turn. Transitions between these discrete behavioral states are relatively abrupt and are manifested by observable discontinuities in behavior, cognition, affect, and attention, as well as by marked shifts in regulatory physiology.

Discrete behavioral states can be identified by operational criteria that make use of observable behaviors and physiological markers. Commonly used markers include affect, motor activity, muscle tone, spontaneous vocalization, heart rate, respiratory rate and pattern, skin perfusion, and attentional deployment (Wolff, 1987). When considered singly, these markers may appear to vary linearly. When considered in the aggregate, however, they reliably define the discrete behavioral states contained within a larger, multidimensional space of potentially available behavioral states. The DBS model provides a powerful perspective from which to view the shifting complexities of children's behavior and to understand the cumulative developmental impact of trauma-induced dissociative states of consciousness.

The work of Wolff, Emde, Harmon, Prechtl, and other researchers indicates that infants arrive in this world with their behavior organized into a set of a half-dozen or so discrete states that cycle around feeding and sleeping. As an infant develops, additional discrete states appear and the sequencing of the states becomes more complex. New states and branching pathways appear at certain points along the larger cycles, permitting the infant to follow different pathways as a result of internal or environmental interactions. The rapidly increasing complexity of these behavioral architectures, coupled with the ambulatory mobility of toddlers, makes the systematic study of this process increasingly difficult after the first year. However, qualitative and quantitative studies of certain discrete behavioral states (e.g., alcohol and drug intoxication, hypnosis, meditation, panic attacks, catatonia, rapid-cycling bipolar illness) continue to document the presence and importance of discrete behavioral states throughout the life span.

The DBS model of dissociation postulates that one of a child's critical developmental tasks is acquiring control over the modulation of behavioral states. The ability to modulate behavioral states is manifested by the child's capacity to match behavioral state appropriately with environmental demands, to sustain a desired behavioral state in the face of disruptive stimuli, to suppress an undesired state, and to reestablish a desired behavioral state when it is disrupted. The acquisition of this capacity is manifested in increasing attention span, regulation of emotion, and self-control over behavior.

A closely related developmental task is the integration of behavior across discrete behavioral states. Behavioral integration is central to the creation of a unified sense of self spanning the different behavioral-state-evoking contexts and situations that a child encounters daily. Metacognitive integrative functions both emerge from and contribute progressively to the integration of knowledge and behavior over time and across contexts. Trauma, in particular, appears to disrupt the development of metacognitive integrative functions.

Within the DBS model, dissociation is viewed as constituting a special category of discrete behavioral states. Dissociative states are characterized by alterations in accessibility of certain types of memories, skills, and knowledge, and by alterations in core aspects of sense of self and identity. There appear to be several different types of discrete dissociative states. Some are commonly present in children and follow a "normal" trajectory over the life span, usually declining in frequency with age.

Pathological dissociation represents a marked deviation from normal trajectories, with an increase in the numbers, types, and frequency of dissociative states in response to social and environmental interactions. Pathological dissociation is characterized by profound developmental disturbances in the integration of behavior and in the acquisition of developmental competencies and metacognitive executive functions. Multilevel developmental disturbances are produced by the segregation or compartmentalization of information, skills, and behavior into discrete dissociative states, such that this knowledge is only erratically (as opposed to reliably) available to the individual. Difficulties with the integration of dissociatively compartmentalized information impair metacognitive executive functions and iteratively disrupt the developmental consolidation of sense of self over the life course.

The DBS model is not complete; it contains gaps and some apparent inconsistencies. Such is the nature of theories and modeling. It has, however, the advantage of explaining a significant percentage of the hard data available and of informing clinical interventions. The applicability of the DBS model is not limited to the dissociative disorders. Indeed, the larger appeal of this model is that it draws upon and illuminates experimental and clinical data from other psychiatric conditions, such as panic attacks, bipolar illness, and periodic catatonia (Putnam, 1988). It also addresses many aspects of normal behavior in daily life. The DBS model is offered both as a guiding clinical model for interpreting symptoms and informing therapeutic interventions, and as a testable experimental model of pathological dissociation.

OVERVIEW OF THE BOOK

To understand dissociative children, it is necessary first to consider the larger clinical picture associated with childhood trauma. Chapter Two provides a brief historical summary of the growing recognition of the long-term negative effects of childhood trauma. Although many forms of trauma have been implicated in the development of pathological dissociation, childhood maltreatment is by far the most important source of trauma for children and adolescents with dissociative disorders. Accordingly, Chapter Two considers the state of knowledge about the effects of maltreatment. In particular, it reviews a diverse list of symptoms and behaviors commonly associated with maltreatment.

Chapter Three extends and integrates the information reviewed in Chapter Two. How can we account for the number, apparent diversity, and dense comorbidity of problems associated with maltreatment? Chapter Three takes two approaches to this question. The first considers how traditional factors, such as the child's age or developmental level, gender, and culture, may interact with such variables as the type and severity of maltreatment experiences and the nature of the family environment. (The reader should recall the discussion above of a developmental-psychopathological framework.) Second, the chapter examines two adult outcomes—borderline personality disorder (BPD) and eating disorders—associated with histories of maltreatment and family dysfunction. Neither BPD nor eating disorders can be said to be "caused" by maltreatment, but maltreatment appears to be an important risk factor for both. The purpose here is to identify four developmental themes (affect dysregulation; problems with impulse control; somatization and biological dysregulation; and disturbances in sense of self and identity) that appear to be common to many of the symptoms, behaviors, and disorders linked with childhood maltreatment.

Chapter Four introduces dissociation. Until recently, discussions of dissociation were largely theoretical and highly speculative. For the first time, we have reasonable measures that provide an empirical view and permit us to test hypotheses concerning the nature of dissociation, its linkage to trauma and maltreatment, and its relation to clinical symptoms and behaviors. Four lines of evidence connecting increased levels of dissociation with many types of trauma are reviewed. The question of whether dissociation exists on a normal-to-pathological continuum or as separate types (i.e., "normal" and "pathological") is raised. I return to this question repeatedly throughout the remainder of the book. Finally, the role of dissociation as a classic psychological defense is considered from the perspective of three clinically identified functions: automatization, compartmentalization, and alteration/estrangement of sense of self.

Chapter Five pursues the question of pathological dissociation, first from the perspective of clinical symptoms, and then from the perspective of the DSM dissociative disorders. Dissociative symptoms are divided into two large categories: amnesias and memory symptoms, and dissociative process symptoms. Amnesias and memory symptoms include experiences of losing time, perplexing forgetfulnesses for basic information, gaps in the continuity of autobiographical memory, amnesias for the source of information and intrusive memories (such as dissociative/posttraumatic flashbacks). Dissociative process symptoms include depersonalization and derealization, passive influence/interference experiences, auditory hallucinations, trance-like states, discrete identity disturbances (such as MPD alter personality states), and unique alterations in cognitive processing that are increasingly being conceptualized as a form of dissociative "thought disorder." The DSM approach to pathological dissociation is critiqued, and the five DSM-defined dissociative disorders are described. The chapter concludes with a discussion of the psychiatric validity of the MPD/DID construct—a topic of considerable debate.

Chapter Six begins to look at the psychobiological mechanisms implicated in pathological dissociation. Because memory symptoms play a cardinal role in the dissociative disorders, the chapter begins with a brief overview of the current understanding of memory in general and of children's memory in particular, particularly as the latter is relevant to clinical and forensic settings. Next the chapter reviews the effects of stress and trauma on memory. The question of how and why traumatic memories differ from nontraumatic memories is considered in the context of the current controversies regarding the existence of special traumatic memories. This discussion is likewise extended to children.

The second half of the chapter is devoted to a detailed discussion of the experimental data on memory performance in dissociative patients. Dissociative memory symptoms can be understood as extreme examples of dissociative-state-dependent memory storage and retrieval phenomena. Certain dissociative-like memory symptoms can even be produced in normal individuals through the creation of distinctly different mental states by means of drugs or mood manipulations. With this background, the chapter revisits the traumatic memory controversy by considering the problem of pseudomemories. It is argued that pathological dissociation probably increases susceptibility to creation of pseudomemories, but that significant trauma is necessary to produce this degree of dissociation.

The first half of Chapter Seven continues the examination of psychobiological mechanisms that are affected by trauma and potentially implicated in pathological dissociation and other trauma outcomes. An effort is made to derive higher-order principles, rather than simply to repeat recent reviews of the raw data. First, I present a table in which symptoms associated with trauma are mapped onto biological stress response systems. This mapping, based on an extensive review of the literature, offers a set of potential biological contributions to many of the trauma-related symptoms reviewed in Chapter Two. A set of general principles concerning the role of various factors in posttraumatic biological functioning is then extracted from what are admittedly preliminary research findings. Next, the chapter examines the differential psychophysiology of the alter personality states of MPD patients. When considered together with the dissociative memory research discussed in the preceding chapter, these studies collectively demonstrate that MPD patients exhibit interesting psychobiological differences across alter personality states that cannot be duplicated by simulating control subjects. The psychophysiological studies provide further evidence that pathological dissociation involves entry into discrete behavioral states, with physiological characteristics and memory storage and retrieval properties that are state-dependent. After a brief look at the fledgling research on the neurobiology and neuroanatomy of dissociation, the second half of the chapter critiques traditional explanatory models of MPD, including autohypnosis, neurological models, social role playing, animal models, and computer-based analogies.

Chapter Eight formally introduces the DBS model of pathological dissociation (discussed briefly above). The centerpiece of the book, the DBS model serves to organize the diverse lines of discussion regarding trauma and psychopathology in the first half of the book, and to inform the clinical discussion that follows. The DBS model is embedded in a developmental-psychopathological perspective and "explains" how severe, early traumatic experiences coupled with pathological parenting can result in pathological dissociation and contribute to persistent problems with affect regulation, impulse control, and consolidation of self.

Chapter Nine examines what is known about factors contributing to the development of normal and pathological dissociation. In addition to considering the traditional demographic variables identified in Chapter Three, the chapter offers a set of predictions based on the DBS model, and discusses research on the relation of normal developmental processes to dissociation. The intent is to get the reader thinking about family interactions and their effect on the child's developmental efforts to self-modulate behavioral states.

Chapter Ten is an interlude. It is organized around the theme that if the DBS model is valid, there should be evidence of its implicit operation in the everyday behaviors of normal life. In this vein, religious experience, drug use/abuse, television, sex, and sports are examined from the DBS perspective.

Chapter Eleven marks the shift to a clinical focus for the reminder of the book. It contains a series of clinical vignettes illustrating a range of dissociative phenomena in children and adolescents. Chapter Twelve reviews child/adolescent dissociative symptoms and behaviors and their differential diagnosis. It discusses an approach to diagnosis that includes information gathering, parent interviews, and child/adolescent interviews. It concludes with a discussion of strategies for the documentation of pathological dissociation, including standardized child and adolescent scales (copies of the scales themselves are provided in the Appendices), psychological testing, and longitudinal observation.

Chapter Thirteen offers general therapeutic principles for working with traumatized and dissociative children and adolescents. This broad approach grows out of my experience in writing and teaching about the treatment of pathological dissociation over the past 15 years. It is clear to me that prescriptive, step-by-step approaches actually cause more problems than they solve, as therapists struggle to assimilate concrete dictates into their personal models of how to conduct therapy with a given person. I elucidate principles and goals, and leave therapists to determine how these are best achieved for a given situation.

Chapter Fourteen begins with a discussion of clinical outcomes for maltreated children in general and dissociative children in particular. There are remarkably few hard data. The chapter continues with a discussion of therapeutic issues that commonly occur in the course of working with dissociative and traumatized children. Specific questions that arise in the therapy of MPD, such as when to work directly with alter personality states, are taken up here. The chapter concludes with a discussion of play therapy approaches to trauma and dissociation.

Treatment of a traumatized and dissociative child must always occur in the context of the child's primary caretaking situation, be it with biological or foster parents, or in a group home or residential setting. Chapter Fifteen addresses the difficult issues that must be confronted within the larger caretaking context. The final chapter reviews the psychopharmacological treatment of trauma and dissociation. It begins with an overview of the principles of pediatric psychopharmacology, and then discusses appropriate target symptoms and relevant medications.

SUMMARY

Pathological dissociation has been a controversial subject for more than a century. Many of the arguments from the past continue in some form today. Critics often focus their attacks on a mythical version of MPD, promulgated in part by the popular media. In the last decade, hundreds of scientific and clinical studies of dissociation have been published. This book seeks to integrate these around a conceptual model that informs treatment and further investigation.

Multiple definitions of dissociation exist. They converge around the idea that dissociation represents a failure of integration of ideas, information, affects, and experience. Clinically, pathological dissociation is approached from two perspectives—the categorical (DSM) approach and the dimensional approach. Each has its strengths and weaknesses, which will become apparent in later discussions.

The history of the clinical recognition of pathological dissociation in children and adolescents parallels that of adults, although it lags behind in numbers of cases and general clinical awareness. Early reports by Kluft and by Fagan and McMahon are credited with stimulating the field. This book examines child and adolescent pathological dissociation from a developmental-psychopathological perspective, which serves as the foundation for understanding the impact of maltreatment and trauma on young children. Embedded within this developmental psychopathological perspective is a mechanistic model of pathological dissociation, the DBS model. The DBS model postulates that early in development, a young child's behavior is organized as a set of discrete behavioral states. Healthy cognitive and affective development requires that the child acquire control (modulation) over these behavioral states. Pathological dissociation reflects a profound disruption in the self-modulation of discrete behavioral states, together with metacognitive failures in the integration of information and sense of self across behavioral states.

Chapter Two

The Nature and Effects of Childhood Trauma and Maltreatment

The recognition that childhood trauma is widespread has increased, but a deeper understanding of children's responses to trauma has been slow to emerge. The failure to appreciate the unique aspects of childhood trauma is a result of a number of factors, but the principal problem remains the reluctance of society to acknowledge the traumatization of children. This blindness—which at times takes the form of a delusional romanticizing of childhood—denies legitimacy and resources to those seeking to understand and treat traumatized children.

Most of what we know comes from the work of a few dedicated professionals working in diverse settings. Until recently, their findings were often ignored or disbelieved by their peers. See, for example, Benedek's (1985) description of a professional audience's hostile, mocking responses to Lenore Terr's (1979, 1983) landmark work with the children kidnapped at Chowchilla, California. Both society in general and the helping professions in particular are just beginning to comprehend the lifelong legacy of childhood trauma.

As yet, there is no larger synthesis of these differing sources of knowledge. Clinicians and researchers working with different types of childhood traumatization are just beginning to come together in professional forums to hear about each other's work. In addition to the unique aspects of the different types of trauma, differences in professional orientation and clinical approach slow—but ultimately enrich—the integration of knowledge. As clinicians and researchers seek to intervene and to study newly emerging sources of traumatization in U.S. society (e.g., the explosion of drug-related community violence in U.S. inner cities), they draw upon information gleaned from earlier work with children exposed to war, disasters, and maltreatment. A more solid integration of knowledge about the effects of childhood trauma will ultimately emerge from current multidisciplinary approaches.

I begin this chapter by briefly reviewing the history of the study of childhood trauma, and briefly outlining the sources of such trauma that are not related to actual maltreatment. I then turn to a more detailed examination of child maltreatment—its definitions, its incidence/prevalence, and matters related to its detection and reporting.

A BRIEF HISTORY OF PROGRESS IN UNDERSTANDING CHILDHOOD TRAUMA AND ITS SEQUELAE

Clinical reports of children living in institutions, particularly orphanages, began to appear in the latter half of the 19th century (Langmeier and Matejcek, 1973; Benedek, 1985). These children—many of them traumatized by the loss of their parents through death or abandonment—demonstrated developmental delays and intellectual deficits. Although these observations were unsystematic by modern standards, they suggested to some that psychological factors might influence physical and intellectual development (Benedek, 1985). Little was described by way of treatment, except for attention to the improvement of the children's hygiene and physical surroundings.

World War II, with its massive decimation of civilian populations, produced large numbers of displaced and abandoned children. Years of suffering—witnessed and experienced violence; the loss of parents, relatives, and friends; malnutrition; and imprisonment—left deep scars on that generation. Studies by Solomon (1942) and by Anna Freud (Freud and Burlingham, 1943) suggested that parental responses to traumatic experiences were critical in shaping a child's reactions to such events. Anna Freud's work indicated that, in the absence of parents or other family members, peer support was important in mitigating the consequence of wartime traumatization (Freud and Burlingham, 1943). Reports on the World War II generation continue to inform us about the long-term effects of such experiences (e.g., Yehuda et al., 1995).

The postwar work of René Spitz (1945, 1946) on "hospitalism" and anaclitic depression in institutionalized children had a profound impact on the field of child development in general and on the field's understanding of the effects of maltreatment in particular. Early work on separation and loss in children, together with John Bowlby's (1958, 1982) seminal conceptualization of the attachment response as a biological function indispensable for human survival, provided a powerful new perspective on the effects of trauma on child development. The concept of attachment has been elaborated by many additional studies of normal, disturbed, and traumatized children. It is one of the most fruitful approaches to understanding normal and abnormal development (Thompson, 1991). Attachment theory has become a mainstay of the developmental-psychopathological approach to the effects of maltreatment on children (Cicchetti and Carlson, 1989).

Today, more attention is being paid to the problems and needs of traumatized children. Experienced researchers are actively working with a variety of types of traumatized children. In addition to studies of maltreated children, investigators are working with refugee children from war zones, and even with children living in the midst of war and ethnic strife. The pioneering work of Robert Pynoos, Spencer Eth, and their colleagues with children who have witnessed homicide, suicide, and rape has produced an appreciation of just how traumatizing exposure to violence can be for child eyewitnesses (Pynoos and Eth, 1984, 1985; Pynoos et al., 1987; Pynoos and Nader, 1988).

NONMALTREATMENT SOURCES OF TRAUMA TO CHILDREN

Community Violence

By virtually all indices, the United States is the most violent country in the industrialized world (Richters and Martinez, 1993; Osofsky, 1995). For adolescents and young adults between 15 and 24, homicide is the second leading cause of death. African-American males are homicide victims seven times more often than same-age European-American males (Richters and Martinez, 1993). Homicide rates are only one index of violence and fail to capture the chronic exposure of citizens and their children to almost daily violence in some inner-city neighborhoods.

In a seminal study conducted under risky conditions, Richters and Martinez (1993; Martinez and Richters, 1993) found that 9% of first- and second-graders and 14% of fifth- and sixth-graders had witnessed a shooting, and that 25% and 43%, respectively, had seen a mugging. The Washington, D.C., neighborhood studied by Richters and Martinez was classified as only moderately violent by official crime statistics. Similar high rates of witnessed violence have been reported in a survey of 6th-, 8th-, and 10th-graders in New Haven, Connecticut (Marans and Cohen, 1993); in a study of African-American children in Chicago (Bell and Jenkins, 1993); and in a study of children seen at a Boston public pediatric clinic (Groves, Zuckerman, Marans, and Cohen, 1993). A study of 2,248 urban public school 6th-, 8th-, and 10th-graders found that 40% had seen a shooting or stabbing in the previous year (Schwab-Stone et al., 1995). My work at City Lights, an alternative school for high-risk adolescents in Washington, D.C., opened my eyes to the extraordinary levels of violence witnessed by many disadvantaged inner-city children (Putnam, 1993a).

Disasters

Floods, hurricanes, tornadoes, earthquakes, and the like are common events. Transportation and technological disasters (e.g., airplane crashes and industrial accidents) are not uncommon. Studies of the effects of disasters on adults show clear increases in psychopathology, compared with control groups or baseline measures (Rubonis and Blickman, 1991). Although these effects are not as well studied in children, studies and reviews suggest that natural and human-made disasters cause considerable acute distress and long-term effects in a substantial percentage of children and adolescents (Belter and Shannon, 1993; Yule, 1993; Garrison et al., 1995).

War and Civil Conflict

The bombings of the World Trade Center in New York City, and of the Federal Building in Oklahoma City, Oklahoma, brought home the fact that terrorist acts do occur and will continue to occur in the United States. In addition to home-based terrorism, the United States often receives influxes of refugee children from war-torn areas of the world (Arroyo and Eth, 1985; Seine et al., 1995). Exposure to war or violent civil strife does not automatically produce psychopathology in children (Jensen and Shaw, 1993). In low- to moderate-intensity situations, especially when children and their family members are not directly involved, children appear to acclimate to the situation. However, longitudinal studies of children exposed to extreme situations find that many develop PTSD or posttraumatic symptoms that persist well into adulthood (Jensen and Shaw, 1993; Hubbard, Realmuto, Northwood, and Masten, 1995).

Domestic Violence

Domestic batterings, stabbings, and shootings are common. It is estimated that 3.3 million children are exposed to acts of violence between their parents (Thormaehlen and Bass-Feld, 1994). Children in such households witness many levels of violence, from explicit threats to sexual and homicidal assaults. Domestic violence is intentional and repetitive, and involves emotional abuse and intimidation. Domestic violence is also associated with many other parental and family problems, which compound the effects of the witnessed violence. Joy Osofsky (1995) has eloquently reviewed the research on the effects of exposure to violence on young children. According to what we know about the effects of witnessing injury and death to loved ones, children exposed to domestic violence probably represent a large—and largely unrecognized—group of traumatized children.

Accidents and Injuries

Accidents are the most common cause of death among children (Marzurek, 1994). Many serious accidents occur, often producing significant posttraumatic symptoms. For example, about 40,000 children under age 15 years are hospitalized for serious burns every year (Herndon, Rutan, and Rutan, 1993). Incidentally, burns are involved in many physical abuse cases, and up to 26% of pediatric burn admissions result from abuse (Renz and Sherman, 1992). In one study, dog bites accounted for about 1 out of every 200 emergency room visits and usually involved children under the age of 15 years (Wiggins, Akeman, and Weiss, 1994). (The second most commonly attacked group is older women.) Dog attacks on children are usually far worse than simple bites; they often involve hideous hand and facial injuries (particularly to the nose), which require extensive reconstructive surgery. Children mauled by dogs frequently develop posttraumatic symptoms requiring lengthy treatment.

Conclusion

The point of this overview is that, as a group, children are frequently exposed to violence and accidents. Clinical research with children exposed to these and similar sources of trauma has contributed to our knowledge. However, for our purposes, the most relevant source of information about the effects of trauma on children is the knowledge gleaned from clinical experience and research with maltreated children. From here on, I focus on child maltreatment and its effects in this book, but research on other sources of childhood trauma is included when it is informative.

CHILD MALTREATMENT

Definitions

The definition of "child maltreatment" remains a problem for social and legal policy makers, clinicians, and researchers (Barnett, Manly, and Cicchetti, 1991). Giovannoni (1989) has explored the evolution of our definitions of child maltreatment as they have emerged in social, legal, medical, and mass media contexts. Although one can point to statutes dating to colonial times, most U.S. social and legal conceptualizations of child maltreatment originated in the 19th century.

Wissow (1995) defines child maltreatment as "the intentional harm or a threat of harm to a child by someone acting in the role of caretaker, for even a short time" (p. 1425). Most authorities divide child maltreatment into neglect, physical abuse, sexual abuse, and emotional abuse; for the purposes of this book, child maltreatment includes the wide range of behaviors and conditions that can be subsumed under these four general categories. Reports of neglect—defined as a caretaker's failure to provide for basic needs and care, medical care, supervision, and/or support—typically outnumber all other forms of abuse combined. Physical abuse involves inflicting bodily injury through excessive force or physically endangering a child through circumstance or activity (Wissow, 1995). Sexual abuse includes both active and passive sexual contact, as well as exposing a child to sexual acts or materials (Wissow, 1995). Emotional abuse—the most difficult category to define—usually involves emotional coercion or disparagement that interferes with a child's social and psychological development (Wissow, 1995).

Incidence and Prevalence

As with many criminal behaviors, it is difficult to be certain of the precise incidence and prevalence of child maltreatment. Several organizations release statistics and reports based on survey data or the collation of child protection agency records. In most instances, the numbers grow yearly and range between 1.4 million (Wissow, 1995) and 2.9 million (U.S. Department of Health and Human Services, and National Center on Child Abuse and Neglect, 1996) children a year. An estimated 150,000—200,000 children experience serious to life-threatening injuries, and between 2,000 and 5,000 die yearly (National Center on Child Abuse and Neglect, 1988; Wissow, 1995). More children die every year from maltreatment than from automobile accidents. Much (probably most) maltreatment goes unreported, and national surveys generally find higher rates of abuse and violence than statistics gathered from agencies indicate (Finkelhor and Dziuba-Leatherman, 1994). Child maltreatment occurs across all economic and cultural groupings, although children in families at lower socioeconomic levels tend to be at greater risk (see Chapter One).

The reported incidences of different types of child abuse vary with age. Neglect is most commonly reported for younger children, in part because it is easier to identify and substantiate neglect for infants and toddlers than for teenagers. A disproportionate number of maltreatment fatalities involve younger children; children under age 5 account for 80% of deaths (Wissow, 1995). Statistics indicate that the incidence of sexual abuse peaks between the ages of 7 and 10 years. However, our data suggest to us that this may be an artifact resulting from averaging distinctly younger and older age groups, and that relatively few cases actually fit the average (Trickett, Reiffman, Horowitz, and Putnam, in press). The highest risk for sexual abuse to females occurs at about 3–4 years of age (Bronfenbrenner Life Course Center, 1996). Physical abuse appears to have two peaks—one during infancy and early childhood, and another during the teenage years. Emotional abuse appears to increase steadily with age (Wissow, 1995).

Different types of abuse frequently co-occur. Emotional abuse frequently accompanies physical abuse, especially when such abuse is inflicted in the context of punishment. Coercion and intimidation are often part of sexual abuse, particularly for older children who understand the improper nature of what is happening. Physical coercion into sexual acts often occurs for older children, particularly when the perpetrator is not the biological father and cannot rely on parental authority and relationship to enforce compliance. As Dante Cicchetti observes, it is usually more accurate to characterize a child's experiences as "maltreatment" than as one type or another of "abuse."

Detection and Reporting of Abuse and Neglect

Mental health professionals are ethically obligated and usually legally mandated to report suspicions or evidence of child maltreatment to the appropriate authorities (Kalichman, 1993). State laws vary as to which individuals are mandated reporters. In some states, all citizens are mandated reporters. In others, certain categories of professionals are not covered by statute (e.g., school psychologists are mandated reporters, but research psychologists are not). It is important for clinicians to know the law for their state.

With the partial exception of physical abuse, most maltreatment is difficult to detect. Clinicians should maintain a high index of suspicion and notify the proper authorities of any reasonable suspicion. Disclosure of maltreatment can be facilitated by routinely asking about such experiences during history taking (Wissow, 1995). Parents can be asked, "Have you ever been involved in a relationship where there was physical violence?" or "When you were a child, did anything ever happen that you considered to be physically or sexually abusive?" (Wissow, 1995, p. 1426). A positive response to either query can be followed up with a question such as "Have you ever had any concern about these things in your present relationship?" (Wissow, 1995, p. 1426). Children can be asked about how they get along with their parents, or can be asked questions such as "Have you ever been afraid that someone is going to hurt you or to do something to you that you didn't want?" Positive responses should be followed up with an open-ended question, such as "Can you please tell me about it?"

If maltreatment is suspected, an appropriate report should be made to the child protection agency in the child's city or county. Forensic investigative interviews with children are the province of trained professionals and should not be conducted by interviewers who are unfamiliar with children's cognitive capacities and the ways in which they can be influenced or misled.

The reliability of children's accounts of sexual abuse and other maltreatment is a topic of heated debate—much of which occurs in the court room. This adversarial context impedes reasoned discussion of what we do and do not know and how we should conceptualize the issues. Lamb, Sternberg, and Esplin (1994) point out that confusion between questions of competency and questions of credibility clouds this issue. "Competency" is the ability to communicate information about one's past experiences, whereas "credibility" concerns the accuracy and truthfulness of that information. Separating these two issues illuminates much of the data we have on the reliability of children's testimony. The topic of the reliability of children's traumatic memories is taken up again in Chapter Six.

Signs and Symptoms of Physical Abuse

Physical abuse may leave key signs and symptoms that health care providers should be alert for. Kempe, Silverman, Steele, Droegemueller, and Silver (1962) began the modern era of medical diagnosis of child maltreatment with their description of the "battered-child syndrome." A decade later, Caffey (1972) added the "shaken-baby syndrome." The descriptions of these two syndromes have done much to alert professionals to physical abuse and have gained wide acceptance in court (Wissow, 1995). The battered-child syndrome usually occurs in children under age 3 and includes subdural hematoma, single or multiple fractures in various stages of healing, soft-tissue injury, multiple bruises or cuts, failure to thrive, and patterns of injury that are not consistent with the explanations given (Wissow, 1995). The shaken-baby syndrome usually occurs in infants and children under 2 years of age and is manifested in subdural or subarachnoid hemorrhage, focal or diffuse brain injury, retinal hemorrhage, cervical spine injury, and rib and metaphyseal long-bone fractures (Wissow, 1995).

In general, signs suggestive of physical abuse include multiple injuries in different stages of healing and/or injuries that fit the shape or pattern of an identifiable object (e.g., a burn in the shape of an iron). The type and age are the injury is often inconsistent with the explanation provided by the caretaker, and the story may change with retelling (Wissow, 1995). Certain disorders (e.g., osteogenesis imperfecta) can be misinterpreted as physical abuse; therefore, evaluation by a trained professional is mandatory even when apparent signs of physical abuse are present.

Physical Diagnosis of Sexual Abuse

Unfortunately, there are seldom definitive physical findings in sexual abuse cases. Children believed to have been sexually abused within the previous 48–72 hours should be examined at a rape treatment center for collection of forensic evidence, such as semen, pubic hair, and fibers (Wissow, 1995). Presence of a sexually transmitted disease (STD) is widely regarded as a significant finding, but certain STDs (e.g., chlamydia and gonorrhea) may be transmitted perinatally. Nonsexual transmission has been postulated (but not proven) to occur for herpes, human papillomavirus, and trichomonas (Wissow, 1995). The relation of genital warts to sexual abuse is controversial, and authorities differ on the upper age limit for latent perinatal infection, after which sexual abuse is suspected (Cohen, Honig, and Androphy, 1990; Gutman, Herman-Giddens, and Phelps, 1993; Wissow, 1995).

Changes in female genital anatomy have been investigated as markers for sexual abuse. Increased hymenal diameter has been suggested as an indicator of genital trauma, but studies show considerable variation in normal anatomy. Hymenal size and configuration may also vary as a result of differences in the examination technique and the child's state of relaxation (Wissow, 1995). It is even suggested that in some cases a traumatized hymen may return to its original diameter within a few weeks to months (McCann, Voris, and Simon, 1992).

One important sign that has been largely overlooked is the presence of vaginal foreign bodies (VBFs). In a seminal review, augmented by a case series, Herman-Giddens (1994) makes a strong case that the presence of a VBF is a likely indicator of sexual abuse. In prepubertal girls, VBFs often produce a classic triad of vaginal bleeding or spotting, discharge, and odor. In retrospect, this was probably responsible for the bloody vaginal discharges observed in the case of Penni (see Chapter Eleven).

In summary, there are no undisputed markers of child maltreatment, particularly sexual abuse. Clinicians should maintain a high index of suspicion for the possibility of maltreatment. When possible abuse or neglect is suspected, the appropriate authorities should be notified. (See the discussion of the physical examination in Chapter Twelve.)

SYMPTOMS AND BEHAVIORS IN MALTREATED AND TRAUMATIZED CHILDREN AND ADOLESCENTS

Development of Research

The course of research on the effects of maltreatment and trauma on children and adolescents follows a familiar path. Beginning with impressionistic case series in the late 1970s to mid-1980s, we are moving into an era of increasingly sophisticated design and methodology (Aber, Allen, Carlson, and Cicchetti, 1989). Although results from early studies were informative, they were constrained by a number of limitations. Clinical samples of convenience (i.e., samples selected on the basis of accessibility rather than representativeness) were commonly studied. Early studies had small samples that contained a heterogeneous mixture of types and severity of maltreatment. Children were typically assessed only once, usually shortly after disclosure of maltreatment, and were rarely evaluated in more than one context. Age/developmental stage and gender differences were often not examined. Home environments were not characterized, and parental psychopathology was seldom included.

Each of these factors (and others) has proven important in understanding outcomes associated with maltreatment and trauma. Current studies address many of these earlier problems—at least in part. Unfortunately, the current funding climate has already seriously curtailed the next level of studies (Thompson and Wilcox, 1995). The youngest generation of investigators is being lost as research grants prove almost impossible to get. Indeed, child abuse research has fallen upon very hard times. These problems are not limited to child trauma research; they are coming to dominate the larger arena of child and adolescent health problems.

As research becomes more sophisticated, so do the conceptual models that help us understand and integrate the findings. No single model dominates the maltreatment field. Early models were psychoanalytically oriented and organized around defensive processes, such as identification with the aggressor. Current models can be divided into those focused around categorical diagnoses (e.g., the model centered around the DSM diagnosis of PTSD) and those postulating disturbances along one or more developmental dimensions—for example, Finkelhor's (1988) traumagenic model, Spaccarelli's (1994) appraisal model, and

Cicchetti's developmental/transactional model (Cicchetti and Carlson, 1989; Cicchetti and Lynch, 1995). Each has its strengths and weaknesses. At this state of our knowledge, it is unrealistic to expect a single model to cover all the bases. As discussed in Chapter One, I favor a developmental-psychopathological perspective.

In terms of understanding the effects of trauma and maltreatment on children and adolescents, present purposes are best served by approaching the data in a series of steps. I begin here by reviewing the various symptoms and behaviors associated with histories of maltreatment and trauma. In Chapter Three, I consider a number of cross-cutting factors that influence maltreatment outcomes, such as age/developmental stage, gender, types and severity of trauma, and the mediating effects of the child's environment. I also consider four common developmental themes that link different adult DSM diagnoses associated with child maltreatment. The overall intention of the discussion in these two chapters is to outline a broad, developmentally-informed, perspective from which to consider the impact of childhood trauma and its relationship to juvenile dissociative disorders.

DSM-Defined PTSD in Maltreated Children and Adolescents

In his remarkable book, *Achilles in Vietnam* (1994), Jonathan Shay juxtaposes passages of Homer's *Iliad* with narratives from Vietnam veterans to highlight the antiquity and the universal nature of posttraumatic symptoms. The definition of a specific set of posttraumatic symptoms as a distinct psychiatric diagnosis, PTSD, awaited the DSM-III (American Psychiatric Association, 1980), although clinical precursors such as "railway spine" and "soldiers' heart" anticipated this formulation by more than a century.

Clinical experience with Vietnam combat veterans was especially instrumental in the creation of the diagnosis. As conceptualized by the DSM, PTSD involves the production of three basic sets of symptoms— reexperiencing, avoidance and numbing, and hyperarousal—as a direct response to an identifiable traumatic stressor (American Psychiatric Association, 1980, 1987, 1994). Reexperiencing symptoms involve intrusive and distressing memories, thoughts, mental images, dreams, and flashbacks related to the traumatic event. Avoidant and numbing symptoms involve attempts to avoid exposure to reminders of the trauma and include attempts at thought stopping, social withdrawal, amnesia for the trauma, and constriction of affect. Hyperarousal symptoms include irritability, explosive anger, hypervigilance, problems with concentration, and difficulty falling and staying asleep.

Classified as an anxiety disorder, DSM formulations of PTSD have proven controversial and faced challenges with each revision (Putnam, 1996c; Brett, 1996; van der Kolk, 1996; Yehuda and McFarlane, 1995). These formulations have focused on whether PTSD is appropriately classified as an anxiety disorder, the difficulty in defining what constitutes a traumatic stressor, problems with the generalization of a combat-based PTSD formulation to other forms of trauma, and the high rates of comorbidity with other primary psychiatric disorders. In particular, PTSD is highly associated with affective disorders, anxiety disorders, conduct disorder, and substance abuse disorders (e.g., Kessler, Sonnega, Bromet, Hughes, and Nelson, 1995); leading critics to argue that the DSM formulation is too narrowly drawn to capture the complexity of posttraumatic responses (e.g., van der Kolk, 1996).

Clinicians and researchers have questioned the appropriateness of applying adult PTSD criteria to children and adolescents (Armsworth and Holaday, 1993; Finkelhor, 1990; Hillary and Schare, 1993; Putnam, 1996c). As a clinical construct, the idea of PTSD is useful in that most studies find that the majority of traumatized children manifest one or more symptoms that fall within the core PTSD symptom sets. However, the majority of traumatized children do not fulfill DSM criteria for PTSD as a disorder (Fletcher, 1996). Traumatized children, especially younger children, may also manifest posttraumatic symptoms that differ from adults and thus do not quality them for a DSM diagnosis (McNally, 1991; Scheeringa, Zeanah, Drell, and Larrieu, 1995; Fletcher, 1996).

Using a sample of children and adults who had witnessed a school-yard shooting, Schwarz and Kowalski (1991) investigated the effects of the increasingly restrictive series of DSM definitions on the diagnostic rates for PTSD in children and adults. Applying each in turn, they found marked differences in the frequencies and patterns of symptoms endorsements and concluded that DSM-III-R and DSM-IV criteria in particular favored the diagnosis in adults over children. Scheeringa and colleagues (1995) applied DSM-IV criteria to 20 severely traumatized infant cases and found that, although all showed many symptoms of impairment, none qualified for a diagnosis. Based on this analysis, they derived a set of alternative PTSD criteria for infants and toddlers, which, when applied to new cases, had better reliability than the DSM-IV.

The DSM-IV definition of PTSD includes three reexperiencing symptom variants for children allowing for traumatic play, dreams without recognizable content, and trauma-specific reenactments to qualify (American Psychiatric Association, 1994). The newly defined criteria for a traumatic stressor allows for disorganized or agitated behaviors in children to substitute for the fear, helplessness, or horror response required of adults. Many child clinicians, however, feel that these additions are not sufficient to bridge the differences between children and adults.

The requirement for three denial or avoidant symptoms has frequently been identified as developmentally inappropriate because these symtpoms are especially difficult to reliably assess in children (Fletcher, 1996; Green, 1993; Schwarz and Kowalski, 1991). Scheeringa and colleagues (1995) required only a single avoidant symptom which they expanded to include constriction of play, social withdrawal, or decreased range of affect. They also included loss of acquired developmental skills, particularly regression in language or toilet training under this category. They added a "new fears or aggression" criterion to cover the commonly observed appearance of new anxieties or agression in acutely traumatized children. Problems with applying the adult notion of a "foreshortened sense of future" to children have also been identified.

Diagnostic criteria based on posttraumatic aberrations of play present a rich opportunity to articulate more developmentally salient criteria for children. In addition to the repetition, reenactment, and affective constriction often described in posttraumatic play, children may exhibit avoidant and dissociative play behaviors (see discussion in Chapter Fourteen). Loss of social, academic, and self-care skills and a variety of behavioral regressions provide yet another opportunity to capture posttraumatic symptoms in children. For example, many acutely traumatized children exhibit a marked age regression in their television program choices. For sexually abused children, inappropriate sexual behaviors (perhaps a form of posttraumatic reenactment?) could be also included. Somatic symptoms may also serve as traumatic reenactments in children and should be considered as alternative criteria (Amaya-Jackson and March, 1993).

Although clinicians may chose, for a variety of reasons, to assign a diagnosis of PTSD to a child who does not fulfill DSM criteria (researchers are not permitted this option), it should be recognized that most traumatized children do not officially qualify as having PTSD. Therefore, it is usually more appropriate to characterize such children as having posttraumatic symptoms or responses rather than as having PTSD. In the following chapters, I will endeavor to speak of posttraumatic symptoms to describe situations where children fall short of the disorder, but nonetheless have significant reexperiencing, avoidance and numbing, and hyperarousal symptoms. We have good reason to believe that many of these children are significantly distressed and impaired and deserve the same level of attention and intervention as those children who qualify for a DSM diagnosis.

Dimensional Assessments of the Effects of Maltreatment

In Chapter Five I provide a detailed dimensional consideration of what I describe there as "primary" dissociative symptoms, and in Chapter Four I examine the lines of evidence linking these symptoms to trauma and maltreatment. The maltreatment effects I describe in this section overlap to a considerable extent with the "secondary" and "tertiary" symptoms set forth in Chapter Five. Although several of the effects discussed below (e.g., depression, anxiety, somatization) correspond to various DSM diagnoses themselves, they are conceived of here as *ranges* of symptoms and behaviors on which maltreated youngsters show more extreme responses than various nonmaltreated populations—not as formal diagnoses.

Depression and Anxiety

Depression and depressive symptoms are common short- and long-term outcomes in victims of childhood maltreatment. At least three major reviews document this association (Browne and Finkelhor, 1986; Beitchman et al., 1992; Polusny and Follette, 1995). This is true for both clinical and nonclinical samples (Polusny and Follette, 1995). A large community study assessing depression with the National Institute of Mental Health (NIMH) Diagnostic Interview Schedule found rates of depression ranging from 13.4% to 21.9% of abused and 3.9% to 5.6% of nonabused subjects (Burnam et al., 1988). The mechanisms underlying the high rates of depression in adults with maltreatment histories are not known. It is likely that biological factors, such as dysregulation of the hypothalamic–pituitary–adrenal (HPA) axis, play a significant role. Psychological phenomena (e.g., guilt and shame) are probably also important. For example, Andrews (1995) found that feelings of shame were significantly related to chronic or recurrent depression in women abused in childhood. Zlotnick, Ryan, Miller, and Keitner (1995) compared 12-month rates of recovery from depression in abused and nonabused women; nonabused women were 3.7 times more likely to have recovered by 12 months.

The existence of significant depression in children was not widely accepted until the early 1980s—the same period when the first reports of high rates of depression in maltreated children began to appear (Blumberg, 1981). Numerous studies of clinical samples have found elevated levels of depression in maltreated children (e.g., Allen and Tarnowski, 1989; Cerezo and Frias, 1994; Mancini, Van Ameringen, and MacMillan, 1995). Comparing sexually abused children at initial intake and again 18 months later, Oates, O'Toole, Lynch, Stern, and Cooney (1994) found that initial depressive symptoms improved in some children. However, at the latter evaluation, 35% still had significant depression and 56% had dysfunctional levels of self-esteem.

In addition to PTSD (which is classified as an anxiety disorder in the DSM), higher rates of agoraphobia and social phobia (Pribor and Dinwiddie, 1992; Saunders et al., 1992), as well as of simple phobias and panic disorder (Burnam et al., 1988; Pribor and Dinwiddie, 1992; Saunders et al., 1992), have been reported for abused than for nonabused subjects. Beyond PTSD, there does not seem to be much specificity for which type of anxiety disorder occurs. In a study of 205 consecutive adult anxiety disorder patients, Mancini et al. (1995) found that 23.4% reported childhood sexual abuse and 44.9% reported physical abuse. Abused patients had significantly higher depression and anxiety scale scores, as well as greater impairments in social functioning, but a history of abuse was not specific for any particular anxiety disorder.

Suicidal and Self-Destructive Behaviors

Arthur Green (1967, 1968) should be credited with first recognizing the relationship between maltreatment and self-destructive behaviors. In the first controlled study, Green (1978) found that physically abused children exhibited significantly more suicidal and self-destructive behaviors than normal and neglected children. Subsequent studies have replicated his seminal observations in children, adolescents, and adults. For example, Rosenthal and Rosenthal (1984) found high rates of abuse and neglect in their study of suicidal preschoolers. Deykin, Alpert, and McNamara (1985) compared rates of prior contact with the department of social services for abuse and neglect in 159 adolescents who had attempted suicide and two nonsuicidal comparison groups treated for medical conditions. Contact with the department was three to six times higher for suicide attempters. Numerous other child and adolescent studies report significant correlations between maltreatment severity variables and suicidal and self-harmful behaviors.

Studies of self-destructive behavior in adults drive this point home. van der Kolk, Perry, and Herman (1991) and colleagues prospectively followed patients with personality disorders or bipolar II disorder for an average of 4 years. They found that histories of childhood physical and sexual abuse were highly predictive of self-cutting and suicide attempts. In a random community sample in New Zealand, Romans, Martin, Anderson, Herbison, and Mullen (1995) found a clear statistical association between sexual abuse in childhood and self-harm. This replicated an earlier community sample study of Canadian women by Bagley and Ramsay (1986). Community sample studies by Jackson, Calhoun, Amick, Maddever, and Habif (1990) and Saunders et al. (1992) report comparable findings. Other investigators have reported similar results in clinical and nonclinical samples (e.g., Briere and Runtz, 1986; Brown and Anderson, 1991; Boudewyn and Liem, 1995). Most studies find significant "dose–effect" relationships between indices of abuse severity and likelihood of self-harm (e.g., van der Kolk et al., 1991; Boudewyn and Liem, 1995; Romans et al., 1995).

Obviously, maltreatment in childhood is only one source contributing to the spectrum of self-harm behaviors in psychiatric patients. Other sources of trauma have been implicated in case reports—for example, rape (Greenspan and Samuel, 1989) and combat trauma (Lyons, 1991). It should be noted that various medical conditions are also associated with self-harm in children, including genetic and metabolic disorders such as Cornelia de Lange syndrome, Lesch–Nyhan syndrome, and familial dysautonomia (N. Putnam and Stein, 1984). Finally, self-harmful behavior also occurs in nonabused depressed children, mentally retarded children, and children with pervasive developmental disorders. Therefore, self-destructive behaviors alone should not be assumed to imply maltreatment.

Sexualized Behaviors

Psychosexual problems are considered the strongest and most specific effect of sexual abuse (Friedrich, 1993; Cosentino, Meyer-Bahlburg, Alpert, Weinberg, and Gaines, 1995; Knutson, 1995). From early clinical reports (e.g., Yates, 1982) to well-controlled empirical studies (e.g., Cosentino et al., 1995), sexually abused children have consistently been found to be highly eroticized, often behaving in grossly inappropriate sexualized ways. These effects have been found across different assessment methodologies—for example parent report (Cosentino et al., 1995), observations of free play with anatomically explicit dolls (Jampole and Weber, 1987; Everson and Boat, 1990), ratings of children's drawings (Hibbard, Roghmann, and Hoekelman, 1987), behavioral interaction tasks (Mausert-Mooney, 1992), and reviews of medical records (Kolko, Moses, and Weldy, 1988).

One of the best instruments for assessing sexualized behavior in young children is the Child Sexual Behavior Inventory (CSBI; Friedrich, Grambsch, and Damon, 1992). Studies with the CSBI demonstrate that when contrasted with nonabused clinical and nonclinical groups, sexually abused children exhibit more sexual behavior problems—for instance, masturbating excessively and openly, exposing their genitals, being indiscriminately affectionate toward strangers, and inserting objects into themselves (Friedrich et al., 1992; Friedrich, 1993; Cosentino et al., 1995). (See the case of Naideane in Chapter Fifteen.) Childhood sexual abuse is also a significant factor in early pregnancy (Stevens-Simon and McAnarney, 1994). (It should be noted that the children of abused adolescents are significantly smaller and less mature, probably as a result of a combination of earlier age, less prenatal care, more substance abuse, and greater levels of stress; Stevens-Simon and McAnarney, 1994).

Critics raise the chicken-and-the-egg dilemma. It is argued (from the audience at professional gatherings, but rarely if ever in print) that a child's sexualized behaviors may have precipitated molestation, rather than being a consequence of it; presumably, such a child seduced an adult perpetrator into doing something that he or she would never otherwise do. This is a difficult question to investigate definitively, and critics will be able to hide behind this "blame the victim" rationalization for some time to come. But the clinical observation that many abused children act out sexually in ways that resemble what was done to them strongly suggests that their behavior is a reaction to their experiences (Cosentino et al., 1995). Furthermore, many studies report evidence of a "dose–effect" relationship between indices of the severity of maltreatment (types of maltreatment, age of onset, duration, etc.) and severity of the behaviors observed (see Chapter Three). This indicates that maltreatment influences a child's behavior both qualitatively and quantitatively. Few clinicians who have actually worked with maltreated children doubt that abuse and neglect make profound contributions to a spectrum of maladaptive behaviors.

Somatization

Somatization—that is, recurrent multiple physical complaints without apparent medical cause—has been strongly associated with histories of childhood maltreatment in adult and child studies. At this stage, a direct cause-and-effect linkage has not been definitively established. A large number of adult studies find that women with histories of physical and/or sexual abuse have more medical complaints than nonabused comparison women. When specific types of somatic complaints are examined, abuse histories are significantly more common in women with pelvic pain, gastrointestinal (GI) distress, and headache (e.g., Walker et al., 1988; Reiter, Shakerin, Gambone, and Milburn, 1990; Wurtele, Kaplan, and Keairnes, 1990; Lechner, Vogel, Garcia-Shelton, Leichter, and Steibel, 1993; Walker, Gelfand, Gelfand, Koss, and Katon, 1995; van der Kolk et al., 1996).

In children, somatization and conversion-like phenomena (e.g., pseudoseizures) are widely regarded as suggestive of possible maltreatment, particularly sexual abuse (e.g., Berman, 1978; Jungjohann, 1990; *Lancet*, 1991; Bowman, 1993). Our longitudinal study of sexually abused girls finds highly significant differences between abused and comparison girls on three independent measures of somatization. Prominent symptoms include headache; chest, joint, and limb pain; and GI distress, nausea, and vomiting (Putnam, Trickett, and Burke, 1995).

A number of factors may contribute to somatization in maltreatment victims. Physiological dysregulation (discussed in Chapter Seven) may underlie some complaints that are currently viewed as psychosomatic. The higher levels of health risk behaviors (e.g., cigarette smoking, substance use) found in maltreated adolescents and adults also take their toll on well-being (Riggs, Alario, and McHorney, 1990). Family factors also play an important role in children's somatization. For example, Livingston, Witt, and Smith (1995) studied the children of adult somatizers and found that these children had 11.7 times as many emergency room visits and missed 8.8 times as much school for medical complaints. Finally, somatization is a well-recognized mode of expression for psychological distress, which maltreated children have in great abundance.

Dissociation has been correlated with somatization in several studies. Walker and colleagues found significantly elevated DES scores in women with chronic pelvic pain and GI distress (Walker, Katon, Neraas, Jemelka, and Massoth, 1992; Walker et al., 1995). Briquet's syndrome—the original 19th-century "hysteria," now classified in the DSM as somatization disorder—has been linked with dissociation. Pribor, Yutzy, Dean, and Wetzel (1993) found that high DES scores in women with Briquet's syndrome were predictive of histories of abuse and greater somatization. Studies of dissociative disorder patients find very high levels of somatic symptoms—especially headache; GI and abdominal distress, nausea, and vomiting; and general pain (Putnam, Guroff, Silberman, Barban, and Post, 1986; Coons, Bowman, and Milstein, 1988; Ross, Heber, Norton, and Anderson, 1989c). Saxe et al. (1994) compared somatization in dissociative and nondissociative inpatients. They found that 64% of dissociative patients met DSM-III criteria for somatization disorder, reporting an average of 12.4 somatic symptoms, compared with 3.1 symptoms in the nondissociative group. There were also significant differences in number of medical hospitalizations and consultations.

Substance Abuse

For the purposes of this book, I consider "substance abuse" to be synonymous with "drug addiction" as broadly defined in Chapter Ten (see the more extensive discussion there). The recognition of the role of childhood maltreatment in substance abuse repeats a familiar pattern in child abuse research. It began with a few clinicians troubled by the high rates of physical and sexual abuse in their substance abuse patients, and the independent recognition by others of the high rates of substance abuse in victims of child abuse (e.g., Benward and Densen-Gerber, 1975; Herman, 1981; Miller, Downs, Gondoli, and Keil, 1987; Root, 1989). These parallel sets of observations stimulated exploratory research (Dembo et al., 1987; Miller et al., 1987; Harrison, Hoffman, and Edwall, 1989; Ladwig and Andersen, 1989; Singer and Petchers, 1989). Results from the first round of studies now inform current research, and a clearer picture of the linkages between childhood maltreatment and substance abuse is beginning to emerge. This story is far from complete, and more research is needed to clarify these linkages. It appears as if substance abusers with histories of childhood maltreatment have different patterns of substance abuse and may require different treatment approaches than substance abusers without such histories.

Substance abuse and child maltreatment are linked in complicated ways. A parental history of substance abuse is a strong risk factor for a child's developing a substance abuse disorder. A large percentage of maltreated children have substance-abusing parents (Famularo, Stone, Barnum, and Wharton, 1986; Miller et al., 1987; Murphy et al., 1991). Obviously, poverty and neglect are common factors. However, the relationship between substance abuse and child maltreatment is often not a simple or direct one. For example, Miller et al. (1987) found that although parental alcohol-related problems increased a child's vulnerability to sexual abuse, the parents themselves were rarely the perpetrators. Rather, it appears that such parents' failure to protect their children leads to extrafamilial victimization in many cases.

One of the most rigorous investigations of these questions to date is the longitudinal study conducted by Dembo et al. (1987, 1990). This research examined the influences of childhood abuse experiences and previous alcohol/drug use on emotional functioning and subsequent alcohol/drug use in several samples of high-risk youths in detention centers. These authors found that females had greater rates of sexual victimization than males (65% vs. 24%, respectively). A history of sexual abuse had a direct effect on likelihood of drug use, whereas a history of physical abuse had both a direct and an indirect effect, with the indirect effect mediated through self-derogation and negative views of self.

Aggression, Conduct Problems, and Criminal Behaviors

Numerous studies have linked histories of physical abuse to aggression (Knutson, 1995). This association is not as clear-cut for sexual abuse, although the linkage between sexual abuse and commission of sexual crimes such as rape and prostitution appears convincing (Shaw et al., 1993; Widom and Ames, 1994). In general, abused and neglected children have higher rates of conduct disorder, oppositional behaviors, and social problems than comparison groups (Dubowitz, Black, Harrington, and Verschoore, 1993; Black, Dubowitz, and Harrington, 1994; McLeer et al., 1994; Merry and Andrews, 1994; Paradise, Rose, Sleeper, and Nathanson, 1994; de Paul and Arruabarrena, 1995; Janus, Archambault, Brown, and Welsh, 1995). Studies of runaways routinely find high rates of physical abuse (Janus et al., 1995). Some have criticized research on the relationship of maltreatment to delinquency as being conceptually or methodologically flawed (Schwartz, Rendon, and Hsieh, 1994). The work of Widom and Ames (1994), using a prospective-cohorts design, is perhaps the best approach to this question, although these authors caution that their reliance on official records may skew the results. I think that it is clear that maltreatment, particularly physical abuse, makes a significant contribution to conduct problems and antisocial behavior. However, some of these effects may be indirect or influenced by non-maltreatment-related variables (e.g., family environment).

Cognitive Sequelae

Important early research focused on the intellectual delays and cognitive deficits found in abused children (Bowlby, 1973; Cohn, 1979; Green, Voeller, Gaines, and Kubie, 1981). Criticisms that these studies failed to control for the effects of poverty, disturbed parenting, and understimulation have been addressed by more recent studies (e.g., Oates and Peacock, 1984; Einbender and Friedrich, 1989; Carrey, Butter, Persinger, and Bialik, 1995). Verbal IQ scores in particular have been found to be significantly lower in maltreated children (Friedrich, Einbender, and Luecke, 1983; Salzinger, Kaplan, Pelcovitz, Samit, and Krieger, 1984; Tarter, Hegedus, Winsten, and Alterman, 1984; Carrey et al., 1995). Carrey et al. (1995) found strong negative correlations between severity of abuse and verbal and Full Scale IQs on the Wechsler Intelligence Scale for Children—Revised (WISC-R).

General language skill development is believed to be disrupted by maltreatment (Cicchetti and Beeghly, 1987; Law and Conway, 1992; Cicchetti and Lynch, 1995). Delays in expressive and receptive language have been found in a number of studies (Cicchetti and Lynch, 1995). These deficits are also influenced by features of the caretaking environment, such as fewer verbal interactions between parents and children, less verbal teaching, and insecure attachment (Cicchetti and Lynch, 1995). Maltreated toddlers talk less about themselves and their internal states (e.g., happy, sad, etc.), particularly negative mood states, than nonmaltreated toddlers; they also make fewer verbal responses to social contingencies (Cicchetti and Lynch, 1995). See the fuller discussion of cognitive deficits in trauma victims in Chapter Six.

Preliminary studies suggest disruption of other cognitive functions in maltreated children. Play—a major symbolic realm for children—is less cognitively and socially mature in maltreated children than in nonmaltreated children (Alessandri, 1991). Differences in play are to some extent correlated with differences in mother–child interactional styles (Cicchetti and Lynch, 1995). Haviland et al. (1995) found evidence of impaired reality testing in abused adolescents, including distortions of reality, uncertainty of perceptions, hallucinations, and delusions. Researchers have speculated at length about the impact of maltreatment on children's mental models of the way that the world works, but unfortunately there has been little direct research on this topic to date.

Attentional and Hyperactivity Problems

Recently, child researchers have begun to link histories of abuse with symptoms of attention-deficit/hyperactivity disorder (ADHD) (McLeer et al., 1994; Merry and Andrews, 1994; Glod and Teicher, 1996). ADHD symptoms typically occur in 25–45% of severely maltreated children, well above the frequently reported base rate of 9% in pediatric patients. Glod and Teicher (1996) used belt-worn activity monitors to study 72-hour activity profiles in maltreated children with and without PTSD. Children with PTSD had activity profiles resembling those of children with ADHD, whereas the profiles of those without PTSD more closely resembled those of depressed children. Some speculate that these ADHD-like symptoms differ from conventional ADHD, and arise from posttraumatic hyperarousal, increased anxiety, and responses to traumatic reminders (De Bellis, Lefter, Trickett, and Putnam, 1994b; Glod and Teicher, 1996). More research on this question is badly needed.

School Problems

Given the types of symptoms and behaviors associated with maltreatment, one would anticipate that school performance would be seriously and complexly disrupted. Posttraumatic stress symptoms such as intrusive thoughts, flashbacks, hyperarousal, and avoidant symptoms, together with dissociation and cognitive deficits, should significantly impair academic achievement. Behaviors such as aggression and hypersexuality might well impede socialization and peer acceptance. Propensities toward substance abuse and risk taking would be expected to make these children unwelcome and to lead to their being regarded as a bad influence on their peers.

Remarkably little research has been done on this question, which is an important one because school represents one of the few positive influences in the lives of many of these children. Results to date are mixed, reflecting differences in what researchers have chosen to measure (see review in Trickett, McBride-Chang, and Putnam, 1994). Grades are often not a good measure, because standards vary greatly from teacher to teacher and are always relative to the overall quality of students in a given classroom. Standardized testing is a better measure, but unfortunately different school systems use different achievement tests, so that comparability is often not possible across school districts. Teacher ratings of a child's behavior, relative to that of other children in the class, provide the most useful measures of the child's academic competencies and behaviors in relation to peers.

In the most comprehensive study to date, we (Trickett et al., 1994) compared 83 sexually abused girls with 64 matched controls on measures of cognitive ability, perceived academic competence, classroom behavior problems, and grades. We found that a history of sexual abuse had a direct negative impact on classroom social competence, learning competence, and overall academic performance. Abuse was positively related to avoidant behavior, but was not related to grades. Abuse was positively related to anxiety, depression, bizarre behavior, dissociation, and hyperactivity. Abuse was negatively related to cognitive functioning. The best predictors of learning problems, avoidant behavior, and poorer overall academic performance were hyperactivity and dissociation.

It is a terrible tragedy that the cognitive and behavioral sequelae of maltreatment wreak such havoc on the academic performance and school behavior of maltreated youngsters. Their academic failures and misbehaviors deny them the kinds of academic and social successes that could help to mitigate their negative home experiences. Instead, they often end up in special placements with other troubled and learning-disabled youths, who become their peer group. As they grow older, they are seen as exhibiting behavior problems and may be expelled or implicitly discouraged from continuing in school. For several years, as noted earlier in this chapter, I served as a consultant to a special school in Washington, D.C., for adolescents who had been expelled from public schools (and D.C. public schools tolerate some pretty disruptive behavior). I did not find "bad kids" there, just very badly treated kids (Putnam, 1993a). If we can find ways to help these youths get more out of school, we would be making a major intervention in their lives.

Development of Self

The development and consolidation of an autonomous "self" is believed to be seriously disrupted in many maltreated children (Cicchetti and Lynch, 1995). Although maltreated infants recognize their rouge-marked faces as readily as nonmaltreated subjects do, they typically display a neutral or negative affect, in contrast to the controls' surprise and delight (Schneider-Rosen and Cicchetti, 1991). Self-assessment, as exemplified by self-esteem and self-competence measures, appears to be significantly and complexly disrupted. Most studies find self-esteem to be significantly lower in maltreated children, but self-competence ratings may be unrealistically exaggerated in younger maltreated children (e.g., Black et al., 1994; Cicchetti and Lynch, 1995). By the age of 8 to 9 years, most maltreated children describe themselves as less competent than their peers (Cicchetti and Lynch, 1995). By adulthood, victims of childhood maltreatment exhibit a wide range of disturbances of self (Putnam, 1990; Cole and Putnam, 1992).

A scattered literature, ranging from psychoanalytic theory to empirical pediatric research, has addressed the issues of disturbances of sense of self in maltreated children and adults. Gender identity is thought to be adversely affected in both males (Watkins and Bentovim, 1992; Lisak, 1994) and females (Cosentino, Meyer-Bahlburg, Alpert, and Gaines, 1993; Price, 1993; Green, 1994). Abuse-related distortions in body image have been postulated to mediate disturbed eating behaviors, although this turns out to be a complex equation (e.g., Byram, Wagner, and Waller, 1995). Kurt Fischer and colleagues have elegantly demonstrated complex disturbances in self-representations in sexually abused adolescent girls (Calverley, Fischer, and Ayoub, 1994). Fischer believes that these disturbances in self-definition reflect a distinct self-representational developmental pathway, rather than a regression to or fixation at earlier levels.

Psychobiological Sequelae

Research has identified or implicated a large number of neurobiological systems in the psychobiology of trauma. Neurobiological systems found to be altered by traumatic experiences include the HPA axis, the sympathetic nervous system, central catecholamines, serotonin systems, the endogenous opiates, and probably the immune system (Charney, Deutch, Krystal, Southwick, and Davis, 1993; De Bellis and Putnam, 1994; Yehuda and McFarlane, 1995; De Bellis, Burke, Trickett, and Putnam, 1996). Elsewhere, we (De Bellis and Putnam, 1994) review research on the psychobiological effects of childhood maltreatment (De Bellis and Putnam, 1994). Several biological systems are known to be altered, and a number of others are likely affected. In the next few years, we should see an explosion of research in this area as a variety of noninvasive biological probes become widely available (e.g., the ability to measure blood hormone levels in saliva) (De Bellis and Putnam, 1994; Putnam, 1996b). The availability of valid animal stress response models—particularly primate studies—also greatly informs research.

In view of the limited research to date, many of the biological data should be regarded as preliminary (Yehuda and McFarlane, 1995). Nonetheless, these studies provide scientifically compelling evidence that stressful and traumatic experiences result in persistent dysregulation of a number of critical biological systems. The long-term consequences of such biological dysregulation is not known, but they may play an important role in the high levels of somatization found in victims of childhood maltreatment. This question is discussed further in Chapter Seven.

SUMMARY

Despite their ubiquity, morbidity, and mortality, the effects of trauma on children are not widely appreciated. Child maltreatment is the single largest source of childhood trauma and the one most closely associated with serious psychiatric sequelae. Maltreatment outcomes are diverse. In children and adolescents, dimensional assessments are usually more informative than the categorical DSM diagnosis of PTSD. Many different symptoms and behaviors are frequently reported, including sexualization, cognitive deficits, problems with the sense of self, suicide and self-destructive behaviors, somatization, depression, and anxiety, as well as dissociative and posttraumatic symptoms. Aggression toward others occurs in a significant minority of cases. Substance abuse is common and may differ in pattern and treatment response from that of substance abusers without a maltreatment history. The multitude of symptoms and maladaptive behaviors associated with maltreatment compromise the development of children, contributing to lifelong suffering and to poor social and occupational attainments.

Chapter Three

Influential Factors and Common Themes in Maltreatment Outcomes

Such wide-ranging effects are attributed to child maltreatment that a few reviewers have concluded there must be no effect (e.g. Burton, 1968). As yet, no psychiatric disorder has been proven to be "caused" by childhood maltreatment, although strong evidence is accumulating for MPD. Those who know and work with child or adult victims of maltreatment are convinced that it contributes to and often causes many adverse outcomes. The diversity of maltreatment outcomes should not be regarded as evidence of no effect, but rather as evidence for extraordinarily pervasive adverse effects.

We are just beginning to sort out the factors that contribute to these effects. This chapter first summarizes what is known about the relative contributions of different factors to the outcomes associated with maltreatment. The chapter concludes with the argument that the differences in reported outcomes suggested by differences in DSM diagnoses are more apparent than real. It is argued that four major developmental themes (disturbances in affect regulation; problems with impulsivity; somatization and biological dysregulation; and disturbances in self-concepts) are common to the psychiatric disorders associated with histories of childhood maltreatment.

FACTORS THAT INFLUENCE
MALTREATMENT OUTCOMES

Age/Developmental Stage

The developmental-psychopathological framework predicts that significant age/developmental stage factors should affect the outcome of maltreatment experiences. In child development, stages are marked by the appearance of new capacities, both physical and cognitive, that alter a child's relationship to others and to the environment. In research analyses, a child's age is often used as a proxy for the child's developmental stage. However, age is actually only a correlate for certain developmental processes. For example, age is correlated ($r\sim.85$) with "Tanner stage," a measure of pubertal physical development. This is a high correlation, but it still leaves a quarter of the variance unaccounted for. Many cognitive-developmental processes show much greater age variations.

Age at the beginning and ending of maltreatment, which roughly encompasses the sequence of developmental stages spanned by the maltreatment, should influence which developmental tasks are most disrupted. To date, only coarse-grained analyses have been attempted. Investigators typically divide samples into younger and older children, depending on the age at the onset of maltreatment. Several studies indicate that there are age/stage effects for some outcomes (Meiselman, 1978; Courtouis, 1979; Finkelhor, 1979; Russell, 1986; Wolfe, Gentile, and Wolfe, 1989); however, studies do not always agree on which ages are most severely affected (Trickett et al., in press). In aggregate, these data indicate that younger children are more vulnerable.

Focusing on the interconnected themes of the development of self and socialization, we (Cole and Putnam, 1992) have sketched out an example of a developmental-psychopathological approach to age/stage issues in incest. Our model emphasizes that age/stage effects are not static. The victim has opportunities to reprocess the experience at developmental transitions and over the life course. Individual differences in development and outcome are understood in terms of alterations in developmental trajectories, as opposed to fixations in time. The model hypothesizes that different developmental tasks should be affected at different time points. The synopsis below summarizes the major points.

During infancy and toddlerhood, major developmental tasks include (1) discovery of the world of people and objects; (2) establishment of secure social relationships within the family; (3) establishment of a basic sense of self; (4) the development of an autonomous sense of awareness; and (5) acquisition of an initial sense of right and wrong (good and bad) (Cole and Putnam, 1992). Highly dependent on their caregivers, infants have a limited repertoire of coping and self-regulation capacities, such as gaze aversion and self-sucking. Infants are easily overwhelmed by intense or chronic stress. Toddlers show somewhat greater capacity for coping with stress in themselves and even make attempts to reduce stress in others (Cole, Barrett, and Zahn-Waxler, 1992). Infants and toddlers have little capacity to understand the nature of maltreatment perpetrated against them, but are strongly affected by physical trauma and by the unavailability, either physical or emotional, of their primary caretakers (Field, 1994). Infants often respond to trauma with dysregulation of sleep and feeding, whereas toddlers evidence profound regression.

The developmental tasks of preschoolers (ages 2–5) involve integration of self with social restrictions. Preschoolers acquire increasing control over their behavior and affect. They move from simple physical exploration of the world to pretend and symbolic play; they also learn to differentiate what is real and what is not. Denial is believed to be a fundamental coping strategy. (Interestingly, denial is also commonly invoked by parents when dealing with an anxious preschooler—e.g., telling the child that an injection "won't hurt.") Dissociative capacity appears to increase rapidly during the preschool years, perhaps in part as a result of increasing capacities for fantasy and imagination. Maltreatment at this age disrupts ongoing self-organization and progression of emotional self-regulation. Maltreatment is believed to produce problems in the child's ability to differentiate affective states, and it may increase reliance on denial and dissociation as coping strategies.

During childhood (the elementary school years), developmental tasks revolve around elaborations of self to include awareness of psychological characteristics, such as thoughts, feelings, and motives. Self-criticism and awareness of shame and pride become evident at about 7–8 years of age. Children become aware of their positive and negative qualities and begin to accept both. Metacognitive processes facilitate integration of self. Now children can reflect on the self as "object."

Friendships also become increasingly important. Children become sensitive to peer evaluations and incorporate the perspectives of others into their own self-appraisals. This widened social world offers new sources of interpersonal support, as well as challenges to self-regulation and impulsivity. Defensive coping is more cognitively organized with capacities for reasoning, reflection, and rationalization. Maltreatment at this age disrupts socialization and has a negative impact on the sense of self through experiences of pervasive guilt, shame, and confusion.

Adolescence is marked by the passage through puberty—a period of physical growth and change exceeded only by infancy. The physical changes of puberty drive psychological readjustments, as the adolescent strives to incorporate his or her developing secondary sex characteristics and the altered responses of others into a new self-image. Social development is characterized by a curtailment of same-sex friendships and the development of relationships with the opposite sex. The loyalty of same-sex friendships gives way to intimacy, mutuality, and exclusivity with the opposite sex. Self-understanding becomes highly introspective, and friendships involve considerable self-revelation. The task of identity formation requires the adolescent to integrate a complex of self-related features into a stable, unified sense of self that is compatible with the views of significant others. Maltreatment disrupts this self-definition process and interferes with exploration of opposite-sex relationships. Various maladaptive "coping" behaviors become increasingly available during the teenage years—for example, substance abuse, running away, suicide and self-destructive behaviors, risk taking, and sexual acting out.

Developmental tasks and transitions in adulthood are driven more by external circumstances than by physical and cognitive development. Developmental psychologists conceptualize adult life in phases. Typically, early adult life is organized around marriage and the birth of children. An expansion phase follows the birth of the last child. There is increased self-reflection on life circumstances and choices: "What will I be when I grow up?" is transformed into "Who have I become?"

Research suggests that maltreatment, particularly incest, has a strong negative impact on adult development—especially for women. Deviation from traditional adult trajectories (e.g., either early childbearing or avoidance of having children) appears to be one consequence. Poor marital adjustments, often involving revictimization, are not uncommon. In addition, a history of childhood abuse increases a woman's likelihood of sexual assault two- to threefold (e.g., see Cloitre, Tardiff, Marzuk, Leon, and Portera, 1996). Finally the stresses of marriage and child rearing can further strain self-boundaries and emotional regulation. Adulthood, however, may permit radical readjustments for a maltreated individual. Victims can leave home and pursue their own interests, and can regulate contact with their perpetrators. Moreover, they can do for their own children what was not done for them—and in so doing can address some of their own developmental deficits.

Gender

Few maltreatment outcome studies have had sufficient numbers and balance of subjects to test adequately for gender effects. However, recent interest in gender influences on child and adolescent psychiatric disorders has stimulated research on this question in maltreated children. Here, I use research on sexual abuse to illustrate these effects for maltreatment in general.

In the area of sexual abuse, most of what we know about maltreatment effects comes from research on females. Although they are lower than for females, prevalence estimates for the sexual abuse of boys vary about as much. For example, a comprehensive review by Watkins and Bentovim (1992) found rates varying between 3% and 31% of boys. Child and adolescent psychiatric inpatient samples find sexual abuse in about half of the girls and 16% of the boys (Watkins and Bentovim, 1992). Community studies of children and adolescents typically find girl–boy ratios ranging from 2:1 to 4:1, which yield male prevalence rates of 2.5–9% (Watkins and Bentovim, 1992). Nonclinical adult male samples (typically college students) have prevalence rates of about 10–15% (Fromuth and Burkhart, 1989). Special populations, such as male prostitutes, may have markedly higher rates.

The vast majority of sexually abused females are abused by males—most frequently family members. When one begins to examine the effects of sexual abuse on males, one finds that there may be a "sex of the perpetrator" effect. That is, some boys are sexually abused by males and others by females. Typically, 5–28% of abused males are abused by females (Watkins and Bentovim, 1992). When boys are abused by a male, the perpetrator is often not a family member (Watkins and Bentovim, 1992). However, when boys are abused by a female, the perpetrator is most often the mother (Watkins and Bentovim, 1992). Thus relationship to perpetrator confounds analyses of perpetrator gender effects.

Many of the outcomes for males are the same as for females—that is, depression, self-destructive behaviors, anxiety, low self-esteem, difficulty in trusting others, a tendency to be revictimized, substance abuse, and sexual maladjustment. However, a number of uniquely male issues have also been identified. Prominent among these are homosexuality concerns, masculinity issues, and sexual aggression toward others.

Homosexuality issues have been noted by numerous investigators (Watkins and Bentovim, 1992; Lisak, 1994). Many researchers believe that these concerns play a role in the notable reluctance of male adolescents to report sexual victimization. Many boys appear to interpret their victimization by males as evidence that they were picked because of some "sign" of homosexuality (Watkins and Bentovim, 1992). Closely related are masculinity issues, in which victims struggle with feelings of masculine inadequacy. Counterphobic hypermasculinity appears to be a common response (Lisak, 1994).

Sexual victimization of others is an outcome for a significant minority of male victims. Studies of adolescents who commit serious sexual offenses (Shaw et al., 1993) and of adults who are sexually aggressive offenders (Seghorn, Prentky, and Boucher, 1987) find high rates of sexual abuse in their childhoods. Seghorn et al. (1987) found that child molesters (victims under 16 years of age) were more than twice as likely as rapists (victims 16 and older) to have been sexually abused themselves as children. Rapists, however, were more likely to have been abused by a family member. These studies and others implicate additional, non-abuse-related factors (e.g., family turmoil and instability) as playing a significant role in the lives of offenders.

Preliminary studies of sexually abused males suggest that there are gender-specific outcomes in addition to the more common general outcomes, such as depression, suicidality, and PTSD symptoms. Research in other areas of developmental psychopathology has found significant gender differences in the prevalence of ADHD, anxiety disorders, conduct disorder, depression, and phobias (Cicchetti and Cohen, 1995a). It would be surprising if there were not gender effects on maltreatment outcomes. This question is addressed for the dissociative disorders in Chapter Nine.

Nature and Severity of Maltreatment

Many studies include analyses attempting to determine whether different types of maltreatment or differences in the severity of a given type of maltreatment affect outcomes. Thus, for sexual abuse, some studies suggest that penetration is associated with more deleterious impacts; others find that duration or frequency effects are more pernicious. Differences in outcome have also been associated with relationship to perpetrator, age of onset, and use of force and coercion. In short, although effects are often reported for severity or type of maltreatment, there are some inconsistencies across studies. To date, investigators have largely considered each type/severity variable in isolation, rather than examining these variables as interactive factors.

Our experience of examining assorted variables related to type and severity of sexual abuse in our longitudinal study suggests that these variables are complexly confounded (Trickett et al., in press). We have found significant intercorrelations among most of these variables—for example, number of different kinds of abuse, age of onset, duration, and relationship to perpetrator. In particular, the presence of a nonbiological father figure perpetrator was associated with much later abuse onsets and shorter durations. When we examined these variables in a hierarchical-regression analysis, relationship to perpetrator emerged as a powerful predictor of pertinent outcome measures, such as presence of a disruptive behavior disorder and sexual acting out. If the field is to get a better handle on "what hurts whom and how," future research must consider maltreatment severity and type (together with other variables, such as race/ethnicity and family environment) in more sophisticated multivariate analyses and structural-equation models.

Race and Ethnicity

Race differences in diagnosis and treatment are rarely discussed in the psychiatric research literature, although investigators find these effects more often than they report. What little research we have available suggests that race factors significantly influence diagnosis and treatment services (e.g., Cuffe, Waller, Cuccaro, Pumariega, and Garrison, 1995; Kilgus, Pumariega, and Cuffe, 1995). Some of these differences may be attributable to the cultural bias inherent in diagnostic systems such as the DSM (see, e.g., Cervantes, 1994). Racial/ethnic distributions of maltreatment victims in the United States have remained relatively constant for the past few years (Bronfenbrenner Life Course Center, 1996): European-Americans account for approximately 55% of cases, African-Americans for 26%, and Hispanic-Americans for about 9%. There do not appear to be statistical interactions between race and age of victim.

When the type of maltreatment is controlled for, preliminary data indicate that race and ethnicity alone make little contribution to outcome. However, race and ethnicity may be interact with the type of maltreatment to influence outcomes. Investigating the scores of a racially mixed sample of abused girls on measures of depression, anxiety and self-esteem, Mennen (1995) found a significant interaction between race/ethnicity and abuse patterns: Latina girls with histories of sexual abuse involving penetration scored higher on all outcomes. We also find race by perpetrator relationship effects; for instance, in our sample, white girls are more likely to have been abused by their biological fathers than are minority girls (Trickett et al., in press).

Family Environment

Until recently, maltreatment outcome research focused almost exclusively on the characteristics of the maltreatment and the age of the child as determinant factors. Types and severity of maltreatment, the age at which it begins, and the developmental periods that it spans are important variables, but research is increasingly implicating non-maltreatment-related family processes as significant to outcome.

For example, in a community sample, Wind and Silvern (1994) examined the roles of retrospectively measured perceived parental warmth, family stress histories, and abuse variables on adult outcomes of 259 working women. They found that each made an independent contribution. Parental warmth strongly influenced the relationship of intrafamilial abuse to depression and self-esteem. PTSD was most strongly influenced by the characteristics of the abuse experience. In a prospective study of neglected and physically abused children and normal controls assessed at two points in time (preschool and school age), Herrenkohl, Herrenkohl, Rupert, Egolf, and Lutz (1995) found that parenting, family environment, and a child's characteristics had significant effects on the child's behaviors. Family characteristics and sociocultural factors were stronger predictors of the child's behavior than was either physical abuse or emotional maltreatment—although these were also significant factors.

A great deal more research is necessary, but these preliminary studies indicate that family factors not directly associated with maltreatment also make critical and complex contributions to maltreatment outcomes. Certain combinations of factors may significantly mitigate the experience of maltreatment, whereas other combinations probably seriously exacerbate its effects. Family factors undoubtedly account for some of the missing variance in outcome that cannot be explained by type/severity variables alone.

ADULT DSM DIAGNOSES ASSOCIATED WITH CHILD MALTREATMENT: COMMON THEMES

A number of DSM disorders have been associated with maltreatment and trauma histories. For example, studies have linked borderline personality disorder (BPD), MPD, eating disorders, somatization disorder, pseudoseizures, and substance abuse (in females) with histories of maltreatment. Indeed, as noted earlier, this wide range of psychiatric diagnoses has led some to suggest that there are no relatively specific abuse effects.

For purposes of scientific argument, I contend that many patients with histories of maltreatment share disturbances in a set of developmental dimensions, regardless of the DSM diagnosis they happen to receive. Using BPD and eating disorders as examples, I initiate a discussion of four core developmental themes that are intrinsic to maltreatment outcomes. This discussion continues throughout the remainder of the book, and these themes serve as a set of "red threads" that can be traced in the data and the DBS model to be presented later. These four common themes include (1) disturbances in regulation of affect and emotion; (2) problems with impulse control; (3) biological dysregulation and somatization; and (4) disturbances in the development and metacognitive integration of self. Each reflects a disruption in a fundamental developmental process that evolves over the life span of the individual. Although there are undoubtedly genetic contributions to each of these dimensions, social and experiential factors are much more important determinants. First, however, I briefly discuss BPD and eating disorders in turn.

Borderline Personality Disorder

BPD became an official diagnosis with the publication of the DSM-III (American Psychiatric Association, 1980). It was the subject of intense clinical and theoretical interest during the late 1970s and early 1980s; little was then known about the relationship of BPD to traumatic antecedents. By the 1980s, the diagnosis of BPD was in widespread and sometimes indiscriminate use. Not uncommonly, individuals (including colleagues) who evoked hostile countertransference reactions were labeled "borderline." Largely ignored during this period were case series of BPD patients with histories of sexual abuse (e.g., Gross, Doerr, Caldirola, Guzinski, and Ripley, 1980–1981; Stone, 1981; Bryer et al., 1987).

A 1989 paper by Herman, Perry, and van der Kolk on childhood trauma and BPD rapidly changed our understanding of this condition (see also Gunderson and Sabo, 1993). Within a few years, a dozen other studies and reviews had confirmed Herman et al.'s observation that a large percentage of BPD patients have histories of childhood trauma (Paris and Zweig-Frank, 1992; Gunderson and Sabo, 1993). The percentage of BPD patients with trauma histories varies from 50% to 81% across different studies (e.g., Gross et al., 1980–1981; Stone, 1981; Herman et al., 1989; Zanarini, Gunderson, Marino, Schwartz, and Frankenburg, 1989; Ogata et al., 1990; Shearer, Peters, Quayman, and Ogden, 1990; Westen, Ludolph, Misle, Ruffins, and Block, 1990; Hulbert, Apt, and White, 1992). In aggregate, these data suggest that at least half and perhaps as many as three-quarters of all BPD patients have experienced significant trauma in childhood. It is also clear that social, developmental, and biological factors make major contributions to BPD (Paris and Zweig-Frank, 1992).

BPD is a common Axis II diagnosis in a number of disorders most closely associated with histories of childhood trauma. Clinical studies suggest that between 30% and 70% of patients with MPD meet criteria for BPD (Fast, 1974; Scialli, 1982; Buck, 1983; Benner and Joscelyne, 1984; Clary, Burstin, and Carpenter, 1984; Horevitz and Braun, 1984; Kirsten, 1990; Armstrong, 1991; Fink, 1991; Bruce and Coid, 1992). Indeed, the overlap between MPD and BPD is the subject of ongoing debate (e.g. Marmer and Fink, 1994). There is also considerable overlap between BPD and eating disorders (Koepp, Schildbach, Schmager, and Rohner, 1993; Skodol et al., 1993; Waller, 1993a, 1993b; Dulit, Fyer, Leon, Brodsky, and Frances, 1994; Gleaves and Eberenz, 1994; Steiger, Stotland, and Houle, 1994). PTSD has likewise been associated with co-morbid BPD (Southwick, Yehuda, and Giller, 1993).

Eating Disorders

Refusal of food by women can be traced back to the Middle Ages, when "miraculous maids" fasted for the greater glory of God (Attie and Brooks-Gunn, 1995); indeed, some have argued that ascetic fasting was the medieval period's expression of anorexia nervosa. The prevalence of modern eating disorders appears to be increasing over recent decades, although the degree and causes of this change are debated (American Psychiatric Association 1993). Affecting 1–4% of adolescent and young adult white middle-class women, eating disorders appear to be increasing fastest in prepubertal children (American Psychiatric Association, 1993). Bulimia nervosa is more common than anorexia nervosa, but most patients exhibit both bulimic and anorexic symptoms sequentially or concurrently at some point. Many authorities conceptualize eating disorders as existing along a continuum, with only a few extreme cases representing the "pure" anorexic or bulimic subtypes.

Early histories of eating disorder patients are often marked by separations, family deaths, medical illnesses, and surgeries. The official American Psychiatric Association (1993) practice guidelines note that between 20% and 50% of bulimic patients have histories of sexual abuse; these sexual abuse rates are often not significantly higher than rates reported for psychiatric patients in general (Lacey, 1990; American Psychiatric Association, 1993). (This should be understood as a telling statistic about the ubiquity of histories of sexual abuse in psychiatric in-patients.) When studies reporting relatively low abuse rates are reviewed, they are often found to have asked only a single question about a history of possible sexual abuse. Clinical and research experience shows that a single question probing for sexual abuse often misses significant numbers of cases (Peters, Wyatt, and Finkelhor, 1986). Thackwray, Smith, and Bodfish (1991) reported that 49% of their bulimic patients spontaneously reported histories of sexual abuse. Some (e.g., Pope and Hudson, 1992) question this relationship, but the balance of clinical studies suggest that about 30–50% of eating disorder patients have histories of sexual abuse or other childhood trauma.

Like BPD, eating disorders are not *caused* by childhood abuse or trauma, but abuse or trauma appears to predispose some individuals toward developing an eating disorder. Some have speculated that a history of sexual abuse may influence the type of eating disorder (Waller, 1991) or the type of personality disturbance that accompanies the eating disorder (Conners and Morse, 1993).

Common Themes in BPD and Eating Disorders

Disturbances in Affect Regulation

Both BPD and eating disorder patients have significant problems with affect regulation. Indeed, unstable affect characterized by marked shifts among depression, irritability, and anxiety, and usually lasting hours to a few days at most, is specifically included in the DSM criteria for BPD (American Psychiatric Association, 1987, 1994). Intense, inappropriate anger (borderline rage), often explosively triggered by minor insults, is common and is also included as a DSM criterion (American Psychiatric Association, 1987, 1994). Thus, two DSM criteria—and many clinical features—attest to pathological dysregulation of affect as a common characteristic of BPD patients.

Although not included under the DSM criteria for eating disorders, affect disturbances are a prominent clinical feature. One manifestation is alexithymia, the inability or impaired ability to describe or be aware of one's emotions or moods (Kaplan and Sadock, 1991). Common in PTSD patients, alexithymia also appears to be a core problem in eating disorders (see, e.g., Cochrane, Brewerton, Wilson, and Hodges, 1993; Schmidt, Jiwany, and Treasure, 1993; Jimerson, Wolfe, Franko, Covino, and Sifneos, 1994; Laquatra and Clopton, 1994; de Groot, Rodin, and Olmsted, 1995). Binge eating is often used by bulimic patients to regulate mood or to indirectly express such emotions as hostility, anxiety or frustration (Arnow, Kenardy, and Agras, 1995; Tiller, Schmidt, Ali, and Treasure, 1995).

Problems with Impulse Control

Problems with impulse control constitute another criterion for BPD in the DSM. That is, BPD patients often manifest impulsive behavior in at least two areas, not including suicide or self-mutilation, that may be self-damaging (American Psychiatric Association, (1987, 1994). Promiscuous sexual behavior, reckless driving, binge eating, gambling, and impulsive spending are classic examples of impulsivity in BPD patients (Hulbert et al., 1992; Hull, Clarkin, and Yeomans, 1993). Impulsivity is also a significant clinical feature of eating disorders, particularly bulimia nervosa (Fahy and Eisler, 1993; Lesieur and Blume, 1993; Newton,

Freeman, and Munro, 1993; Wolfe, Jimerson, and Levine, 1994; McElroy, Keck, and Phillips, 1995). Some have suggested that there may be a subgroup of highly impulsive eating disorder patients, who have a significantly worse prognosis.

One form of impulsivity shared by important subgroups of BPD and eating disorder patients (as well as of PTSD and dissociative patients) is self-injurious behavior (Lacey, 1993; Dulit et al., 1994; Shearer, 1994; Wolfe et al., 1994; Zweig-Frank, Paris, and Guzder, 1994; Brewerton, Stellefson, Hibbs, Hodges, and Cochrane, 1995; Herpertz, 1995), particularly self-mutilation. Self-mutilation and other self-destructive behaviors are significantly associated with histories of maltreatment in children, adolescents and adults, as already discussed in Chapter Two. Research finds that BPD or eating disorder patients with higher DES scores have higher rates of self-injury than those with lower levels of dissociation (Herman et al., 1989; Demitrack, Putnam, Brewerton, Brandt, and Gold, 1990; Anderson, Yasenik, and Ross, 1993; Murray, 1993; Saxe et al., 1993; Shearer, 1994; Zweig-Frank et al., 1994).

A high rate of substance abuse is another form of self-directed, self-destructive behavior shared by BPD and eating disorder patients (Jonas, Gold, Sweeney, and Pottash, 1987; Koepp et al., 1993; Lacey, 1993; Miller, Abrams, Dulit, and Fyer, 1993; Holderness, Brooks-Gunn, and Warren, 1994). Substance abuse is also common in PTSD and dissociative patients. A history of childhood maltreatment is a common finding in a large percentage of substance abuse patients (see Chapter Two). I believe that substance abuse serves in traumatized individuals as a mechanism of affective and behavioral state regulation (see discussions in Chapters Eight, Nine, and Ten).

Biological Dysregulation and Somatization

Biological derangements and dysregulation are primary features of eating disorders and contribute to their high lethality. Physical complications include all of the effects of malnutrition, especially cardiovascular compromise. Prepubertal children may have delayed physical development and arrested sexual maturation, whereas prolonged amenorrhea is a common feature in menarcheal women. Numerous biochemical and endocrinological abnormalities (e.g., lymphocytosis, abnormal liver functions, hypoglycemia, hypercortisolemia, hypercholesterolemia, hypercarotenemia, and decreased metabolic rate) are common. Dysregulation of the HPA axis is well studied in the eating disorders; patients manifest significant abnormalities in the secretion of adrenocorticotrophic hormone and cortisol (Gold et al., 1986). Brain imaging reveals abnormalities in about half of cases (American Psychiatric Association, 1993). What is cause and what is effect remain to be disentangled.

The patholophysiology of BPD is obscure. Disturbances in serotonin function appear to be the best-replicated findings, and these have been correlated with aggressive and self-destructive behaviors (Hollander et al., 1994; McBride et al., 1994; Rosenberg, 1994). Attempts at pharmacological dissection of BPD into subtypes have not been successful. In view of the high rates of substance abuse and other health-risking behaviors found in BPD, surprisingly few studies have examined somatization. Nor have researchers explored possible physiological shifts underlying the recurrent behavioral oscillations that are so characteristic of BPD patients (e.g., Melges and Swartz, 1989).

A history of childhood maltreatment, particularly sexual abuse, results in significantly higher levels of somatization (see Chapter Two). I believe that the increased somatization found in child maltreatment victims is a reflection of the biological dysregulations found in trauma patients. This is a working hypothesis that is not proven at this time. In the interest of stimulating research, I suggest that BPD patients with maltreatment histories will show significant physiological dysregulation in stress response systems, and that this will be found to be related to affective and attachment shifts and to impulsive behaviors.

Disturbances in Self and Identity

Disturbances of identity constitute yet another core feature of BPD patients. The DSM-III-R criterion is a persistent and marked disturbance of identity, as indicated by uncertainty in at least two of five areas (self-image, sexual orientation, long-term objectives or career choice, type of friends wished for, or values endorsed) (American Psychiatric Association, 1987). The DSM-IV criterion is less specific, calling for only a persistent and marked instability in sense of self or self-image (American Psychiatric Association, 1994). A fluctuating, diffuse, or fragmented sense of self is a classic clinical feature of BPD patients. Indeed, the similarities in the disturbances of self found in BPD and MPD patients constitute the major focus of disagreement among clinicians about the overlap of these conditions.

Body image disturbance is a core feature of eating disorder pathology (American Psychiatric Association, 1994). Dissatisfaction with physical appearance is usually the manifest problem and is significantly related to eating-disordered behaviors in both clinical and nonclinical samples. However, other disturbances of self (e.g., problems with self-esteem) are common. Extreme disturbances in body perception are reported in some emaciated anorexic patients, who describe obese self-reflections in a mirror. Many eating disorder patients have concurrent BPD and thus manifest identity diffusion and fragmentation problems (e.g., Koepp et al., 1993; Rossiter, Agras, Telch, and Schneider, 1993; Skodol et al., 1993; Steiger, Leung, Thibaudeau, Houle, and Ghadirian, 1993; Waller, 1993a, 1993b; Dulit et al., 1994; Gleaves and Eberenz, 1994; Sohlberg and Norring, 1995).

SUMMARY

Efforts to account for the heterogeneity of maltreatment outcomes are incomplete. Although studies find effects related to specific maltreatment variables, these are often highly interrelated and difficult to disentangle. Non-maltreatment-related features of the family environment also contribute a significant amount to the outcome variance. However, when one examines apparently divergent adult DSM disorders associated with child maltreatment, four common dimensions emerge: disturbances in affect regulation; problems with impulse control; somatization and biological dysregulation; and disturbances in self-representation. These dimensions serve as developmental "red threads" to be traced throughout the rest of the book.

Chapter Four

Introduction to Dissociation

Modern understanding of the nature of pathological dissociation is largely shaped by its significant linkage with trauma and with posttraumatic psychiatric sequelae. Most research on dissociation is concerned with the nature of this relationship and the role pathological dissociation plays in trauma-associated disorders. However, the reader should recall that some forms of dissociation are considered normal, and are present to a greater or lesser extent in most individuals. (Chapters Nine . and Ten take a longer look at normative dissociation).

This chapter serves as an introduction to dissociation. It begins with an examination of the measurement of dissociation, and continues with a look at the lines of empirical evidence linking elevated levels of dissociation with traumatic experience. The chapter then describes the debate concerning whether a continuum model or a typological model is better suited to dissociation. It concludes with a psychological discussion of the "defensive" functions of dissociation.

MEASUREMENT OF DISSOCIATION

The significant advances made over the last decade in understanding dissociation result primarily from our increased ability to define and measure dissociative behaviors and symptoms operationally. Many clinicians made significant contributions to the phenomenological description of dissociative disorders and to the development of the DSM-III criteria for these disorders during the 1970s. The first questionnaire to screen for dissociation was the General Amnesia Profile (GAP), developed by Cornelia Wilbur and David Caul (1978). Never published, the GAP was circulated as a handout. A number of GAP-type items are included on the Dissociative Experiences Scale (DES). The GAP simply recorded "yes" or "no" responses to amnesia questions; there were no norms or cutoff scores to guide clinicians.

By the early 1980s it was evident that a better measure was needed to advance the field. I was pondering this issue when I presented my research on MPD to a graduate school psychology colloquium at American University in 1982. Afterwards Eve Bernstein Carlson, a first-year student, approached me and observed, "What you really need is a scale to measure dissociation." I agreed. The development of a reliable and valid dissociation scale, the DES, became the topic of Eve's doctoral dissertation (Bernstein and Putnam, 1986).

The DES operationalizes measurement of dissociation by inquiring about a set of dissociative experiences and symptoms, identified by experienced clinicians as central to MPD and other chronic dissociative conditions. Two official forms of the DES exist: the DES and the DES-II. (There are also a number of unauthorized versions with different questions and answer formats.) Both versions contain the same questions, but they have somewhat different answer formats. All questions share a standard format of neutrally inquiring whether the subject has had a given type of experience, and if so, what percentage of the time that experience has occurred. For example, question 3 inquires, "Some people have the experience of finding themselves in a place and having no idea how they got there. Mark the line to show what percentage of the time this happens to you."

The subject answers by indicating the percentage of time, ranging anywhere from 0% to 100% of the time. The response scale for the DES is a 100-mm analogue line anchored at the ends by "0%" and "100%." For each question the subject simply marks the line to indicate the percentage of time that he or she has had that kind of an experience. To score the answer, the clinician measures the distance in millimeters from 0% to the subject's mark, and the number of millimeters is the score for that question. In practice, we round off to the nearest 5 mm, and the DES becomes a 20-point scale.

The 100-mm analogue line has been criticized by some as unduly cumbersome to score. (Once an evaluator gets the hang of it, this is not really a problem. I can score a DES in under 90 seconds.) A few have substituted the ubiquitous Likert format used in psychological measures. Eve and I tested descriptor-anchored and unanchored Likert formats in early trials, and found that Likert formats discriminated poorly between high and low responders. The 100 mm analogue line was chosen over Likert and other formats because it yielded better discrimination and produced sufficient variance among subjects.

Others have criticized the "percentage of time" construct, pointing out that this is an ambiguous referent to be quantifying. We have always acknowledged that this does not make perfectly logical sense. Paradoxically, we are screening for individuals who have problems with their sense of time. However, when one appreciates a dissociative patient's preoccupation with time, the use of the "percentage of time" format makes more clinical sense. (Actually, this is no more ambiguous than the usual Likert format of asking whether something happens "never," "a little," "a lot," "all the time," etc.) In many respects the proof of the pudding is in the eating. Studies examining the reliability and validity of the DES find that it works remarkably well (Carlson and Putnam, 1993; van IJzendoorn and Schuengel, 1996).

We soon learned that U.S. clinicians are slow to adopt the metric system; apparently few of them own a millimeter ruler. Consequently, the DES-II was developed (Carlson and Putnam, 1993). (We considered naming it the "DES Lite" or the "EZ-DES.") Subjects answer the DES-II by circling a numerical percentage (e.g., 0%, 10%, 20%) for each question. Our initial reliability and validity study established that the DES and DES-II were highly correlated in normal and clinical samples (Carlson and Putnam, 1993) . Ellason, Ross, Mayran, and Sainton (1994) subsequently replicated our findings with a larger sample. In their study, the DES and DES II were correlated at r (178) = .96 in the combined sample and r (87) = .95 in MPD patients. Clinically, the DES and DES-II are interchangeable. I prefer the DES for research purposes.

A manual containing a reproducible copy of the DES-II and information on the clinical and research uses of the DES, together with normal and clinical values and references, is available as a journal article (Carlson and Putnam, 1993). A reproducible copy of the DES-II is available in Appendix One. Copies of the scales and manual are also available from me. The DES and DES-II are public domain documents. No specific permission or copyright release is necessary for reproduction, distribution, or use.

Scale development has been extremely important to research in dissociation and PTSD. Although the DES and DES-II are now established as tools of empirical research, it should not be forgotten that the item content of these measures is directly derived from clinical experience. We can anticipate improved second-generation measures in the near future. For example, the DES-T, a simple eight-item measure derived from the DES and discussed later in this chapter, focuses exclusively on pathological dissociation (Waller et al., 1996). Importantly, dissociation measures tailored to specific developmental periods and different cultures are becoming available and promising to extend research to new arenas.

In addition to dissociation scales, several structured diagnostic interviews have been developed. The two most notable are the Structured

Clinical Interview for DSM-IV Dissociative Disorders—Revised (SCID-D-R; Steinberg, 1994) and the Dissociative Disorders Interview Schedule (DDIS; Ross et al., 1989b). Both have been validated and are widely used clinically and for research. The SCID-D-R and DDIS are essential to establishing DSM diagnoses in research studies. A number of studies have cross-validated the DDIS and the original SCID-D with the DES (Ross et al., 1990; Steinberg, Rounsaville, and Cicchetti, 1991; Draijer and Boon, 1993).

In the aggregate, these scales and diagnostic interviews have transformed our understanding of dissociation and the dissociative disorders. They are not perfect, and further work is necessary. Nonetheless, they provide important benchmarks in our continuing efforts to understand the nature of dissociation.

LINKAGE OF DISSOCIATION TO TRAUMA

Among the reasons why Pierre Janet is so highly esteemed by modern practitioners is that he was the first to recognize the critical association between pathological dissociation and trauma (Putnam, 1989b; van der Hart and Friedman, 1989). Clinical reports of the psychological problems of World War I veterans also drew causal connections between traumatic experiences and a range of posttraumatic and dissociative symptoms (Kardiner, 1941). Between the world wars, classic studies of dissociative amnesias by Abeles and Schilder (1935) and Kanzer (1939) reinforced this association.

During World War II, multiple studies delineated what were then known as the "wartime amnesic syndromes," although civilian cases were sometimes included (Putnam, 1985a). These cases were primarily psychogenic amnesia and fugues. Abreaction, facilitated by hypnosis or barbiturates, was the treatment of choice (Putnam, 1992). Despite the success of battlefield psychiatry in World War II with abreactive treatment of dissociative and conversion symptoms, the significance of the association between trauma and pathological dissociation was lost to the larger community of civilian psychiatrists and psychologists. For example, until the late 1970s, MPD was widely viewed as being caused by irreconcilable psychological conflicts rather than by actual trauma.

Several empirical literatures document the significant association between overwhelming traumatic experiences and pathological levels of dissociation. This research can be grouped into four lines of evidence: (1) high levels of reported trauma in patients with dissociative disorders; (2) "dose–effect" relationships between indices of trauma severity and dissociation scores in samples of patients without dissociative disorders;

(3) significantly higher levels of dissociation in traumatized samples than in nontraumatized clinical and nonclinical comparison groups; and (4) peritraumatic dissociation as a predictor of the subsequent development of PTSD (Putnam and Carlson, in press). When these data are considered together, it is difficult to dispute the conclusion that trauma "causes" pathological dissociation.

Levels of Trauma in Dissociative Disorder Patients

Every study of MPD patients that has systematically assessed trauma histories has found a high percentage of cases (i.e., 85–100%) with reported traumatic childhoods (e.g., Putnam et al., 1986; Coons et al., 1988; Loewenstein and Putnam, 1990; Ross et al., 1991; Putnam and Carlson, in press). Critics have faulted these studies for the retrospective nature of their reporting and their lack of external documentation of trauma (Frankel, 1993). In response, clinical investigators have sought to do a better job of documenting trauma histories, although this is an extremely difficult task for adult patients with long-past abuse histories. Recent studies have been able to obtain documentation for children and adolescents (Hornstein and Putnam, 1992; Coons, 1994a). In a heroic effort (aided by the forensic nature of their sample), Swica, Lewis, and Lewis (1996) were able to meticulously document the childhood maltreatment of six men convicted of violent crimes. Many subjects reported no conscious recall or denied the maltreatment that Swica et al. found documented in the subjects' records. None invoked their maltreatment in an effort to escape punishment for their crimes.

Relationships between Severity of Trauma and Dissociation

Dissociation is significantly correlated with indices of trauma severity in a number of studies (e.g., Chu and Dill, 1990; Branscomb, 1991; Carlson and Rosser-Hogan, 1991; Sandberg and Lynn, 1992; Anderson et al., 1993; Kirby, Chu, and Dill, 1993). The magnitudes of these correlations are similar to those reported between trauma indices and posttraumatic symptoms (i.e., Pearson's $r = \sim.25-.45$). Although usually statistically significant, such correlations between single indices of trauma and measures of dissociative or posttraumatic symptoms do not account for a large percentage of the variance. In part, this reflects the problem with the single-variable quantification of trauma discussed in Chapter Three. The relatively low correlations also reflect the fact that non-trauma-related factors, such as disturbed family environments, make important contributions to pathological dissociation. (See Chapter Nine for further discussion.) Nonetheless, these data document a reliable effect between dissociation and trauma.

Dissociation Levels in Traumatized versus Nontraumatized Groups

Many studies have compared traumatized and nontraumatized samples on dissociation measures. In every published study of which I am aware, the traumatized sample has obtained significantly higher scores than the nontraumatized comparison group (for a table listing 14 such studies, see Putnam and Carlson, in press). Although most of these studies have compared maltreated subjects with nonmaltreated normal controls, samples of combat veterans with PTSD are also well represented (e.g., Loewenstein and Putnam, 1988; Branscomb, 1991; Bremner et al., 1992; Marmar et al., 1994; van der Kolk et al., 1994).

Peritraumatic Dissociation as a Predictor of PTSD

The fourth line of evidence entails the clinical recognition that significant dissociation proximal to a traumatic event predisposes an individual to the subsequent development of PTSD. Arieh Shalev described this in the mid-1980s in his research on combat stress reaction among Israeli soldiers. Subsequent studies by Charles Marmar, Daniel Weiss, and their colleagues have confirmed Shalev's observation in Vietnam veterans with PTSD and in emergency service workers responding to the 1989 San Francisco Bay Area freeway collapse (Bremner et al., 1992; Marmar et al., 1994; Weiss, Marmar, Metzler, and Ronfeldt, 1995). Similarly, Koopman, Classen, and Spiegel (1994) found that the level of acute dissociative symptoms in response to the 1991 Oakland/Berkeley firestorm was predictive of subsequent PTSD. Additional studies are underway. Clinical assessment of peritraumatic dissociative symptoms should become a routine practice of clinicians responding to acutely traumatized individuals.

Cognitive and Biological Correlates of Pathological Dissociation

In the near future, we will add a fifth line of evidence. Preliminary research suggests that certain biological markers associated with severe stress and trauma are significantly correlated with dissociative symptoms. For example, Stein, Koverola, Hanna, Torchia, and McClarty (in press) reported strong correlations between DES scores and decreases in left hippocampal volume in adult women with histories of childhood sexual abuse. We have found significant correlations between DES scores and cerebrospinal fluid levels of neurotransmitters and their metabolites (Demitrack et al., 1993).

CONTINUUM VERSUS TYPOLOGICAL MODELS OF DISSOCIATION

The debate about whether individuals suffering from pathological dissociation constitute a discrete "type" or, alternatively, represent one extreme of a continuum of dissociation is as old as the field. Pierre Janet held the former point of view, that is, he maintained that pathological dissociators are a group of individuals who are fundamentally different from normal individuals. Janet (1930) believed that a combination of constitutional vulnerability, suggestibility, and powerful emotional events contributed to this propensity. By contrast, his colleagues, William James and Morton Prince, conceptualized dissociation as a continuum ranging from minor, "normal" phenomena such as absorption to pathological conditions such as fugue states and MPD. Prince, for example, was a strong believer that clinical dissociation was a form of hypnosis, which he characterized as a spectrum running from "light" to "deep" hypnotic states. In his final review of dissociation theory, Prince (1927) observed: "Let us take the two extreme types of hypnosis, the so-called lighter and deeper states (mere figures of speech, by the way), and tabulate the phenomena as determined by observation. Between the two extreme types, every degree and variety of dissociation, inhibition and integration occurs" (p. 162).

By and large, the continuum theory carried the day, although some hypnosis researchers cautioned that certain phenomena were better conceptualized as distinct discontinuities from normal consciousness than as deeper states of hypnosis/dissociation (e.g., Balthazard and Woody, 1989; Frankel, 1990). When Eve Bernstein Carlson and I drafted the DES, we adopted the prevailing continuum model of dissociation. However, even then I was sufficiently cognizant of this issue to recognize that, should it be necessary, it was possible to go from dimensional (continuum) data to categorical (typological) models more easily than vice versa.

The subsequent widespread adoption of the DES generated large data sets from clinical and nonclinical samples. Making use of data that we collected and that our collaborators and colleagues contributed, Eve and I poured over countless plots of DES score distributions and examined subscale profiles in different diagnostic groups. It was apparent that the distribution of DES scores for some diagnostic groups (e.g., patients with PTSD) were better explained by the existence of two or more discrete dissociative types than by a dissociative continuum. We presented our observations and conjectures at several meetings of the International Society for the Study of Multiple Personality Disorder (later renamed the International Society for the Study of Dissociation). In the early 1990s we began work on this question, using a large data set collected from seven clinical sites (Carlson et al., 1993; Putnam et al., 1996a).

Our exploratory efforts were interrupted by Niels Waller, a dynamo of a statistician. Niels was reviewing the DES for the Buros Institute of Mental Measurement's yearbook, and raised questions about the validity of our factor analyses (Waller, 1995). Eve and I immediately sent him the seven-site data set for a reanalysis that controlled for skewness in the distribution of certain item scores (Carlson and Putnam, 1993). To make a long story short, Niels applied a set of taxometric statistical analyses and concluded that a taxonic or typological model fit better— particularly for clinical samples—than a continuum model (Waller et al., 1996).

A taxonic or typological model basically returns to Janet's 19th-century clinical formulation that certain people experience certain dissociative states that are, by and large, not encountered by the majority of the general population. It postulates that there are at least two distinct types of dissociation, normal and pathological. There is a discrete group of people—whom we label "pathological dissociators"—who are profoundly different from the rest of the population. One of the important contributions of Waller's analyses is an eight-item subscale of the DES, the DES-T (the T is for "taxon"). The intention was to make the DES-T as compact as possible. DES-T items were required to be highly discriminative for pathological dissociation. One purpose was to serve as empirically generated diagnostic criteria. The other reason for compactness was to demonstrate that a tighter definition of pathological dissociation yields better empirical data. In an effort to test this approach further, we have distributed the DES-T to investigators collecting DES data. The items that make up the DES-T are listed in Table 4.1.

The DES-T drops DES items that ask about experiences of absorption and enthrallment (e.g., item 17, which refers to becoming so absorbed in television or a movie that one is unaware of events happening around one). (Some amnesia and identity items were also dropped for the sake of compactness; see discussion in Waller et al., 1996.) Absorption appears to be normally distributed throughout the population in a trait-like fashion and does not correlate significantly with psychopathology. DES absorption items account for most of the correlations with hypnosis and absorption scales. The DES-T only retains items that in-

TABLE 4.1. DES Items That Make Up the DES-T

Item no.	Description
3	Finding oneself in some place but unaware of how one got there
5	Finding new things among belongings—do not remember buying
7	Seeing oneself as if looking at another person
8	Do not recognize friends or family members
12	Feeling that other people, objects, and the world are not real
13	Feeling that one's body is not one's own
22	Feeling as though one were two different people
27	Hearing voices inside one's head

Note. From Waller, Putnam, and Carlson (1996).

quire about profound amnesia (e.g., item 3) and profound depersonal-ization (e.g., item 7). These are the dissociative experiences that are rarely endorsed by normal individuals or general psychiatric patients.

Thus we have two competing models of dissociation. The first is the traditional model that dissociation is a spectrum ranging from normal forms to pathological forms; the second is the Janetian view that there are distinct types of dissociation. In the continuum (dimensional) model, pathological dissociation occurs when an individual experiences more frequent and/or "deeper" states of dissociation. In the taxon (Janetian or typological) model, pathological dissociation represents a different type of dissociative experience.

Which of these two models is correct? I am not certain yet. Each accounts for some of the data. The dimensional model must be invoked to explain certain findings, and the typological model must be invoked to account for other results. I tolerate this apparent inconsistency by recalling that there are well-established examples of dual explanations in science—for example, the particle and wave theories of light. Neither theory alone is sufficient to describe all of the physical phenomena of light, but together they permit highly accurate predictions of a range of photic phenomena.

DISSOCIATION AS A DEFENSIVE RESPONSE TO OVERWHELMING TRAUMA

Janet (1901) first highlighted the "unconscious" defensive psychological functions served by dissociation to reduce anxiety and psychic conflict. In the modern era, Ludwig (1983) reformulated these functions in a classic article. He proposed that dissociation serves adaptive and defensive purposes, including automatization of behaviors; efficiency and economy of effort; resolution of irreconcilable conflicts; escape from the constraints of reality; isolation of catastrophic experiences; cathartic discharge of feelings; and the enhancement of herd sense. Others have suggested additional functions, including analgesia and detachment from the self (Putnam, 1991a).

For heuristic purposes, I group the defensive functions of dissociation into three overriding categories: (1) automatization of behavior; (2) compartmentalization of information and affect; and (3) alteration of identity and estrangement from self. These defensive processes, which reflect the multidimensional nature of dissociation, operate independently and in concert to produce the psychological and clinical phenomena that we call dissociative behaviors. In an acute traumatic situation, they function together to reduce extreme psychological—and probably physical—pain.

Automatization of Behavior

Normal Automatization

One of the everyday benefits of "normal" dissociation is the capacity of the mind to divide attention into two or more streams of consciousness; this allows an individual to perform more than one mental task at a time. Driving in rush-hour traffic while carrying on a conversation or planning future activities is a common example. In close quarters at highway speeds, driving is no simple task, and misjudgment can have tragic consequences. Yet DES studies indicate that a large percentage of the general population report dissociating while driving. For example, a sample of 100 individuals certified as "normal" (by structured interview) reported that about 20% of the time when driving a car, they suddenly realized that they did not remember what had happened during all or part of the trip (DES item 1).

How can a person safely do this? "Automatization" involves the redirection of conscious awareness away from a repetitive or procedural activity. Sufficient cognitive resources remain available for the person to continue to perform the routine activity at an acceptable level, but attention and awareness are redirected toward tasks demanding more focused awareness. Often automatization involves withdrawal of attentional resources from a boring external activity and reallocation to a more stimulating internal activity (e.g., fantasy).

For routine automatization to be safe, there must be metacognitive mechanisms that can rapidly switch full attention back to the primary procedural task—such as when some "bloody fool" swerves into the person's lane on the freeway. The emergency jolt of adrenaline that surges through the person's body instantly refocuses his or her full attention on the life-threatening situation. As "driver," the person snaps back into the immediate situation as it develops. Whatever the person may have been saying, thinking, or fantasizing about is suspended; indeed, the content of those reveries may not be available to recall at a later point. Failure to perform this attentional shift in an emergency can be fatal—an obvious evolutionary selection pressure.

Routine automatization is a dynamic process, waxing and waning across parallel mental activities. Allocation of attentional resources to any given stream of consciousness varies as a function of external and internal demands. Automated behaviors may range from minor mental overflow activities (e.g., doodling while talking on the telephone) to complex tasks (e.g., driving an automobile). Automatization increases efficiency of some procedural activities (e.g., typing speed) that become "inhibited" by self-conscious scrutiny. In amateurs, creative and athletic abilities, such as playing a musical instrument or serving in tennis, are often facilitated by the suspension of consciously directed performance. However, when one listens to the pros—that is, symphony musicians or professional tennis players—they report that their full and focused conscious attention hardly wavers. When it does, they make mistakes.

Automatization is not a form of magic or an untapped mental power. In everyday circumstances, it merely permits a boring procedural task to continue at an acceptable performance level while a person's attentional resources are focused on more appealing or demanding tasks. Compared with focused mental activity, this has costs in efficiency. Laboratory studies of divided mental activities suggest that there is interference between parallel tasks, decreasing efficiency and increasing error rates (Delignieres and Brisswalter, 1994; Pashler, 1994; Russell and Weeks, 1994; Curran and Hintzman, 1995). There may also be qualitative deficits in task performance, such as a failure to recognize and take advantage of transient opportunities that present themselves. Certainly the lore concerning the acquisition of proficiency in arts and skills indicates that nothing less than fully focused attention will suffice.

Dissociative Automatisms

"Dissociative automatisms" are episodes of automatic behavior not controlled by conscious thought (Kaplan and Sadock, 1991). Given the earlier discussion of continuum versus typological models of dissociation, this question must be asked: Are automatisms extreme examples of a spectrum of automatic behaviors, or do they represent a different type of automatic behavior? I favor the latter explanation. Behaviorally limited automatisms are also associated with epileptic processes, particularly ictally and postictally in complex partial seizures (Bye and Foo, 1994; Devinsky et al., 1994). Seizure-related automatisms are typically simple, are frequently gestural, and often include oral/lingual components (Bye and Foo, 1994; Devinsky et al., 1994).

More complex dissociative automatisms are reported in connection with acute stress in individuals with posttraumatic and dissociative disorders (Bisson, 1993; Erdreich, 1994). These are complex behaviors and occasionally include criminal acts (e.g., Shaw, 1992; Erdreich, 1994). Janet's famous description of dissociative fugues involving railway travels and hotel bookings is often quoted to illustrate how complicated, and yet completely ordinary, dissociated behavior can be. (The original is quoted on p. 14 of Putnam, 1989a.)

Dissociative automatic behavior can be life-saving. In a life-threatening situation, an individual may be called upon to perform heroic feats in order to survive or to save others. Escapes from a death trap, such as an airplane crash or a burning building, often produce dissociative automatization. Anecdotes abound, although for obvious reasons the systematic study of such behaviors is difficult. When asked immediately afterward about their thoughts and actions in the situation, people often have little to say. Clinically, it is evident that after an overwhelming traumatic event that elicits a strong automatized response, there is usually little recall of the actions or events. In time, a more complete story may emerge.

Situations of extreme grotesquery or horror—for instance, rescue personnel performing triage on gruesome casualties in a major disaster—may induce depersonalization and automatization. It is theorized (but not proven) that in cases of repetitive trauma, such as repeated physical or sexual abuse, automatization occurs when a child is repeatedly forced to perform a painful or distasteful act. It is believed that automatization of such abuse-elicited behavior provides a psychological way of complying with the demands of the perpetrator without the child's having to be fully aware of what is happening or what he or she is doing.

In dissociative patients, automatic behaviors of many types can occur both under stress and in apparently normal, everyday situations. The threshold for automatization of certain types of behavior is probably much lower in dissociative disorder patients than in normal individuals. MPD patients, with their array of alter personality states, provide dramatic examples of divided mental processes in action. MPD patients often report multiple, independent streams of consciousness representing the "separate" mental activity of alter personalities. This has never been objectively verified, but division of mental functions probably occurs to a much greater extent than in normals. It is also clear that MPD alter personality states are far from completely autonomous entities, and that they share common information and behaviors at multiple levels. Chapters Six and Seven discuss the empirical investigation of alter personality state separation in MPD patients.

Compartmentalization

A second core defensive function of dissociation is "compartmentalization," the separation of areas of awareness and memory from each other. Compartmentalization may be alternatively conceptualized as a failure of integration of experience and knowledge. This complicated process appears to be mechanistically related to state-dependent learning and memory retrieval, which are discussed in more detail in Chapter Six.

All of us periodically experience state- or context-dependent compartmentalization of our ability to recall information. For example, many people identify with the experience of being at work and planning to do something when they go home (e.g., finding a book or report necessary at work). Yet at home, they completely forget about their intention and only remember it when they return to work. Concrete reminders, such as notes to oneself or the proverbial string tied around a finger, serve as memory aids to bridge context- or state-dependent compartmentalization. State-dependent memory is also commonly illustrated by the apocryphal story of the drunken man who must get drunk again to recall where he put his car keys during his last binge. As we shall see in Chapter Six, these folklore examples are supported by laboratory research on dissociative- and drug-state-dependent learning and memory retrieval.

Defensively, compartmentalization permits the isolation of overwhelming affects and memories. Dissociative-state-dependent compartmentalization provides an individual with a mechanism to store and recall emotionally loaded information separately from other information, in cases where intense psychological conflict might result if the two sets of information should become associated. This helps the individual to avoid painful cognitive dissonance. By compartmentalizing overwhelming experiences and feelings, a child can both know that he or she is being terribly maltreated by a parent and can simultaneously idealize that parent. As Ludwig (1983) observed, dissociation permits an individual to avoid facing irreconcilable conflicts. Compartmentalization also allows one to hold different views of one self and different versions and interpretations on one's own life history—a more common process than is generally recognized (Weingartner, Putnam, George, and Ragan, 1995).

In most instances, dissociative compartmentalization is far from perfect. Trauma-related emotions and memories intrude periodically into normal awareness (e.g., intrusive memories and flashbacks). Patients often say that traumatic intrusions are the most painful and disruptive symptoms they experience. Sometimes unexpectedly blotting out normal awareness, intrusive memories and flashbacks are exceedingly disruptive and disorganizing for an individual engaged in important tasks.

Certain situations, such as exposure to trauma-related stimuli—or, conversely, a decrease in normally distracting stimuli, such as occurs while an individual is lying awake in bed at night—can increase the individual's susceptibility to intrusive memories and affects. When faced with such situations, vulnerable individuals often use drugs and alcohol to ward off intrusions. At times this can be self-defeating, as drug-altered states of consciousness sometimes increase awareness of dissociatively compartmentalized material (Krystal, Bennett, Bremner, Southwick, and Charney, 1995). Research measuring intrusive cognition in the laboratory—for example, studies using the variant of the Stroop color-naming paradigm in which the latency in naming the color of trauma-related words is measured—independently verifies what patients have been telling us about the ability of trauma-related cues to trigger intrusive cognitions, imagery, and affects (see, e.g., McNally, 1995; Litz et al., 1996).

A possible consequence of dissociative compartmentalization seems to be the relatively "unprocessed" nature of traumatic material. Painful experiences that have been dissociatively sequestered do not seem to have been nearly as psychologically transformed by time as other memories have been; they have a "raw," emotionally "fresh" quality. This is difficult to capture objectively, but nonetheless it is a common clinical feature.

When dissociatively compartmentalized memories are accessed and worked with therapeutically, there is often a vivid immediacy to the recall experience. It feels as if "it" just happened, or indeed sometimes as if "it" is still happening. Clinically, it is believed that the "unprocessed" nature of compartmentalized traumatic memories makes them powerful "unconscious" influences that shape the individual's behavior in ways that are largely out of awareness. For example, see van der Kolk and Kadish's (1987) account of Mrs. D.'s initially perplexing reenactments of the Cocoanut Grove nightclub fire, which she did not recall surviving.

In MPD patients, the profound degree of memory compartmentalization personified by the alter personality states often appears to serve as a protective response that preserves stress-sensitive abilities from disruption by overwhelming affects and memories. Such abilities (e.g., musical and artistic talents) may be accessible only through specific alter personality states, which are insulated from other alter personality states flooded with traumatic memories and affects. The breaching of alter-personality-state-dependent compartmentalization during treatment may disrupt these abilities, contributing to the sense of psychological deterioration that sometimes accompanies the early stages of therapy. With successful treatment, abilities and talents that once were unique to specific MPD alter personality states become available to the individual as a whole, although they may never be the same pure and "single-minded" experiences that they were when compartmentalized within a single state.

Alteration of Identity and Estrangement from Self

Alterations of self and identity constitute a core symptom of pathological dissociation. All of the dissociative disorders include forms of identity alteration. In dissociative amnesia, important personal information too basic to be "forgotten" (e.g., one's name) is not available to volitional recall. In dissociative fugue, dissociative amnesia may be accompanied by the adoption of a secondary identity, which is often antithetical to the primary identity. While a secondary identity exists, there is usually amnesia for the details of the primary identity. When the primary identity returns, there is often a reciprocal amnesia for the events related to the secondary identity.

Depersonalization is characterized by the persistent or recurrent experience of feeling detached from one's self and mental processes. Subjectively, this is an extremely distressing experience, although the individual's torment is often not apparent to an observer. MPD is, of course, centered around the existence of alter personality states with very different senses of identity. The DSM "catchall" category of DDNOS (see Chapter Five) contains heterogeneous examples, including culture-specific conditions in which the individual's usual identity is replaced by a new identity attributed to a power, spirit, or deity (American Psychiatric Association, 1994).

Although dissociative alterations of identity take a variety of forms, the defensive dynamics behind these alterations—in concert with the alterations in memory retrieval—serve to protect the individual (if only transiently) from a psychologically unacceptable experience. Often the alterations of identity are selective, as commonly occurs in dissociative amnesia or dissociative fugue. In these time-limited disorders, an individual may dissociate only those aspects of identity that link him or her with a specific event. Generally, full awareness of primary identity returns spontaneously or with relatively nonspecific therapeutic interventions.

More chronic identity disturbances, such as depersonalization disorder and MPD, represent complex processes. The defensive aspects, while sometimes transparent to an outside observer, can be dynamically opaque to the individual. They typically become more and more elaborated with the passage of time. The first alter personality states of MPD patients are often reported to have arisen in the context of an overwhelming traumatic event and to have had immediate survival value. However, their persistence often leads to psychological elaborations in directions that are apparently at odds with their initial adaptive purposes—for example, the transformation of protective alters into internal persecutors (Putnam, 1989a). Clinically, it is apparent that many of these long-term elaborations are maladaptive and problematic.

Dissociation and PTSD

The terms "PTSD" and "dissociation" are sometimes used loosely as if they were essentially synonymous. Certainly they are clinically related, but pathological dissociation and PTSD do not always occur in the same patient by any means. As a group, patients with PTSD score higher than patients without PTSD on dissociation measures (e.g., see Loewenstein and Putnam, 1988; Branscomb, 1991; Carlson and Rosser-Hogan, 1991; Bremner et al., 1992). Their average score on the DES is about 30, compared with an average score of 10 for normals and 44 for MPD patients. It is also established that dissociation, as measured by the DES and peritraumatic dissociation instruments, can prospectively predict the development of PTSD in acutely traumatized individuals.

However, when we inspected the distribution of DES scores in a sample of PTSD patients, we found that they divided roughly half and half into patients who scored an average of 17 and those who scored an average of 44 (Putnam et al., 1996a). This finding suggests that there may be two forms of PTSD with respect to pathological dissociation. It remains to be determined whether this is a clinically meaningful difference, but experience with BPD patients suggests that it will be. BPD patients with higher levels of dissociation have significantly more suicide attempts and self-mutilation than those with lower DES scores (e.g., Shearer, 1994; Zweig-Frank et al., 1994). These findings support the typological model of pathological dissociation.

SUMMARY

The development of valid and reliable measures of dissociation and structured diagnostic interviews for dissociative disorders has greatly advanced our state of knowledge about normal and pathological dissociation. One of the most important findings to emerge is the strong linkage between trauma and pathological dissociation. This is supported by four independent lines of evidence (to which a fifth should soon be added), and it holds for many types of trauma. Empirical research has also reopened the century-old debate about dissociative types versus a dissociative continuum. Although this question remains to be settled, it has stimulated exciting new research and helped to refine our concepts of measurement.

Clinically, dissociation is often conceptualized as a defensive process that protects the individual in the face of overwhelming trauma. However, research on the role of peritraumatic dissociation in the subsequent development of PTSD, and on the existence of many maladaptive forms of dissociation, demonstrates that there is a high price to pay for dissociative defenses. For heuristic purposes, dissociative defenses are conceptualized as performing three major tasks: automatization of behavior in the face of psychologically overwhelming circumstances; compartmentalization of painful memories and affects; and estrangement from self in the face of potential annihilation.

Although often mentioned in the same breath, dissociation and PTSD are not synonymous. Not all dissociative disorder patients have PTSD, and only half of PTSD patients have significant dissociation as measured by the DES.

Chapter Five

Pathological Dissociation

WHEN IS DISSOCIATION PATHOLOGICAL?

All models and theories of dissociation postulate the existence of both normal and pathological forms of dissociation; they differ on what makes dissociation pathological. As discussed in Chapter Four, the continuum model holds that dissociation is manifested as a normally distributed spectrum of dissociative experiences and behaviors. Pathological dissociation occurs when an individual exceeds a certain threshold for the degree of the dissociative behavior (e.g., forgetting information related to personal identity) and/or for the length of time that the dissociative behavior persists. In either case, the amount of dissociation is sufficient to cause demonstrable impairments in the individual's social and/or occupational functioning. Different social groups may have different culturally accepted thresholds.

The taxon model requires that normal and pathological dissociation be of different types. That is, pathological dissociation involves experiences that are never (or exceedingly rarely) experienced by normal people. The cognitive organization of pathological dissociators is fundamentally different from that of normal individuals.

As yet, the validity of either model has not been determined. We have approached this question statistically (Waller et al., 1996). A convergent approach is to examine the developmental trajectories of normal and pathological dissociation to see what occurs. Such developmental studies are in progress (Putnam, 1996d; Putnam and Trickett, 1997).

From a developmental perspective, the continuum model predicts that pathological dissociation occurs in one of two ways. In the first instance, the individual does not show a normal, age-related decline in dissociation with time (see the discussion of age/stage effects in Chapter Nine). Pathological dissociation occurs when the individual's degree of dissociation becomes markedly discrepant from that of peers. In the second instance, the individual's level of dissociation increases with development—perhaps as a cumulative result of life experiences—and eventually exceeds a culturally sanctioned threshold.

The taxonomic model predicts that the developmental trajectories are fundamentally different for normal and pathological dissociative outcomes. There are clear separations in such developmental dimensions as memory organization, metacognitive self-monitoring, and identity, leading to fundamentally distinct cognitive organizations.

It is worth keeping these questions in mind in this chapter, which considers pathological dissociation from the twin perspectives of (1) dissociative symptoms and (2) the DSM dissociative disorders. Like other discussions in this book, this reflects a juxtaposition of dimensional versus categorical approaches.

DISSOCIATIVE SYMPTOMS

Several reviews of historical MPD cases establish that most of the symptoms reported today were described in 18th- and 19th-century patients, and vice versa (Putnam, 1989a; Bowman, 1990; Hacking, 1991; Goff and Simms, 1993). A few features, notably the average number of MPD alter personality states, appear to have changed over time (Putnam, 1989a; Goff and Simms, 1993). These differences are probably more apparent than real, and are likely to reflect differences in the conceptualization of the syndrome rather than differences in the patients. In this vein, Hacking (1995) observes that the 19th-century conceptualization of MPD as "dual personality" made it difficult for clinicians to see more than two personalities.

Our understanding of the nature of dissociative symptoms, their relationship to traumatic antecedents, and their role in a patient's life has changed dramatically in the modern era. We have a better idea of which symptoms are pathognomonic for MPD and other dissociative disorders, and which are idiosyncratic to a given individual or can be attributed to other sources of stress or pathology. This broader perspective results from the vista provided by the statistical description of large numbers of cases. A century ago, even authorities such as Morton Prince and Pierre Janet had only a handful of cases from which to generalize. Modern studies frequently include dozens to hundreds of cases. This broader viewpoint has permitted us to identify and distinguish a set of core dissociative symptoms, and to separate these core symptoms from frequently associated posttraumatic symptoms and from other symptoms (e.g., somatic, and affective).

Richard Loewenstein (1991a) was the first to sort the myriad of symptoms described in MPD patients into meaningful clusters. The power of his approach goes beyond its heuristic intentions. Although there remain inevitable disagreements about the details of such lumping and splitting, dissociative symptoms are now approached in a more systematic manner, and interventions are targeted toward specific symptom clusters. If experience with PTSD serves as a guide, it is likely that certain symptom clusters in MPD and other dissociative disorders will prove easier to treat than others (Solomon, Gerrity, and Muff, 1992).

I have modified the symptom clusters proposed by Loewenstein (1991a) into sets of primary dissociative symptoms, frequently associated posttraumatic symptoms, secondary symptoms, and tertiary symptoms. Table 5.1 details this scheme. Primary dissociative symptoms reflect the direct effects of dissociation on cognition and behavior; these are divided into (1) amnesias and memory symptoms, and (2) dissociative process symptoms. Associated posttraumatic symptoms—for example, avoidance, physiological reactivity, hyperarousal, flattened affect, detachment, and other PTSD-like symptoms besides those pertaining to dissociation—share a common trauma-related origin with the dissociative symptoms. Although they are not primarily dissociative in nature, they are included in this table because they frequently co-occur with pathological dissociation.

Affective symptoms, somatization, and certain disturbances of self (e.g., low self-esteem) commonly noted in trauma victims are—in my opinion—secondary responses to dissociation and to associated posttraumatic stress symptoms. This hierarchical symptom organization implies that treatments directed toward secondary symptoms are only palliative until the underlying primary dissociative and trauma-related symptoms are addressed.

Finally, I believe that pathological dissociators exhibit tertiary behaviors (e.g., substance abuse, self-destructive behaviors, promiscuity, etc.) that reflect maladaptive coping responses toward the primary and secondary symptoms. The intrinsic maladaptiveness of these tertiary behaviors is usually reflected in underlying disturbances in core developmental processes (i.e., affect regulation, sense of self, metacognitive self-monitoring judgments, etc.). Resolution of substance abuse or other tertiary maladaptive behaviors is usually not possible until the underlying primary, dissociative postraumatic, and secondary symptoms are addressed.

I now discuss the primary dissociative symptoms in detail.

TABLE 5.1. Symptom Clusters in Pathological Dissociation

Primary dissociative symptoms

Amnesias and memory symptoms

Time loss, blackouts, and amnesias
Fugue episodes
Perplexing fluctuations in skills, habits, and knowledge
Fragmentary autobiographical recall
Difficulty in determining the source of recalled information
Difficulty in determining whether remembered experiences actually
    occurred
Dissociative flashbacks

Dissociative process symptoms

Depersonalization
Derealization
Passive influence/interference experiences
Dissociative auditory hallucinations
Trance-like states
Alter personality states (in MPD and fugue patients)
Switching behaviors
Dissociative "thought disorder"

Associated posttraumatic symptoms

Avoidance
Intrusive thoughts
Physiological reactivity
Hyperarousal
Flattened effect
Detachment

Secondary symptoms

Depression
Anxiety
Somatization
Low self-esteem

Tertiary symptoms

Substance abuse
Suicidal and self-destructive behaviors
Promiscuity and other sexualized behaviors

Amnesias and Memory Symptoms

Time Loss, Blackouts, and Amnesias

As described in Chapter Six, many dissociative memory symptoms can be accounted for in terms of state-dependent learning and memory retrieval. Blackouts and time loss, in the absence of substance abuse or organic problems, are hallmarks of dissociative pathology. There are two basic ways in which blackouts, amnesias, and time loss experiences come to these patients' attention. Some repeatedly discover evidence indicating that they have done things that they cannot recall (e.g., friends describe events for which the patients have no recollection). In the second instance, a patient "wakes up" or "comes to" in the middle of an event and has little or no idea of how of he or she came to be there. In either case, amnesia may be less than total—a "grayout." Or it may dynamically wax and wane, so that an individual recalls less information at some points in time than at others (Loewenstein, 1991b). Every mental status examination of every psychiatric patient should include a few basic probes for time loss and fugue experiences.

Patients will have different ways of conceptualizing and describing dissociative experiences of time loss. Some, especially children and younger adolescents, may believe that everyone has such experiences. Older adolescents come to understand that experiences of time loss are not normal. In some instances they may develop paranoid ideas that others are causing these experiences. Patients often have personal ways to describe time loss experiences (e.g., "flicking," "skipping time," "memory lapses"). When asking about such experiences, a clinician should include a generic example of time loss. Here are some examples:

> "Have you ever had the experience of finding that a lot of time has gone by, and it is much later than you thought, or even a different day?"
>
> "Have you ever had the experience of looking at a clock and noting that it is a certain time—for example, nine o'clock in the morning? And the next thing you know, it is much later—say, three o'clock in the afternoon—and you have little or no recollection of what you did between nine in the morning and three in the afternoon?"
>
> "Have you ever come to or just found yourself in the middle of doing something, and you had no recollection of when or why you started to do that thing?"

If a patient acknowledges having an experience of this type, the clinician should ask for specific examples. Adult and older adolescent dissociative patients are generally able to provide two or three such instances, which can be explored in greater depth. For each example, the therapist should inquire about substance abuse or other mitigating factors. Some MPD patients primarily report experiences of "coming to" in the middle of doing something. Others may only report examples of finding evidence for unremembered behavior. In my experience, men more often provide examples of finding evidence of unremembered behavior than of "coming to." Evidence may consist of patients' being told about the events, finding that they have done something that they don't remember doing, or finding possessions that they do not recall acquiring. Often a person's behaviors, or the results or possessions, are "out of character" for the individual and perplex or trouble him or her.

Fugue Episodes

Fugue episodes involve travel during a time loss episode, so that an individual finds himself or herself somewhere else than the person remembers being. Although lengthy, dramatic fugues are the stuff of soap operas and adventure stories, most real-life examples are prosaic and involve trips to the mall, night life, or business related events. Again, the individual may find evidence that the event has occurred or may "come to" in middle of the experience.

REGINALD

Reginald was a 17-year-old African-American male, with whom I worked from 1987 to 1989 as a consultant to a special Washington, D.C. school for disturbed children (see Putnam, 1993a). Early in our work, I was able to discern that he had MPD. As often happens in therapy with adult MPD patients, one of the major rapport-building entrees into Reginald's dissociative symptoms came about when we were first able to discuss his frequent amnesic experiences, especially fugue episodes. Reginald referred to his sense of coming and going caused by the switching among his alter personality states as "flicking." At times he blamed "flicking" on other people and entertained paranoid ideas about their control over him. In particular, he was very disturbed by the experience of finding himself somewhere doing something without any idea of why or how he came to be there. My questions about these experiences initially fed his paranoid concerns, but we were able to get beyond these by examining a particular incident in detail.

Reginald had been cruising the Georgetown area of D.C.—a social scene for teenagers—and wandering through clothing and music stores. He had some recall of being in a store examining jackets and internally debating making a purchase. Seemingly an instant later, he found himself standing in an intersection cursing a motorist, who was furiously honking back at him. He felt extremely angry—as if he wanted to kill the man in the car—but he had no idea what had happened. Shaken, he regrouped himself on the sidewalk, discovering that he was now many blocks from Georgetown and had no recollection of leaving the store. Later he realized that his jacket and wallet were missing. It was a frightening and demoralizing experience. Not only had he not purchased a new jacket (the object of his trip to Georgetown), but he had lost his old jacket and the money to replace it.

Gently and supportively, I asked about this experience. After getting a basic—if disjointed—outline of the events, I deferred my other questions about exactly what Reginald could recall, and focused instead on his feelings of confusion and his demoralization. He struggled with a range of adolescent explanations. Was this time travel? Had he stumbled into another dimension? Was this a CIA plot? Mind control? Science fiction, conspiracy theories, and the logic of thriller movies are often invoked by teenage boys to explain their dissociative experiences. Only after Reginald was helped to voice these concerns—and I responded that there were understandable explanations (though I did not discuss these in detail)—did he begin to share accounts of his amnesias and fugues. Talking about such experiences upset him. We could not stay on the subject long. I did not try to cover all the bases with each of the examples, but instead focused on different aspects of each. I identified recurrent elements of these experiences, and we found a common language to discuss what was happening to him.

In many respects, this was a socialization process of the sort that goes on in all psychotherapies. In this process, the therapist and patient seek to develop a shared understanding of the patient's psychological experiences, for the purposes of examining and changing maladaptive patterns of behavior. A skeptic might have concluded that I was leading and shaping Reginald's understanding. Indeed, simply by identifying and substituting my terminology for certain experiences (e.g., "switching" for "flicking"), I was changing his conceptualization and articulation of his symptoms. But this communicative process is common to areas of medicine far beyond the realm of psychotherapy and should not be construed as iatrogenesis. Reginald and I were creating a sharable conceptualization of what was happening with him—a version that would permit us to talk about his experiences and to identify areas for change.

Perplexing Fluctuations in Skills, Habits, and Knowledge

Fluctuations in the level of basic skills, in habits, and in recall of knowledge are classic forms of memory dysfunction in dissociative patients.

Typically, dissociative patients describe suddenly "drawing a blank" when asked to do something that they are very familiar with. Paradoxically, it seems as if overlearned information and skills are especially susceptible to intermittent failures of memory retrieval.

CARLA

Carla, an electroencephalographic (EEG) technician with MPD, would suddenly be unable to recall how to wire up patients—a task she usually excelled at. When this happened, she was adept at getting other technicians to help her without revealing the nature of her problem. On occasion, she was forced to fake the wiring or to feign an asthma attack to excuse herself. She lost one job after the neurologist, made suspicious by the bizarre quality of the EEG, inspected the pattern of the electrodes.

The missing information may be so familiar to an individual that others find it inconceivable that the patient could have "forgotten" it. They may misinterpret such problems as evidence that the patient is lying or is under the influence of alcohol or drugs. The intermittent availability of the skill or information, or the dramatic fluctuations in personal habits, contribute to the suspicious character of these symptoms. Dissociative patients attempt to compensate or cover for their sudden memory deficits in a variety of ways. Some of their deceptions are clearly bogus and contribute to the "phony" character of their behavior.

Gaps in Autobiographical Memory

Fragmentary autobiographical recall is a memory problem in dissociative disorder patients that has long been noted clinically. Evidence of difficulty with such recall has been documented by studies (e.g., Schacter, Kihlstrom, Kihlstrom, and Berren, 1989; Kopelman, Christensen, Puffett, and Stanhope, 1994a; Kopelman, Green, Guinan, Lewis, and Stanhope, 1994b; Bryant, 1995; Weingartner et al., 1995). Among the most dramatic examples occurs in dissociative amnesia (previously called "psychogenic amnesia" in the DSM-III and DSM-III-R). Dissociative amnesia is characterized by the loss of important personal information that is too extensive to be explained by ordinary forgetfulness. Typically individuals with this condition cannot recall large chunks of information relevant to their identity. Episodes of dissociative amnesia are highly associated with acute traumatic experiences (Putnam, 1985a; Loewenstein, 1991b).

In normal individuals, decline in the recall of autobiographical memories for earlier-life experiences can be fitted to a power function

(Rubin, 1986). One common effect, "childhood amnesia," is defined by the recall of fewer memories from before 5–6 years of age than would be predicted by this function (Wetzler and Sweeney, 1986). In normal individuals, childhood amnesia is a relative process, in that there are usually some memories available; there are just fewer than the "expected" number of memories. After their early years, most individuals show a predictable decrease in the recall of autobiographical memories with increasing time from an event. Age-dependent reminiscence effects have also been identified, such that at different stages in one's life, memories from specific earlier stages are overrepresented compared with memories from other periods.

In contrast, dissociative disorder patients often describe abrupt, age-demarcated gaps in autobiographical recall from which no memories can be retrieved. These gaps do not fit with the time-dependent rate of decline in autobiographical recall seen in normal subjects. For example, a dissociative patient may report not being able to recall "anything" from before age 16 years. Another dissociative patient may report missing all memories from ages 8–10 years, but may report adequate recall before and after those years. Whether dissociative discontinuities in autobiographical memory are actually as sharply delineated as patients report is difficult to test. However, such clinical reports clearly reflect psychological processes other than normal forgetting.

Impaired autobiographical recall, like other dissociative effects on memory, dynamically waxes and wanes; it is also, to some extent, alter-personality-state-dependent in MPD patients. Some MPD patients report large gaps of lost time spanning years and years. Others have the ability to retrieve memories from across their life span, but describe selectively missing memories for specific types of events (e.g., absolutely no memory for birthdays or holidays).

ANDREW

Andrew was the first psychiatric patient ever assigned to me. I was a junior medical student rotating through psychiatry. A young teenager, Andrew had been involuntarily committed following a serious suicide attempt. He did not look depressed to me (but then who was I to question the diagnosis?). We met daily in a bright, fluorescent-lit, tile-walled room on a locked ward. As far as I could determine, Andrew's major concern was that "I don't have memories." He repeatedly insisted that he wanted to have memories "just like everyone else."

I did not understand what he meant. At first I thought that he was really saying that he did not have any "happy" memories. My supervisor agreed and suggested that I explore such areas as school and friendships. But Andrew kept insisting that he did not have *any* memories, and that he wanted and needed to have memories. This did not make sense to me. Of course he had memories. He clearly remembered who I was from session to session. Despite the scatter of his subscale scores on testing, the psychologist assured us that there was no evidence of brain damage. His EEG and neurological workup were normal. We could not find anything wrong with his memory. What did he mean? In the end, my supervisor advised me to ignore this complaint and to focus instead on his depression—which I tried, without much success. Andrew wanted to talk about his missing memories. He desperately wanted to "remember" his life. Many years later, while describing the phenomenon of childhood amnesias in MPD patients to someone, I suddenly recalled those first awkward sessions with Andrew—and finally understood.

Source Amnesia and Difficulties in Determining the "Reality" of Memories

Dissociative disorder patients have difficulties identifying the source of "remembered" experiences. Unfortunately, this is not a well-recognized problem and is seldom taken into account by well-meaning therapists seeking to validate their patients' experiences. Chapter Six includes a discussion of the experimental data pertinent to this problem of "source amnesia." Clinically, one finds that dissociative disorder patients have difficulty determining whether a given memory represents something that they directly experienced or something that they read, learned, or were told about in some other fashion. They also have difficulty in determining whether something they remember as happening actually happened or whether they just thought or imagined that it happened. This does not necessarily mean that it did not happen. It means that dissociative patients have difficulties in differentiating memories of direct experiences from memories acquired from nonexperiential sources.

These problems with evaluating and making judgments about the source of recalled information reflect a fundamental metacognitive deficit. On the DES-II in Appendix One, questions 15 and 24 inquire about these problems. (Two related questions, 14 and 18, tap the experience of becoming so involved in a memory or fantasy that it feels as if it is happening.) For example, item 15 says, "Some people have the experience of not being sure whether things that they remember happening really did happen or whether they just dreamed them." Normal individuals and most psychiatric patients report that this happens about 10% of the time. MPD patients typically report that this happens over 50% of the time.

It should be emphasized that patients' difficulties in identifying the source of remembered information and determining whether recalled information reflects actual events do not mean that such patients necessarily lie or confabulate. Many are very clear about their difficulty and acknowledge their uncertainties about whether or not the memory in question is real or not. In my experience, it is more often therapists who are unwilling to tolerate the ambiguity of such memories, and who too quickly rush to "validate" their patients in the naive belief that if the patients "remember" something, it must have happened.

Dissociative Flashbacks

"Flashbacks" are spontaneous occurrences of vivid memories, images, or somatic sensations, associated with altered states of consciousness. Dissociative flashbacks are a hallmark (and DSM criterion) of PTSD (American Psychiatric Association, 1994). They are well documented clinically for many kinds of trauma. A few diehard skeptics about PTSD insist that they are as likely to be productions of the imagination as actual memories (Frankel, 1994). This view is not widely held by clinicians who actually work with traumatized individuals.

Flashbacks are also associated with hallucinogen use. Flashbacks may occur when an individual enters into an altered state of consciousness (e.g., with light anesthesia, alcohol, or psychoactive medications). It is not known whether a common mechanism is involved, but the DBS model (see Chapter Eight) predicts that flashbacks may occur in any situation in which a traumatized individual experiences an emotionally intense or markedly altered state of consciousness.

Flashbacks can be painful, frightening, and disorganizing. They occur in a variety of forms, ranging from intrusive sensations to vivid imagery that blots out awareness of the present. Flashback memories, images, and feelings may not be historically accurate. However, a remarkable number of cases are reported in which flashback elements correspond to actual circumstances. In some cases, there may be a symbolic component to the intrusive imagery or somatic sensation that underlines the patients' dynamics. See, for example, the choir member's urinary urgency, the pastor's limp, and the soldier's headache as described by Lindy, Green, and Grace (1992).

Dissociative Process Symptoms

Depersonalization and Derealization

"Depersonalization" is the sense of unreality of the self, or parts of the self. "Derealization" is the sense of a loss of reality of the immediate environment. Depersonalization and derealization frequently, but not always, occur together. In addition to depersonalization's being considered a distinct DSM-III-R/DSM-IV dissociative disorder, both depersonalization and derealization are associated with a number of psychiatric and neurological conditions, including panic disorder, schizophrenia, BPD, obsessive–compulsive disorder, substance abuse, and epilepsy (Steinberg, 1991). Transient episodes of depersonalization are common responses to trauma and life-threatening experiences (Putnam, 1985a; Steinberg, 1991).

Although distressing, depersonalization and derealization do not impair insight or basic reality testing. Chronically depersonalized individuals often report developing a sense of emotional numbness. In depersonalization disorder, the onset of symptoms is usually abrupt and may occur with awakening from sleep. Offsets tend to be more gradual, with symptoms dissipating over several days. Patients who suffer bouts of chronic depersonalization may become phobic about stimuli that they associate with the triggering of an episode. Prolonged, unremitting depersonalization has led to suicide in some instances. Patients with depersonalization disorder complain that others do not take their experience seriously. Observers unfamiliar with the intense dysphoria produced by depersonalization are often at a loss to understand why a seemingly normal individual is bitterly complaining about how he or she feels.

Depersonalization is a common symptom in MPD. Often it takes the extreme form of an out-of-body experience in which the person feels as if he or she were standing outside and watching himself or herself as if watching another person. In some cases of depersonalization disorder, the person feels split into the observer and the observed. A few depersonalization disorder patients report internal dialogues between two or more internal "parts"; however, no overt alter personality states are evident.

Depersonalization may be accompanied by profound sensory distortions, such as dimly seeing the world as if looking through smoke or fog, or hearing voices sound as if they are muffled and far away. A sense of being enclosed in and cut off from the "real" world by a bubble or a glass cage is also a common complaint. Depersonalization disorder can usually be differentiated from MPD by the lack of significant functional amnesias and by the absence of overt identity disturbances (see "The DSM Dissociative Disorders," below).

Passive Influence/Interference Symptoms

Richard Kluft (1987a) was instrumental in highlighting the role of passive influence/interference symptoms in MPD. Other have subsequently verified his observations (Ross, Heber, Norton, and Anderson, 1989d; Fink, 1991; Ellason and Ross, 1995). Passive influence/interference symptoms were once considered pathognomonic for schizophrenia; now we know that they are actually much more frequent in patients with MPD and other dissociative disorders. These symptoms include feelings, thoughts, impulses, and acts that feel as if they were involuntarily imposed upon a patient from an outside source (i.e., "made" feelings, thoughts, and actions). Passive influence/interference experiences are behind the "struggles for control" that go on in MPD patients. Sometimes these are acted out physically as such patients struggle against themselves.

Dissociative Auditory Hallucinations

Auditory hallucinations are especially common in MPD patients (Putnam et al., 1986; Putnam, 1989a; Hornstein and Putnam, 1992). In the vast majority of cases, auditory hallucinations take the form of voices heard *within* an individual's head, as opposed to being perceived as coming from external sources. The voices may argue with each other, comment on the patient's behavior in the third person; berate or belittle the individual; or provide support, solace, and advice. In addition to being internalized, dissociative hallucinations differ from schizophreniform auditory hallucinations in being distinctly heard and having distinct and consistent "personality" attributes. That is, the patient may hear several distinctly different voices, and each voice has a distinct age, gender, and personality characteristics.

THE DUTCH GROUP

In 1992, I had the opportunity to meet with a group of Dutch citizens who experienced auditory hallucinations in the absence of a formal thought disorder. Most had never been psychiatric patients; they had found each other through a national organization founded by and for people with persistent auditory hallucinations. It was obvious to me that several suffered from pathological dissociation. One woman told a particularly interesting story of a voice that proved helpful whenever she suffered a fugue episode. She might suddenly find herself in an unknown section of Amsterdam, lost and bewildered. Overwhelmed and panicked, she would become impulsively suicidal. At these moments, a gentle and loving woman's voice would talk her through the process of getting home, telling her which streetcars to take and when to get off. She said that the voice was associated with the image of a protective angel, and reminded her of a picture in a religious storybook she had treasured as a child.

Unfortunately, most of the internal voices heard by MPD patients are hostile and pejorative. They can be so loud and intrusive that an individual has great difficulty concentrating and thinking. One MPD patient characterized this experience as "mental jamming"—a metaphor that many such patients identify with. The majority of patients recognize that their internal voices are hallucinations and do not confuse them with real voices. They understand that others do not hear their voices, are not responsible for causing them, and do not experience hallucinations themselves. Many report that they can ignore the voices except when they are stressed. Because auditory hallucinations are associated with psychosis, MPD patients are reluctant to reveal their existence, even to their therapists. This is somewhat less true for children who are not as socialized to what is considered "crazy." Our group's (Hornstein and Putnam, 1992) data indicate that auditory hallucinations are somewhat less common in patients with a diagnosis of DDNOS. However, this generalization should be taken with caution, because (as discussed below) DDNOS covers a very heterogeneous group of patients, undoubtedly including a substantial percentage of patients with unrecognized MPD.

"Trance" Symptoms

Trance-like states, in which individuals "space out" and lose contact with the environment, are common in both children and adults with dissociative disorders. With the exception of depersonalization disorder, where they are infrequent, trance states do not appear to be specific for any dissociative disorder. Adults often have some awareness of their "spacing-out" episodes, but most children do not self-report these experiences. The confusion of dissociative trance-like states with "hypnotic trance" has mistakenly led some to conclude that dissociative disorders are a form of self-hypnosis (see Chapter Seven). In children, these spacing out episodes may be confused with *petit mal* seizures or ADHD. A certain amount of "spacing out" is normal for all children and declines with age. Dissociative "spacing out" is considerably more frequent, produces notable gaps in performance and recall, and is often associated with stress.

Alter Personality States

The alter personality states of MPD patients excite more fascination and evoke greater disbelief than any of their other symptoms. These states have been so sensationalized and stereotyped by the popular media and by skeptics about MPD that it has become almost impossible for them to be taken seriously as psychiatric symptoms. Once considered the hallmark of MPD, they were downgraded to "identities" in the DSM-IV in an unsuccessful bid to shed the notoriety attached to them. (The intent behind this name change is understandable; after all, look what "hypnosis" did for mesmerism.)

An elaborate mythology has grown up around alter personalities. Unfortunately, certain MPD therapists and patients have fed this mythology themselves, and thus it is not easily dispelled. "Professional" MPD patients—that is, those who trade on their disorder for fame and fortune—have cultivated the myth of the multiple as superperson ("Me and my personalities are worth any ten of you singles"). The mass media stereotype of an MPD patient is a woman harboring an internal collection of delightfully different people ranging from wide-eyed little kids to kung fu masters and nuclear physicists. Skeptics tend to focus concretely on the impossibility of there being 10 or 20 or 100 separate people inside that woman's body (e.g., Sarbin, 1995). By and large, this stereotype will not go away.

Alter personalities are real. They do exist—not as separate individuals, but as discrete dissociative states of consciousness. When considered from this perspective, they are not nearly so amazing to behold or so difficult to accept. A fair reading of the MPD literature shows that authorities have long subscribed to this thesis: "Only when taken together can all of the personality states be considered a whole personality" (Coons, 1984, p. 53). Paradoxically, it is the critics who implicitly accept the view that the alter personalities are separate people.

The reported numbers of MPD alter personality states are given great play by critics. As usual, these critics rarely consult the research. Although cases with dozens or scores of alters have been reported, the mode is 3 and the median typically 8–10 (see, e.g., Putnam et al., 1986; Coons et al., 1988; Ross, Norton, and Wozney, 1989f; Kluft, 1991). The differences in alter personality states' self-concepts can be striking, but authorities routinely stress that these are more apparent than real (e.g., Putnam, 1989a; Kluft, 1991). Various typologies have been offered, but few systematic data exist. Types of MPD alters, such as childlike personality states, angry alters, protectors, and persecutors, are found often enough to warrant further investigation.

Switching Behaviors

"Switching" refers to the transition from one discrete behavioral state to another. Switches are common in a number of psychiatric conditions, including panic attacks, rapid-cycling bipolar illness, periodic catatonia, and MPD. Switches typically occur rapidly, lasting from seconds to a few minutes (Putnam, 1988). They are important clinical features of dissociative disorders, signaling the emergence of alter personality states in MPD. Various types of switches have been described, including rapid switches, switches that pass through one or more unstable intermediate states, and switches that require an intervening period of sleep.

Dissociative switches are frequently manifested by discontinuities in train of thought; sudden, inexplicable shifts in affect; and changes in facial appearance, speech, behavior, and mannerisms. Following a switch, dissociative patients may exhibit evidence of disorientation. So-called "grounding" behaviors (e.g., touching the face, marked postural shifts, and rapid scanning of the immediate environment) may also mark switches. In many cases, dissociative switches may be associated with an upward rolling of the eyes or rapid blinking.

Dissociative "Thought Disorder"

Clinicians have long noted that patients with MPD or other dissociative disorders have peculiarities in their thinking. Initially, these were ascribed to the effects of hypnosis on cognition and subsumed under the label "trance logic." "Trance logic" refers to a kind of concreteness of thinking and an ability to tolerate mutually contradictory propositions without a seeming awareness of their logical dissonance. However, recent studies using projective techniques are finding evidence of a unique cognitive organization that can be distinguished from that of normals and schizophrenic patients—the two groups with whom pathological dissociators are most frequently compared on psychological testing.

Psychologist Judith Armstrong has creatively investigated this question (Armstrong, Laurenti, and Loewenstein, 1990; Armstrong and Loewenstein, 1990; Armstrong, 1991, 1996). Developing a protocol that tracked dissociative behaviors and clarified subjective experiences, Armstrong demonstrated that many transient "psychotic" phenomena in dissociative patients actually reflect dissociative process symptoms, such as hallucinations, passive influence/interference experiences, and switching. She also found that dissociative patients resembled schizophrenics on some Rorschach subscales and normals on others. Dissociative patients were similar to schizophrenics on measures of distortions in reality and inaccuracy in perceptions of others (Armstrong and Loewenstein, 1990; Armstrong, 1991). They were significantly different from schizophrenics on self-observation, awareness of complexity and ambiguity, and greater sensitivity to inner and outer complexity. In some instances, they scored better than normals on the self-observation and internal complexity scales. They also exhibited traumatic sensitivity to the ambiguities of Rorschach stimuli, in some cases treating the inkblots as if they were literal representations of traumatic events. In such instances, they exhibited behavioral regression and concreteness of thinking.

The typological model holds that the cognitive organization of people with pathological dissociation is different from that of normal individuals. Preliminary studies support this possibility. However, the generic traumatic responses that pathological dissociators share with PTSD patients complicate the characterization of the dissociative cognition. Study of the cognitive effects of pathological dissociation offers an important avenue of future investigation. (See the section on psychological testing in Chapter Twelve.)

What Does It Feel Like to Dissociate?

Dissociative experiences have been well chronicled in the popular press. Indeed, critics claim that the mere abundance of these accounts is essentially responsible for the creation of MPD (e.g., Merskey, 1992). I will leave the reader to consider such accounts in the original sources. The following is an account of a personal experience.

FRANK

When I was 6 years old, I had a minor surgical operation that involved several days' hospitalization (according to the standards of the time). The procedure was uneventful, and everything went well. Although the hospitalization was rarely discussed subsequently in my family, I have continuous memories for a number of events. These included (1) having a preoperation enema and being surprised by the amount of feces; (2) holding the anesthesia mask to my face and feeling as if I were falling backwards into a spinning black hole (the story of my holding the mask was told several times by my parents as an example of how brave I was); (3) the postanesthesia experience of slipping in and out of consciousness while my father sat by my bed reading to me from Hemingway's *The Old Man and the Sea*; and (4) the experience of suddenly waking that night, with all the adults gone and the other children in the room asleep, and feeling alone and frightened. What I did not recall, until confronted with a highly salient cue years later, was a minor traumatic experience that occurred when my blood was drawn for routine tests.

At age 14 years, I had blood drawn for allergy studies. The nurse rolled a tray into the room containing a glass syringe with a long needle. (Now, I would guess it to have been a 20-cc syringe with a large-bore needle.) The sight of that syringe and needle triggered a flashback to the episode in the hospital when I was 6. In a visual rush, I recalled being pinned down by a man with a white coat, while the man drew my blood with a similar huge syringe and long needle. I saw it happening, even as I simultaneously saw the allergy nurse's surprised reaction to my panic. I had a foot in two worlds. The simultaneity of the past and present experiences was overwhelming—and the past was more vivid than the present. There was a detached, observing part of me that, as a 14-year-old, recognized that I was behaving inappropriately. But I could not help myself or stop it. I could hear myself blurting out the story in a confused fashion. The nurse seemed to understand that I was reacting to something in the past, and made a comment to my embarrassed mother about its being a shame what some people did when they drew blood from children.

I can reconstruct the hospital experience now. Undoubtedly some of the details are incorrect, and others have changed or been added with time. In particular, my medical education has led to deductions about what may have happened. Having drawn blood from children many times myself, I can even empathize (just a little) with the lab technician or medical student involved. In short, he (wearing a white coat) rolled a procedure tray into the room, which prominently displayed a huge syringe with a long needle among the medical paraphernalia. There were four of us children in the room, and I had learned that most of the coming and going of doctors and nurses did not concern me. I recall thinking or saying, "I'm glad that's not for me," and then being horrified when he stopped at my bed. Like many children (and some adults), I equated the size of the syringe and length of the needle with how much it was going to hurt. He told me to hold my arm out, look at the wall, and count to 10. He said that he was not going to stick me with the needle until I reached 10. Of course, I felt the needle at 1. He lied. As much as anything, I think that this betrayal changed the situation for me. I fought back, and he subdued me by pinning me down. I do not recall how it ended, but I assume that he got the necessary blood. As far I can tell, I did not remember this experience until confronted with an analogous situation and similar syringe some 8 years later.

Introspection, once valued, now unjustly has a bad reputation—especially among academic psychologists. Yet introspection remains the most direct source of information about mental life. Examining this experience, I am most impressed by the sense of mental multiplicity inherent in the parallel streams of consciousness. The sensory vividness of the flashback–abreaction component was also very compelling. Indeed, during the abreaction, the present seemed dim and far away. The sense of two simultaneous but differentially vivid "here and nows," together with a detached aspect critically observing my own behavior, produced an overall disorientation and the loss of a centrality or locus of self. I was mentally divided and caught in the grip of an emotional torrent of memory. Until it ran its course, I was not in control of my behavior. Afterward, I could volitionally recall the event, and it had lost its power over me. In short, I briefly came "apart" (dis-integrated) in the face of a uniquely personal "traumatic reminder" (the glass syringe). I was, however, subsequently able to reintegrate my sense of self and experience (i.e., "get it together"), and to include that previously dissociated memory in my life history.

THE DSM DISSOCIATIVE DISORDERS

DSM Criteria

The DSM-IV recognizes five dissociative disorders: dissociative amnesia, dissociative fugue, depersonalization disorder, dissociative identity disorder (DID), and dissociative disorder not otherwise specified (DDNOS) (American Psychiatric Association, 1994). Several of the dissociative disorders listed in the DSM-III and DSM-III-R were renamed in the DSM-IV. These include the renaming of MPD as DID, and the renaming of psychogenic amnesia and psychogenic fugue as dissociative amnesia and dissociative fugue, respectively.

The DSM (American Psychiatric Association, 1952) included the diagnosis "dissociative reaction." This was changed to "hysterical neurosis, dissociative type" in the DSM-II (American Psychiatric Association, 1968) and assigned the DSM code number 300.14, which MPD/DID carries today. The dissociative disorders became a separate diagnostic category in the DSM-III (American Psychiatric Association, 1980) and have been retained and expanded in subsequent revisions. Thus the frequent comment that MPD was "first created" in the DSM-III is incorrect. It was in fact included under the dissociative reaction and hysterical neurosis categories of the two earlier versions.

Although I served on both the DSM-III-R and DSM-IV dissociative disorder work groups, I have strong reservations about the diagnostic criteria specified by the DSM for MPD/DID. More stringent, better-operationalized criteria for MPD can readily be devised. For example, the NIMH research criteria focus on the observable phenomena manifested by the alter personalities of MPD subjects (Loewenstein and Putnam, 1990; Hornstein and Putnam, 1992). The specification of distinctness and consistency of the alter personality states presents just one of several opportunities to delineate diagnostic criteria more crisply. Current DSM-IV criteria do not even require a therapist actually to witness any signs or symptoms of pathological dissociation (American Psychiatric Association, 1994). A DSM diagnosis of DID can be made entirely from the patient's report. Such vague criteria were initially favored by some to stimulate the diagnosis of MPD, which was believed to be underrecognized (e.g., Kluft, 1991). Unfortunately in some instances, this looseness has pushed the diagnostic process in the wrong direction. Thus, I have chosen in this book to refer generally to this disorder as MPD rather than as DID.

Epidemiology of the Dissociative Disorders

General Issues

We know very little about the epidemiology of the dissociative disorders. This is largely a result of the failure of epidemiologists to include measures for pathological dissociation in recent studies. Dissociative disorder researchers have little expertise in epidemiology; consequently, the incidence and prevalence figures they provide are of limited value and should be regarded as "guesstimates."

Enthusiasts' early hyperbole concerning an MPD "epidemic" (e.g., Boor, 1982) haunts us all, because skeptics claim this as "proof" of the iatrogenic nature of modern cases. Changes in the rate of diagnosis of a disorder do not say much one way or the another about the validity either of the disorder itself, or of individual applications of the diagnosis. As I have pointed out elsewhere, there are sufficient examples of valid increases in the frequency of a given diagnosis that it is ridiculous to point to this alone as evidence of iatrogenesis (e.g., Putnam, 1993b, 1996a; McHugh and Putnam, 1995).

Eating disorders and obsessive–compulsive disorder are two psychiatric conditions now known—largely as a result of epidemiological studies—to be considerably more prevalent than previously believed. Diagnosed cases of bipolar disorder increased dramatically after the introduction of an effective treatment, lithium. A cogent formulation of a heretofore unrecognized disorder can also stimulate the frequency with which a diagnosis is made. "Battered-child syndrome" and "shaken baby syndrome," discussed in Chapter Two, are excellent examples. The descriptions of both (Kempe et al., 1962; Caffey, 1972) were followed by marked increases in the number of child abuse cases recognized by physicians.

In short, the frequency with which a diagnosis is made may be influenced by a number of factors, including improvements in our ability to look systematically for it, an increased awareness resulting from a new treatment, and new or better clinical formulations.

Research

The best epidemiological data to date come from a study conducted by Ross, Joshi, and Carrie (1989e) using the DES to survey a large, stratified sample of the general population in Winnipeg, Manitoba, Canada. Ross (1991) subsequently followed up approximately 40% of the sample with his group's diagnostic interview, the DDIS (see Chapter Four). He reported that 3.1% of the interviewed sample met DDIS criteria for MPD and that 11.2% met criteria for one of the dissociative disorders. Niels Waller reexamined Ross's original DES data, using the DES-T as an index of pathological dissociation (Waller and Ross, in press). Waller's calculated base rate for pathological dissociation in the Ross sample was 3.3%. If pathological dissociation were to be equated with MPD, the two different estimates would be congruent. More sophisticated epidemiological studies must be conducted—but tools such as the DES-T make this relatively easy.

Among current sources of data are studies of consecutive admissions to psychiatric units. Several such studies have employed the DDIS or SCID-D to diagnose dissociative disorders in patients admitted to psychiatric facilities. Saxe et al. (1993) screened 110 consecutive psychiatric admissions to a state psychiatric facility with the DES and administered the DDIS to all who scored over 25. They found that 15% of all admissions had MPD. Latz, Kramer and Hughes (1995) studied 175 women consecutively admitted to a state hospital with the DES and DDIS, and found that 12% had MPD. In Canada, Horen, Leichner, and Lawson (1995) screened 48 consecutive admissions with the DES and administered the DDIS to subjects scoring 25 or higher. They reported a 17% prevalence for dissociative disorders, with 6% of subjects meeting criteria for MPD. In France, 30 consecutive victims of "intrafamily rape" were given the SCID-D at a forensic center in Tours (Darves-Bornoz, Degiovanni, and Gaillard, 1995). Fourteen percent met criteria for MPD. Screening consecutive admissions to two units in Zurich, Switzerland with the DES, Modestin and colleagues (Modestin, Ebner, Junghan, and Erni, 1996) found dissociative symptom levels similar to U.S. studies, but a somewhat lower rate (5%) of dissociative disorders as diagnosed by the DDIS.

These studies suggest that between 5% and 15% of psychiatric inpatients meet criteria for MPD. Many more qualify for a diagnosis of another dissociative disorder or of PTSD. Better data are required before we have a good picture of the true prevalence of dissociative disorders, but these studies support the contention that dissociative disorders are not vanishingly rare among psychiatric inpatients.

Dissociative (Psychogenic) Amnesia

Dissociative amnesia (formerly psychogenic amnesia) is an acute and generally time-limited dissociative disorder characterized by an inability to recall important personal information. The nature and scope of the unavailable information are too extensive for it to be explained as ordinary forgetting (American Psychiatric Association, 1994). This information loss must occur in the absence of MPD/DID, dissociative fugue, PTSD, acute stress disorder, or somatization disorder. Nor may the amnesia be associated with the direct effects of a psychoactive substance or a general medical condition. The loss of information must cause significant impairment or distress in an important area of function (e.g., social, marital, or occupational).

The DSM-IV classifies amnesia into five basic types: "localized," "selective," "generalized," "continuous," and "systematized." Localized amnesia is the failure to recall events that occurred during a delimited period of time (e.g., failure to recall anything that happened during a traumatic experience). Selective amnesia is the failure to recall some information or events from a period of one's life (e.g., inability to recall certain combat-related happenings). Generalized amnesia is the loss of all memory of one's life. Continuous amnesia is the ongoing failure to encode and recall events as they occur, from a specific point in the past up through the present. Continuous amnesia is rarely dissociative in origin and usually reflects significant brain damage. Finally, systematized amnesia is memory loss for particular classes of information (e.g., information about certain people or places).

By far the best review of the subject is Loewenstein's (1991b) chapter on psychogenic amnesia and fugue. Early studies and reviews considered psychogenic (dissociative) amnesia the most common form of dissociative disorder. However in the last few decades the numbers of published cases of MPD have exceeded the total for psychogenic amnesia by a considerable margin. Eight case series of psychogenic amnesia, with samples of 30–144 patients, were published between 1935 and 1962. With the exception of scattered case reports, no further clinical series were forthcoming until the Coons and Milstein (1992) study.

This comprehensive evaluation of 25 cases challenged a number of common beliefs about psychogenic amnesia. Coons and Milstein (1992) found that most of their patients' amnesia did not have a sudden onset and that the amnesia was frequently chronic as opposed to transient. In part, this was a result of how they chose to define their sample (i.e., they ignored the "sudden onset" stipulation of DSM-III-R criterion A). However, it suggests that there may be more than one type of psychogenic (dissociative) amnesia. Their sample resembled MPD patients in having high rates of childhood abuse (though lower than those for MPD patients), multiple symptoms (e.g., depression, headaches, somatization, depersonalization, and auditory hallucinations), and high rates of recurrence.

Differential diagnosis includes the other dissociative disorders; dementia, delirium, and organic amnesic syndromes (e.g., Korsakoff's psychosis, amnestic stroke, transient global amnesia, etc.), seizure disorder; posttraumatic amnesia due to brain injury; psychoactive substance abuse amnesia; PTSD; somatoform disorders; and malingering or amnesia for criminal behavior (Loewenstein, 1991b). Clinical evaluation should include a complete history (to the extent of the patient's ability to provide it), including childhood; a full mental status examination; cognitive testing; and baseline clinical laboratory testing and toxicology screening. A dementia workup, including EEG, magnetic resonance imaging (MRI) and neuropsychological testing, is often indicated.

Dissociative (Psychogenic) Fugue

The DSM defines dissociative fugue as unexpected, sudden traveling away from one's home or usual place of work, with inability to recall the past (American Psychiatric Association, 1994). There is confusion about aspects of identity, and some individuals may assume a new identity. These symptoms must cause impairment or distress in some important area, and must not be due to another dissociative disorder, the direct results of a medical condition, or the direct effects of a psychoactive substance.

Fugues can be caused by a variety of organic insults, including epilepsy, strokes, and tumors, as well as by a variety of medications and drugs of abuse (Good, 1989; Kopelman et al., 1994b; Kopelman, Panayiotopoulos, and Lewis, 1994c). The differential diagnosis is essentially the same as that of psychogenic amnesia. A thorough medical and neurological evaluation is mandatory. A combination of psychogenic and neurogenic factors is probably more common than realized (see, e.g., Kopelman et al., 1994b). The incidence of fugues is unknown.

Psychological precipitants include occupational, marital, financial, and legal problems; anticipated stresses such as combat; and suicidal ideation (Loewenstein, 1991b). Fugues may also occur after profound loss (e.g., death of a loved one). Recurrent fugues are probably not uncommon in some individuals, but repeated episodes should increase suspicion for MPD. Classic dissociative fugues typically last a few days, but can continue for months in some cases. An individual in a fugue state may appear a bit odd, but is usually able to function and interact with others appropriately. Recovery of memory and primary identity is usually sudden and spontaneous, leaving the individual bewildered and panicked.

The secondary identity assumed during the fugue state may be partial (i.e., the person retains some elements of the primary identity) or complete. It is often psychologically at odds with the primary identity, supporting dynamic interpretations that fugues represent a psychological defense against overwhelming experiences—particularly those associated with the assumption of risk or responsibility. There is often reciprocal amnesia between primary and secondary identities; that is, while in one identity, the individual has little or no recall of the other identity.

Depersonalization Disorder

Depersonalization disorder is characterized by recurrent or persistent feelings of being detached from or outside of one's thought processes and/or one's body (American Psychiatric Association, 1994). Reality testing remains intact. The depersonalization must cause significant impairment or distress in social, occupational, or other areas. The depersonalization must not be directly associated with another disorder (e.g., schizophrenia, another dissociative disorder, or PTSD), or related to a medical condition (e.g., epilepsy) or to effects of a psychoactive substance (e.g., marijuana).

Depersonalization is a ubiquitous symptom—perhaps the third most common psychiatric symptom after depression and anxiety (Putnam, 1985a). Surveys of normal subjects report widely varying rates, ranging from 8.5% to 70%. Transient episodes of depersonalization appear to be relatively common in adolescents and to decline with age.

Depersonalization is linked to trauma in a number of ways. First, high rates of depersonalization are reported in survivors of sustained traumatic experiences, such as concentration camp inmates (Putnam, 1985a). Second, studies of acute trauma victims find high rates of depersonalization proximal to the traumatic experience (Putnam, 1985a; Cardeña and Spiegel, 1993). Finally, depersonalization is a common symptom in trauma-related disorders, such as PTSD and MPD.

However, depersonalization also occurs in many instances where there is no evidence of traumatic antecedents. It is a common symptom in epileptic patients, especially in association with dominant-hemisphere lesions (Devinsky, Putnam, Grafman, Bromfield, and Theodore, 1989). It is also frequent in anxiety patients and in schizophrenics. The clinical literature is dotted with case reports of depersonalization associated with medication side effects or drug abuse (Steinberg, 1991). Depersonalization has also been associated with intensive meditation or immersion in cult religions (Castillo, 1990).

Dissociative Disorder Not Otherwise Specified

DDNOS is defined as a category in which the principal symptoms are dissociative, but the individual does not meet criteria for another dissociative disorder (American Psychiatric Association, 1994). The most common clinical presentation is symptomatically similar to MPD/DID, but without separate and distinct alter personality states. The DSM-IV also includes derealization without depersonalization under DDNOS. Dissociative states induced by prolonged or brutal torture, interrogation, or indoctrination likewise fall within DDNOS. The DSM-IV further includes a variety of culturally specific possession or dissociative trance states—for instance, *ataque de nervios* (Latin American), *latah* (Malaysian), *pibloktog* (Inuit), and *amok* (Indonesian). Finally, Ganser's syndrome (i.e., the giving of inappropriate or approximate answers) is subsumed under DDNOS.

With such a wide range of conditions lumped under this diagnosis, few generalizations can be made about it. Research studies find high rates of childhood trauma in DDNOS cases (e.g., Hornstein & Putnam, 1992). Clinicians working with these patients feel that many can be described as having MPD without externalized alter personality states. DDNOS patients often report a strong subjective sense of internal division.

Dissociative Identity Disorder (Multiple Personality Disorder)

DID—again, generally referred to herein by its original name of MPD—is defined by the presence of at least two different personality states or identities, each with its own fairly consistent pattern of viewing, relating to, and thinking about the self and the environment (American Psychiatric Association, 1994). Two or more of these personality states must recurrently control the individual's behavior. The DSM-IV added a psychogenic amnesia criterion (C), which requires that the individual exhibit an inability to remeber significant personal information that is too extensive to be explained as ordinary forgetting. As in the other dissociative disorders, this disturbance cannot be due to the effects of psychoactive substances or a general medical condition.

Although I have serious reservations about the appropriateness of the DSM criteria, I believe in the validity of the overall MPD diagnostic construct. For many years, I have said that the validity or existence of MPD must be argued in the same fashion as that of other psychiatric diagnoses (e.g., Putnam, 1986a). Perhaps the best articulation of the requirements for psychiatric diagnostic validity is the paper by Robins and Guze (1970; see also Robins and Barrett, 1989; Andreasen, 1995). They stipulate that valid psychiatric diagnoses must satisfy three basic forms of validity: "content validity," "criterion-related validity," and "construct validity." Content validity is the most fundamental form of validity. It requires that clinicians be able to give a specific and detailed description of the disorder. Criterion-related validity requires that laboratory tests (e.g., biological, radiological, or reliable psychological tests) be consistent with the disorder. Construct validity (or discriminant validity) requires that the disorder be delimited from other disorders.

All of these validity requirements have been robustly met by research on MPD. The clinical phenomenology is well delineated and has been widely replicated by different investigators, using different kinds of methodology, drawn from different populations and age groups (e.g., Putnam et al., 1986; Coons et al., 1988; Ross, 1989; Schultz, Braun, and Kluft, 1989; Loewenstein and Putnam, 1990; Ross et al., 1990; Hornstein and Putnam, 1992; Coons, 1996). The core pathological process, dissociation, can be detected and measured by reliable and valid scales. The disorder can be identified by reliable and valid structured diagnostic interviews (see the discussion of these in Chapter Four). These measures satisfy the reliability requirements imposed by Robins and Guze (1970) on psychological tests as sources of criterion-related validity. Finally, by means of these measures or certain other psychological tests, MPD patients can be robustly discriminated from other psychiatric patients and from normals. This fulfills the construct validity requirement (e.g., Ross et al., 1989d; Steinberg et al., 1991; Carlson et al., 1993; Draijer and Boon, 1993; Steinberg, 1994; van IJzendoorn and Schuengel, 1996).

The MPD construct is further bolstered by other sources of validity that are often absent for other psychiatric disorders. For example, MPD is found in many diverse cultures (e.g., Martinez-Taboas, 1989; Coons, Bowman, Kluft, and Milstein, 1991; Boon and Draijer, 1993; Sar, Yargic, and Tutkun, 1996). By means of translated dissociation scales and structured interviews, MPD can be discriminated from other psychiatric disorders in those cultures. This demonstrates the cross-cultural universality of this form of pathological dissociation.

MPD is one of the oldest Western psychiatric diagnoses. We have clearly described cases dating back two or more centuries. In addition to the contributions of Pierre Janet, Morton Prince, and others, we have descriptions of early MPD cases by such important historical figures as Benjamin Rush, father of U.S. psychiatry (Carlson, 1981). Thus MPD is consistent across time and cultures; such a claim can be documented for few other psychiatric disorders. And, as this book demonstrates, MPD and other forms of pathological dissociation are found in children and have features that fit with developmental data and theories.

Criticisms of the existence of MPD often appear to be directed more at the mass media stereotype described earlier than at the actual condition. One wonders what it is that critics fear most—MPD per se, or what it says about the human condition. To make progress in the deadlock that has developed, we must move arguments about the validity of MPD to the higher level of proof inherent in the Robins and Guze (1970) model or a similarly accepted model of psychiatric diagnostic validity (McHugh and Putnam, 1995).

SUMMARY

Pathological dissociation can be considered from a symptomatic (dimensional) or a DSM disorder (categorical) point of view. Dissociative symptoms can be grouped into two broad categories: amnesias and memory symptoms, and process symptoms. Amnesias and memory symptoms take a number of forms, including amnesias for complex behaviors, perplexing forgetfulness for well-known information, gaps in autobiographical recall, and problems with identifying the source of remembered information. Dissociative process symptoms include depersonalization and derealization, passive influence/interference symptoms, hallucinations, trance-like states, and fugue and MPD's alter personality states.

The DSM concept of pathological dissociation has evolved from the early inclusive concept of a dissociative reaction in DSM-I to five distinct dissociative disorders in DSM-IV: dissociative amnesia, dissociative fugue, depersonalization disorder, DDNOS, and MPD/DID. The first four disorders are rarely challenged, but the existence of MPD/DID has been more or less continually under attack for more than a century. I perceive many of these attacks as misdirected at a mass media stereotype that does not resemble the actual clinical condition. Future debate would be advanced considerably if critics made use of the prevailing standards for the validity of psychiatric diagnosis.

Chapter Six

Trauma, Dissociation, and Memory

As discussed in Chapter Five, disturbances of memory—such as amnesias for complex behaviors, perplexing forgetfulness for well-rehearsed information, and amnesias for the source of information—are cardinal features of pathological dissociation. Understanding the mechanisms of these dissociative memory disturbances is a key to understanding pathological dissociation. As a background for discussing the effects of pathological dissociation on memory, I first provide a review of what has been learned about normal memory from numerous experiments with normal individuals and neuropsychiatric patients. This includes what has been learned about children's memory.

The next step is to examine research on the effects of stress and trauma on memory. These effects are not exclusively dissociative in nature, although amnesias are common in many trauma victims. Traumatic memories are the subject of heated controversies, but recent research is beginning to shed some light on the subject. Within this context, the literature on the effects of stress and trauma on children's memory is reviewed. With this background, the small experimental literature on memory deficits in MPD patients can be examined in depth. Finally, I consider the issue of pseudomemories, which stands at the center of the acrimonious traumatic memory debate.

A BRIEF OVERVIEW OF MEMORY

The Reconstructive Nature of Memory

The study of memory is one of the most active and fascinating areas of neuropsychology—and highly relevant to clinical work. As the debate about "false memories" has driven home, memory is anything but a simple tape recorder or video camera that faithfully records events.

Most memory researchers subscribe to the idea that memory is either partially or wholly reconstructive. That is, the act of recalling an event involves the active linking of previously encoded event-related information with mental models, perceptual biases, associated memories, information, and emotions. This conceptualization is attributed to Frederic Bartlett, who introduced the concept of a "schema" to psychology (Martin, 1994). The schema concept permeates modern cognitive science and is a basic building block across a range of memory models (Martin, 1994).

Multiple Memory Systems

Memory is composed of multiple systems (Tulving and Schacter, 1990). There appear to be at least two distinct memory systems—the "explicit" and the "implicit" memory systems, which are also referred to as the "declarative" and "procedural" memory systems, respectively. These two memory systems are further divided into subsystems by different authorities. The explicit and implicit memory systems are considered distinct because deficits in one are frequently independent of deficits in the other (Squire, 1986). Memory researchers often speak of these two systems as "dissociable," meaning that they can be separated from each other (Shanks and St. John, 1994). Memory research is a rapidly evolving field, and concepts are often short-lived. There is, however, good evidence for drawing basic distinctions between explicit and implicit memory functions.

"Explicit" memory refers to memory for facts and events that involves effortful recall on the part of an individual. When individuals explicitly recall facts or events, they have an awareness of the source of that information—that is, where and how they acquired that information. For example, if a driver's first awareness of the function of an automobile distributor comes when his or hers fails on a lonely road one dark and stormy night, it is likely that the driver will recall this experience when explaining the function of the distributor at a later date.

Most conventional memory studies use tests (e.g., learning and later recalling lists of words) that tap the explicit memory system. However, studies of patients with certain kinds of brain damage show that individuals with significant impairments on explicit memory tests can nonetheless continue to learn and "remember" other kinds of information. For example, patients with Korsakoff's syndrome, an organic amnesic disorder seen in chronic alcoholics, can learn to solve a complex puzzle. Yet each time they are presented with the puzzle, they deny ever having seen it before. They do not recall their training sessions, but they show an improvement with practice that equals that of normal controls. This type of learning and memory is called "implicit" memory. Implicit memory is usually tested indirectly, by showing that an individual's performance improves with prior exposure to relevant information—even when the person has no direct recall of that exposure.

"Priming" is a classic example of implicit memory (Tulving and Schacter, 1990). The prototypical priming experiment involves exposing a subject to target information (e.g., lists of words or line drawings of common objects), and later (from seconds to months) asking the subject to name or categorize the target objects when they are presented in a "degraded" form. Target objects are typically degraded by removing specific amounts of information (e.g., letters from w—ds or pixels from a computer image). Priming is said to have occurred when the subject identifies the previously encountered targets at a significantly higher rate or significantly faster than nonstudied control items. For example, in the Szostak, Lister, Putnam, and Weingartner (1997) study of MPD subjects discussed later in this chapter priming was tested by using line drawings of common objects and backward reading of words previously presented forward as explicit memory targets.

Memory disturbances are integral to a number of psychiatric and neurological conditions besides PTSD and dissociative disorders (Tariot and Weingartner, 1986). Patients with Alzheimer's dementia exhibit dramatic deteriorations in recent memory and ability to learn new information. Studies suggest that Alzheimer's patients have deficits in encoding new information and difficulty in retrieving information encoded prior to the illness. Unlike patients with Alzheimer's, patients with Korsakoff's disease can retrieve and use previously encoded information, but they cannot encode new explicit memory information. Yet they are able to learn complex skills and procedures—although they have no memory of doing so. Patients with depression often manifest memory problems that superficially resemble those of Alzheimer's patients but in fact reflect other neuropsychological mechanisms. Depressed patients have the most difficulty learning information that requires them to make sustained or elaborate efforts, but they do well when the task is organized and requires little effortful processing on their part (Tariot and Weingartner, 1986).

Children's Memory Capacities and Competencies

"Daddy, why don't you and Mommy remember things?" my then almost 4-year-old asked me. Children think that adults have bad memories (ask them!). Adults, particularly parents, have a dim view of children's memories—especially teenagers'. Who is right?

Traditional views of a child's memory regarded it as quite limited in capacity and longevity, and as fragmentary and unorganized (e.g., Myers and Perlmutter, 1979). Recent research has demolished these myths, demonstrating that children's memories are actually quite good—but that they differ from those of adults in some respects. Pioneering work by Katherine Nelson, Robyn Fivush, and others has shown that even young children can give accurate accounts when asked open-ended, free-recall questions (see, e.g., Fivush and Schwarzmueller, 1995; Ornstein, 1995).

The development of different memory capacities from infancy to adulthood is an understudied topic, well deserving of broader support. Currently most studies limit their focus to the forensic implications of a child's memory as it affects the child's ability to testify (e.g., Goodman, Hirschman, Hepps, and Rudy, 1991; Ornstein, 1995). Information about children's memory competencies is important for understanding what one is told or not told by children in clinical settings.

Concerns about children's competencies typically involve questions of whether they can distinguish between fantasy and reality and between truth and falsehood. Children's ability to distinguish between fact and fantasy is generally better than is commonly believed, and by 6 years of age their performance is comparable to that of adults on many laboratory tasks (Lindsay and Johnson, 1987). Adults, with their wider range of experience, have advantages in determining whether or not something could have occurred, but school-age children are able to distinguish between internal fantasies and external events. Older children, and even adults, remain susceptible to being influenced by their fantasies (Harris, Brown, Marriott, Whittall, and Harmer, 1991), but by school age, fabrication of material is not related to incompetency to distinguish fact from fantasy (Lamb et al., 1994).

Much of the difficulty in assessing the validity of a child's report is related to problems with language and communicative abilities. The vocabularies of children are more limited than those of adults and children use fewer adjectival and adverbial modifiers. They also have less experience to use as a basis for comparisons, and fewer shared analogies or metaphors to invoke as explanations. Furthermore, children have limited external perspective-taking capacities and a less sophisticated "theory of mind" with which to understand the kinds of information others (particularly strange adults) may need to understand what they are saying. Children also "logically" associate information in different ways than adults do, producing "looser" accounts and incorporating (from an adult perspective) extraneous material. Individual and cultural factors further affect children's communicative abilities. Collectively, these factors contribute to the brief, sparsely detailed accounts that young children typically provide when asked about an experience.

The statement is often made that children are more "suggestible"—that is, accepting of misleading information—than adults. One implication of this statement is that adults are relatively resistant to suggestion effects. However, research demonstrates that adults too can be manipulated by suggestive questioning (e.g., Loftus, 1979). Studies of children's suggestibility have led to mixed results. Preschoolers appear to be especially susceptible to misleading information, particularly postevent contamination of memories through deceptive suggestions made after the event and before tested recall (Ceci, Ross, and Toglia, 1991). Other data indicate that, within limits, stress enhances resistance to suggestibility (Goodman et al., 1991; Ornstein, 1995).

Additional factors influence "suggestibility," including children's wishes to comply with authority figures questioning them. Children frequently interpret the repetition of a question by an adult as indicating that the prior answer was unsatisfactory (Fivush and Schwarzmueller, 1995). In many respects, however, school-age and older children are not significantly more suggestible than adults. People of all ages can be misled by suggestive questioning, especially when the memories involved are old, the questions are confusing, and a subject feels intimidated or compelled to accept a questioner's version of events (Lamb et al., 1994).

Finally, the "immaturity" of children's memories is frequently invoked as preventing their accurate recall of experiences and events. As always in debates involving generalizations about memory, one must remember that memory is not a simple or a unitary process. There are different kinds of memory—and these memory capacities are differentially influenced by age, stress, and the time elapsed between encoding and retrieval. We know little about the maturational processes of different memory systems.

TRAUMA AND MEMORY

The issues subsumed under the topic "traumatic memories" are now among the major psychiatric controversies of our time. In academia, traumatic memories and the so-called "false memory syndrome" are the subjects of symposia, scholarly articles, professional meeting themes, public debates, and special journal issues. In the popular media, traumatic memories provide material for magazine and newspaper stories, talk shows, and television specials. It is difficult to determine whether much useful information has been generated in either setting; this would be a fascinating social process to watch if it weren't so painful for some people. Despite the current acrimonious and litigious climate, I remain optimistic that a meaningful resolution is gradually emerging from the increased scientific scrutiny generated by professional disagreement.

Memory and Cognitive Functions in Traumatized Individuals

Critics of the concept of traumatic memory operate under the assumption that traumatized individuals have normal memory systems, and therefore that failure to recall traumatic material is accounted for by "normal forgetting" (e.g., Loftus, Garry, and Feldman, 1994; Hembrooke and Ceci, 1995). However, there are ample data establishing that traumatized individuals have significant disturbances in memory and cognitive functions.

Following World War II, high rates of explicit memory deficits were documented in concentration camp survivors (Bremner, Krystal, Southwick, and Charney, 1995a). Studies of Korean prisoners of war and Vietnam combat veterans, using standard measures of memory, found significant deficits in verbal, visual, and short-term memory (Zetlin and McNally, 1991; Bremner et al., 1993a, 1995a; Uddo, Vasterling, Brailey, and Sutker, 1993). Using the variant of the Stroop test that measures latency in naming the color of trauma-related words, numerous studies demonstrate cognitive deficits that are correlated with degree of traumatic stress (Bremner et al., 1995a). In Chapter Two, I review evidence that childhood maltreatment affects cognitive processes in children and adults. In the aggregate, these and other studies demonstrate that cognition and memory are significantly affected by traumatic experiences. Thus, assumptions of the normality of cognitive and memory functions in traumatized individuals are not justified.

Early studies with pneumoencephalography in concentration camp survivors found significant amounts of cerebral atrophy (reviewed in Thygesen, Hermann, and Willanger, 1970). Modern MRI studies find decreases in hippocampal volume that are often significantly correlated with deficits in memory function in combat-related PTSD (Bremner et al., 1995b, 1997). Adults with histories of childhood physical and sexual abuse likewise show significant reductions in hippocampal volume, compared with controls matched on a case-by-case basis for age, gender, race, handedness, education, and alcohol abuse (Bremner et al., 1995b). Stein et al. (in press) found that reductions in left hippocampal volume of adults with histories of sexual abuse were highly correlated with DES scores. Neuroimaging research provides strong evidence that stressful and traumatic experiences produce functional neuroanatomical as well as psychological and physiological sequelae (Rauch et al., 1996).

The Nature of Traumatic Memories

The controversies surrounding traumatic memories have to do with the disputed existence of certain clinical phenomena observed in and reported by individuals with histories of traumatic experiences. These phenomena include (1) the hypervividness of recalled traumatic experiences; (2) the intrusion of traumatic memories into awareness; (3) amnesias for traumatic memories; (4) flashbacks and triggered recall of traumatic memories by environmental or cognitive stimuli; (5) the recovery of previously unavailable traumatic memories; (6) the creation of pseudomemories through suggestion, hypnosis, social contagion, and the like; and (7) nonverbal or "body" memories of traumatic experiences.

In their simplest (and most common) articulation, the essence of most traumatic memory controversies is the disputed existence of one or more of these seven phenomena. One side says that something happens, and the other side says that it doesn't. There are some voices seeking a middle ground, which is about where I think many things will end up when the data are in. In professional settings, this debate has turned into a classic standoff between clinicians and experimentalists. The latter discount the observations of the former as "unscientific," and the former criticize the experiments of the latter as not representative. In the popular media, the game is "victims and villains." These roles are periodically reassigned to suffering victims or accused parents, according to prevailing beliefs. The overall debate has been marked by hostile, antithetical positions, as illustrated by the positions taken on the first and third of the phenomena listed above—the hypervividness of traumatic memories, and amnesias for traumatic memories. (The issue of pseudomemories is discussed separately later.)

Hypervividness of Traumatic Memories

The idea that memories for traumatic experiences are different from memories for normal experiences is at the center of the controversy. Among the ways in which traumatic memories are said to differ from normal ones is in the intensity and vividness of the recalled events. An example is the concept of the "flashbulb" memory—that is, the notion that memories formed during states of high arousal have a "live quality that is almost perceptual" (Brown and Kulik, 1977, p. 74). Opponents contend that high levels of arousal actually impair accuracy of recall. Tromp, Koss, Figueredo, and Tharan (1995) review the literature and conclude that neither the flashbulb concept nor the impairment position is supported by the data. In general, results from studies of actual high-arousal personal events (as opposed to laboratory simulations) indicate that memories of stressful experiences are more accurate, detailed, and persistent (Tromp et al., 1995). However, recall of traumatic events is far from perfect and is subject to alteration by postevent processing, such as therapy (e.g., Foa, Molnar, and Cashman, 1995).

Until recently, memories for "stressful" experiences were largely studied by simulation experiments with college students—for instance, showing a movie of an accident or staging an event, and rating the accuracy of recalled details. Critiques of these experiments conclude that the simulation paradigms are rarely personally stressful and thus lack ecological validity (e.g., Tromp et al., 1995; van der Kolk and Fisler, 1995). Surveys of memories for shocking public events (e.g., John F. Kennedy's assassination, the *Challenger* disaster) find that recall is subject to change with time (Tromp et al., 1995). However, when asked about especially vivid memories, people rarely include shocking public events on their personal lists. Instead, injuries, illnesses, athletic experiences, births, marriages, deaths, holidays, and love affairs rank high (Tromp et al., 1995). Thus, most laboratory studies to date have contributed little to our understanding of the nature of memories for actual traumatic experiences.

Studies of memories for actual trauma, however, are not definitive and produce apparent contradictions. As has been theorized, studies find that traumatic memories in PTSD subjects are sometimes represented in a multimodal and/or nonverbal fashion, including olfactory, visual, auditory, and kinesthetic components that are not typically found in normal memories (Elliott and Briere, 1995; van der Kolk and Fisler, 1995; Williams, 1995). Traumatic memories are also often reported to be an integral part of nightmare and dream content (van der Kolk and Fisler, 1995). Traumatic memories are not easily verbalized. Subjects may initially deny being able to describe what happened to them (Krystal et al., 1995; van der Kolk and Fisler, 1995).

Considerable clinical experience supports the belief that some traumatic memories have a graphic, hyperdetailed quality to them. For example, Lt. General Harold G. Moore has described being mistakenly bombed in Vietnam: "The fearsome sight of those cans of napalm is indelibly imprinted in my memory. It was only three or four seconds from release to impact and explosion, but it seemed like a lifetime" (Moore and Galloway, 1992, p. 189). Studies of recall for stressful but essentially nontraumatic experiences (e.g., invasive medical procedures) consistently find that memories for this type of experience are detailed and resistant to experimenter manipulations, compared with memories for neutral experiences (Ornstein, 1995). However, studies of recall for actual traumatic experiences (e.g., rape) find that some of these memories are also less clear and vivid; contain less meaningful order; and are less well remembered, less thought about, and less talked about than other unpleasant memories (Tromp et al., 1995). Why some memories for trauma appear to be unusually vivid while others seem "blurred" is not known. It does, however, suggest that trauma cuts both ways with respect to the perceived clarity of recall.

The study of the nature of memories for truly traumatic events is difficult, because each person is a single-case study. Attempts to find commonalities depend on validly capturing highly subjective features of the recall process (e.g., vividness of the mental imagery, multisensory representation of the experience) that are independent of the content and meaning of the event for the individual. It is likely that many interactive individual factors—ranging from personality characteristics to the degree of brain damage—influence the ways in which traumatized individuals recall past events. It is not surprising that this debate has not been settled yet, or that defenders of both extremes can produce examples that fit their conceptions.

Amnesias for Traumatic Experiences

Perhaps the hottest of the controversies concerns amnesias for traumatic events. Clinically, amnesia for psychologically overwhelming experiences is well documented. For example, at least a dozen studies from World War II describe significant numbers of soldiers with partial or complete amnesia for combat experiences (see reviews in Putnam, 1985a; Bremner et al., 1995a; van der Kolk and Fisler, 1995). Similar amnesias have been documented for natural disasters, accidents, kidnapping, and torture (van der Kolk and Fisler, 1995). Amnesias for childhood maltreatment, particularly sexual abuse, are widely reported in clinical studies (van der Kolk and Fisler, 1995).

It is only in the area of child abuse that skeptics seem to doubt the existence of traumatic amnesias. (It is curious that they have not challenged veterans' groups on this point, but choose to target only women and children.) The argument between those who believe that some percentage of maltreated individuals have partial or complete amnesias for their experiences, and those who believe that traumatic events should be (if anything) especially well remembered, has evolved into a national public debate. To those of us caught in the line of fire, it often feels more like a war. But—as in war—these heated exchanges are generating a torrent of new research, and data are rolling in.

It will be a while before all of the results are sorted out and a consensus is achieved, but an outline of the characteristics of amnesias for childhood trauma is beginning to emerge. Studies of clinical and nonclinical populations reliably find that a minority of subjects with histories of abuse report that there were periods in their lives when memories for the abuse were partially or completely unavailable (Herman and Schatzow, 1987; Briere and Conte, 1993; Feldman-Summers and Pope, 1994; Williams, 1994, 1995; Elliott and Briere, 1995). Reports of past partial or complete amnesia for abuse experiences is associated with more severe abuse in many of the studies (Herman and Schatzow, 1987; Briere and Conte, 1993; Elliott and Briere, 1995), but not in all (Williams, 1995). Subjects reporting having had partial or complete amnesias for abuse were generally much younger at the time of the abuse than those reporting continuous memories of it (Herman and Schatzow, 1987; Briere and Conte, 1993; Elliott and Briere, 1995; Williams, 1995). Subjects who report recovering memories for abuse experiences are generally more symptomatic than those who report continuous memories (Briere and Conte, 1993; Elliott and Briere, 1995). Non-abuse-related family factors, such as degree of maternal support for a child, also appear to play important roles in whether or not an individual develops amnesia (Williams, 1995).

Contrary to critics' assertions, many subjects recall previously unavailable traumatic memories in nontreatment settings—frequently in the context of a triggering event, such as another traumatic experience (Andrews et al., 1995). There is much more to be learned about who develops partial or complete amnesia and why, but the studies cited above have firmly established the clinical existence of partial and complete traumatic amnesias in a percentage (10–42%) of childhood abuse victims. All of the 25 studies reviewed by Scheflin and Brown (1996) demonstrate the existence of partial or full amnesia in a subset of trauma victims. These amnesias resemble those reported by combat veterans and presumably share a common traumatic mechanism.

Neural Mechanisms Postulated for Traumatic Memories

One reason why the concept of special traumatic memories is taken seriously by neuroscientists is that a number of well-described neuromechanisms may account for some of the clinical phenomena. Fear conditioning, behavioral sensitization and kindling, and long-term potentiation (LPT), individually and/or in combination, could explain many of the symptoms and behaviors in traumatized individuals with PTSD and pathological dissociation. Each of these mechanisms is the subject of many basic-science animal studies and some clinical research—and it is beyond the scope of this book to do more than briefly introduce each.

In fear conditioning, a neutral stimulus (e.g., a buzzer or light) is paired with an aversive stimulus (e.g., electric shock to a foot). With repeated pairings, the neutral stimulus becomes emotionally significant causing laboratory animals to "freeze" when they hear the buzzer alone. Now, when the buzzer sounds, the animals' heart rate and blood pressure increase and their pain sensitivity decreases. Fear conditioning has been proposed as a mechanism to explain the powerful effects of traumatic reminders on individuals with PTSD. Analogies have been drawn between fear-conditioned freezing behavior and dissociative responses (e.g., Ludwig, 1983).

"Behavioral sensitization" and "kindling" refer to an increased behavioral or physiological reactivity to repeated presentations of the same stimulus (Post, Weiss, and Smith, 1995). These phenomena are of interest to PTSD researchers because the behavioral and physiological reactivity increases with repeated presentations. Sensitization and kindling involve "memory-like" neural mechanisms, which are retained over an animal's lifetime. Kindling can be produced by periodically delivering tiny electrical pulses to certain brain areas (e.g., the amygdala and hippocampus). Kindling can also be produced by repeated administration of cocaine, by repeated painful stimulation (e.g., tail pinching), or by repeated sexual stimulation (e.g., periodic penetration of a rat's vagina with a glass rod). Kindling often shows cross-sensitization, in that seizures elicited by one stimulus (e.g., electric pulses) facilitate kindling by another stimulus (e.g., cocaine). Some have postulated that repeated traumatization (e.g., incest) could produce kindling-like vulnerability to repeated stressors. However, laboratory research suggests that it is very difficult to kindle primates—at least as compared with rats.

LTP is a neural mechanism best studied in hippocampal brain slices. In LTP, a single burst of electrical stimulation can increase (or decrease) the responsiveness of other neurons to stimulation for periods of many hours. LTP has been associated with memory mechanisms in basic research studies.

Each of the mechanisms described above is influenced by many of the neurotransmitters and hormones stimulated by stress and trauma (e.g., catecholamines, cortisol, corticotropin-releasing hormone). Over the years, many investigators have speculated that traumatic memories may in fact be different from normal memories because they are encoded in the context of high levels of trauma-activated neurotransmitters and hormones. (For a more detailed discussion, see Krystal et al., 1995.)

Effects of Trauma and Stress on Children's Recall

Some researchers purport to study traumatic memories in children by using medical analogues. For example, Ornstein (1995) baldly asserts, "Indeed, a visit to the doctor for a check-up provides a reasonable, although admittedly not perfect, analog for sexual abuse, which obviously cannot be studied in an experimental fashion" (p. 582) Let us be clear about this, however: This medical examination analogy is, in effect, equating a pelvic examination with a rape (D. A. Zarin, personal communication, 1996). A pelvic examination is not equivalent to a rape by any reasonable clinical measure. Simply compare the incidence of PTSD for rape (e.g., Breslau, Davis, Andreski, and Peterson, 1991; Resnick, Kilpatrick, Dansky, Saunders, and Best, 1993; Resnick, Yehuda, Pitman, and Foy, 1995) with the incidence of PTSD for pelvic examinations. Rape is a formidable source of PTSD, with rates of 51–80% percent in victims. I am unable to locate even a single-case report of PTSD attributable to a pelvic examination (or to a voiding cystourethrogram), although pelvic exams have an enormously higher base rate than rape.

Statements such as the quotation above are tragically mistaken and demonstrate how wide the gap is between trauma experts and some experimental psychologists. One does not find recognized authorities on trauma endorsing these types of experiments as valid analogues of maltreatment. There are simply too many critical differences between what happens in a doctor's office or hospital and what happens in rape or incest. Medical examination studies may be useful to assess the effects of that kind of stress on children's recall, but they simply do not approximate the critical variables of sexual abuse incidents.

In general, medical examination and procedure studies find that stress enhances recall of salient information—although peripheral, less salient information is recalled less well (Goodman et al., 1991; Lamb et al., 1994; Ornstein, 1995). Studies by Pynoos and colleagues of children who have witnessed rape or murder also find that such children are generally accurate reporters; although retrieval of peripheral details may be impaired, central elements of traumatic experiences are well recalled (Pynoos and Eth, 1984, 1985; Pynoos et al., 1987; Pynoos and Nader, 1988). Thus there is agreement between laboratory and clinical studies that stress increases recall for salient detail, but impairs recall for other information.

Young children are more susceptible to delayed-recall effects

(Brainerd and Ornstein, 1991). In situations involving repetitive events, children (and adults) tend to have difficulty differentiating between events related to a specific instance and those associated with related experiences. This is especially pertinent to situations such as incest, which may occur dozens to hundreds of times over the course of years. Errors of omission are more common than errors of commission. Erroneous information is often traceable to other examples of the same experience (Oates and Shrimpton, 1991; Lamb et al., 1994).

What is missing from both the clinical and experimental literature is an understanding of the effects of repetitive, invasive physical and sexual acts inflicted by a primary caregiver in a family environment in which the child is threatened if he or she reveals any details. Many authorities on trauma believe that this cumulative experience is qualitatively different from single-event stressful experiences and leads to differences in memory processes. This is not proven, but the well-replicated finding of non-normality of cognition and memory in trauma victims—both adults and children—strongly suggests that trauma alters basic cognitive systems in profound ways.

Another confounding variable that is rarely addressed is the fact that both clinical and experimental studies tend to focus on stress at the time of encoding of the memory. However, traumatic memories must often be recalled under stressful conditions, such as interrogation by police, child protective service investigators, or a cross-examining attorney. Little is known about the combination of stress effects at time of encoding and again at subsequent retrievals. All of this suggests that research on this topic has a long way to go, and that overgeneralizations from either the clinical or the experimental literature are risky.

DISSOCIATIVE DISTURBANCES OF MEMORY

A positive effect of the "false-memory" debate is the scientific investigation of the effects of dissociation on memory processes. A number of eminent scientists are now studying dissociative patients, especially patients with MPD. In the same manner as memory researchers study other patients with memory problems (e.g., the famous patient H. M.), memory researchers are interested in MPD as a window into basic memory mechanisms. Their lack of interest in MPD as a psychiatric diagnosis sets them apart from the bitter debate between believers and skeptics. It will be interesting to see what they make of this disorder.

To date, research on the memory disturbances in MPD has been limited to a few intensive case studies. All of these investigations should be regarded as preliminary. To some extent the results confirm clinical observations, and to some extent they appear to contradict the clinical findings. The studies use different approaches and tend to focus on somewhat different questions, so that there has been little replication of one by another. At this point, it is difficult to know which findings can be generalized and which are unique to the MPD patients studied. Here I discuss the experimental data in the context of three general sets of clinical phenomena: (1) interpersonality amnesias, directional awareness, and compartmentalization; (2) impaired and depersonalized autobiographical recall; and (3) source amnesias.

There have been three general approaches to the study of dissociations of memory. The first uses psychophysiological measures, particularly electrodermal activity (EDA). EDA is the change in skin electrical conductance produced by sweating and emotional reactions. Investigators have attempted to determine whether physiological responses to stimuli that are emotionally relevant for one alter personality state generalize to alter personality states that claim not to be aware of the emotional nature of the stimulus. The second approach uses a variety of neuropsychological tests, often adapted from studies of organic amnesias, to determine whether information learned in one alter personality state is available (explicitly or implicitly) to other alter personality states. The third approach involves the study of memory dysfunctions in normal individuals during dissociation-like states created by drugs or alcohol.

Interpersonality Amnesia, Directional Awareness, and Compartmentalization of Memory

"Interpersonality amnesia" refers to the long-standing clinical observation that MPD patients in certain alter personality states report no recall of the events experienced in other alter personality states. Interpersonality amnesia is manifested, for example, when an individual takes a trip in one alter personality state and later, in another such state, finds himself or herself at the destination with no recall for the events of the journey. Interpersonality amnesia is a major form of unremembered behavior in MPD patients.

"Directional awareness" refers to the observation that MPD patients in certain alter personality states claim to be aware of their subjective experiences while in other alter personality states, whereas in the other states the individuals claim to have amnesia for experiences in the former states. That is, alter personality state A claims awareness of the activities of personality state B; B, however, reports no awareness of the activities of state A. In one study, over 85% of clinicians reported evidence of such directional awareness in their MPD patients (Putnam et al., 1986).

Finally, "compartmentalization" refers to MPD patients' frequent reports that information that is learned or otherwise accessible to the patients in certain alter personality states may not be available to them in other alter personality states. Compartmentalization is believed to account for the sequestration of certain abilities, skills, and knowledge to specific alter personality states of MPD patients.

Prince and Peterson (1908) were the first to investigate interpersonality amnesias. Using a predecessor of the polygraph or "lie detector" to measure changes in skin electrical activity, they attempted to determine whether the EDA responses of one alter personality to emotionally laden words were present when other alter personality states were in executive control of the patient's behavior. They found that increased EDA occurred for emotion-laden words even when the alter personality tested claimed to be unaware of the experience that produced the emotional response to that word (Prince and Peterson, 1908; see also Zahn, Moraga, and Ray, 1996).

Several decades later, Ludwig, Brandsma, Wilbur, Bendfeldt, and Jameson (1972) used EDA to investigate the transfer of information across alter personality states. They found that a classically conditioned EDA response to a specific stimulus was transferred across alter personality states. However, EDA responses to stimuli that were emotionally charged for one personality were absent for other personalities. Their findings contrast with the results of Prince and Peterson (1908), and demonstrate that contradictory results can occur both across MPD subjects and across pairs of alter personality states within an MPD subject.

Using a blaring tone, we (Putnam, Zahn, and Post, 1990) investigated whether habituation to a noxious stimulus would transfer across the alter personalities of MPD patients, or whether each alter would have to habituate independently. Habituation was measured by EDA to the noxious tone. MPD patients manifested essentially the same habituation curves as simulating control subjects; that is, habituation in one alter personality state carried over to other alter personality states. Zahn et al. (1996) have critiqued the methodology of these and related psychophysiological studies, and conclude that it will be difficult to use psychophysiology to prove or disprove the existence of interpersonality amnesia.

Neuropsychological studies have explored the questions of interpersonality amnesias and compartmentalization (Silberman, Putnam, Weingartner, Braun, and Post, 1985; Dick-Barnes, Nelson, and Aine, 1987; Nissen, Ross, Willingham, Mackenzie, and Schacter, 1988). In the first of these studies, we (Silberman et al., 1985) compared the ability of

9 MPD patients and 10 age- and gender-matched simulating controls to keep highly similar information separate. Subjects learned two separate lists of 20 words each that shared the same overall category (e.g., types of fruit, furniture, or flowers). The words on the two lists often had the same meaning. For example, list 1 might contain "couch," "lamp," and "dresser," and list 2 would have "sofa," "light," and "bureau."

After a few hours elapsed, subjects were asked to recall words from each list separately. This was a free-recall memory task. Then they were provided with a list of 60 words containing the 20 words from list 1, the 20 words from list 2, and 20 words that shared the same category but were not on either list. This last set of words was included to measure the degree of random intrusions. Subjects were asked to pick out the words from lists 1 and 2 and to identify which list they came from. This was a recognition memory task. We were interested in the degree of leakage by group and by task—that is, in whether the two groups (MPD patients and simulating controls) would differ on how many words from list 1 were misrecalled as being on list 2 and vice versa, for both the free-recall and recognition tasks.

This experiment was conducted both within a given alter personality state and between two different alter personality states. That is, in the "within-state" condition, an individual in one alter personality state learned both lists and tried to keep them separate. In the "between-state" condition, a subject learned list 1 while in one alter personality state and list 2 while in a second alter personality state. The pairs of alter personality states were chosen, in part, because it was claimed that they were amnesic for each other.

Each control subject was tested as himself or herself and as a simulated alter personality. The simulated alter personalities of the controls had fabricated identities (e.g., names, ages, races, genders, hobbies) chosen by the control subjects. Controls, who were matched in gender and age with the MPD subjects, were encouraged to elaborate and rehearse their simulated alter personalities as often as possible over a several-week period. Many of the controls had great fun and put on a good act. During the experiment, the tester treated the controls and simulated alter personalities in the same fashion as the alter personality states of the MPD subjects.

The results were interesting. In the within state condition, there was no difference between controls and MPD subjects in their ability to compartmentalize information. However, in the between-state condition, the MPD subjects were significantly better at keeping the two lists of words separate. MPD patients improved their compartmentalization between states, whereas the performance of the simulating control subjects was markedly worse between states than within states.

Indeed, in many types of experiments, there is a notable deterioration in the performance of simulating control subjects when they attempt simultaneously to simulate an alter personality state and to do a complex mental task. Simulating controls exhibit a sort of "pat your head—rub your tummy" effect; they either unconsciously drop their simulation as they concentrate on the task, or do poorly on the task as they focus on maintaining their simulation. However, it should be noted that despite the improvement in compartmentalization shown by our MPD subjects during the between-state part of the experiment, they still manifested considerable leakage of information from one alter personality to another. In other words, their degree of compartmentalization of these neutral words was far from perfect.

Other interesting findings included evidence for a qualitative difference in the mental mechanisms associated with effective compartmentalization in the MPD subjects. Somewhat paradoxically, the degree of within-state compartmentalization was significantly correlated with the degree of between-state compartmentalization for the MPD subjects, but not for the simulating controls. The MPD subjects also did better on the recognition task than on the free-recall task, suggesting that the cuing structure provided by the list of words helped them to keep the information separate.

Working with a single MPD patient, Dick-Barnes et al. (1987) used a paired-associate (word list) learning task, a perceptual–motor task, and an attention task to determine whether learning and practice in one alter personality state would improve the performance of other alter personalities. They found that transfer of learning across personalities occurred with both the paired-associate learning and perceptual–motor tasks; errors made by one alter personality state were the same as the errors made by another personality state. However, the attentional task yielded somewhat different results. In this experiment, each personality had to respond (i.e., push a button) when two sequentially presented visual stimuli were matched. Visual event-related potentials were recorded from two occipital leads, and the waveforms analyzed. At standard time points on the waveforms were there were significant differences in the shapes of the waveforms among the three alter personalities tested.

Nissen et al. (1988) approached the questions of interpersonality amnesia, directional awareness, and compartmentalization by intensively studying eight alter personalities of an MPD patient with a variety of neuropsychological tests. They found evidence both for transfer of information between reportedly mutually amnesic alter personality states, and for interpersonality amnesia and compartmentalization of information. On several learning and memory retrieval tasks, learning by one alter personality clearly improved the performance of other personalities relative to chance levels. However, on other tasks—particularly tasks using complex or ambiguous stimuli—there was little or no evidence of transfer of information across alter personality states. Nissen et al. made the salient observation that "the degree of compartmentalization in this patient appears to depend on the extent to which that knowledge is interpreted in ways that are unique to a personality as well as the extent to which processes operating at the time of retrieval are strongly personality-dependent" (1988, p. 131).

Using an array of explicit and implicit memory tests, we (Szostak et al., 1997) studied a pair of alter personality states in each of three patients with MPD. With each pair, we investigated the influence of learning (implicitly and explicitly) on subsequent performance under four learning/test conditions. Two of these four conditions were within-state conditions (i.e., personality A learned the material and later A was tested; B learned the material and later B was tested). The other two were between-state conditions (i.e., A learned the material and later B was tested; B learned the material and later A was tested). The learning/test trials were spaced about 3–4 days apart. After this set of trials was completed, the same four learning/test trials were repeated a second time with new information to determine how consistent the findings were.

Again, the findings were interesting and contained a mixture of confirmatory and contradictory results. We found evidence for significant alter-personality-state-dependent compartmentalization in the between-state conditions for most learning/test trials. That is, information learned by one alter personality was not readily available to the other personality. This compartmentalization effect was strongest for the implicit memory tasks, but was apparent in some patients for explicit memory tasks also.

However, the results were not always consistent between MPD patients, or in some cases even within a given patient between the first and second replications. The more structured the memory task (e.g., a recognition task vs. a free-recall task), the less alter-personality-state-dependent compartmentalization was seen. Memory tasks with ambiguous stimuli (e.g., a fragmented-pictures implicit learning task) produced the greatest degree of compartmentalization. These findings are congruent with the observation of Nissen et al. (1988) quoted above.

Thus, there is experimental support for the clinical observation that *between states,* the alter personalities of MPD patients appear to compartmentalize information to a significantly greater degree than simulating control subjects. However, the experimental data also indicate that the degree of compartmentalization is considerably less than complete. Information learned in one personality state is often partially available to other personality states, whether or not a patient reports any subjective awareness of this. Thus the alter personalities of MPD patients do not have completely separate memories and awareness—a fallacious claim sometimes made in the mass media. They only have a relative increase in compartmentalization of their awareness of and differential access to learned information.

What I am here calling "compartmentalization" is probably a mixture of volitional, effortful, and somewhat conscious tasks and nonvolitional, unconscious processes. Compartmentalization takes places largely out of awareness. There may be different compartmentalization mechanisms for implicit and explicit memory or for short- and long-term memory. Compartmentalization probably plays an important role in creative states of mind, wherein an individual suspends or blocks out background mental activity and "single-mindedly" focuses his or her attention in the immediate moment. Compartmentalization also permits an individual to maintain side-by-side, mutually contradictory responses to the same stimulus or situation. Which of a given set of mutually exclusive responses is activated at a particular time appears to be influenced by contextual cues. Clinically, one often sees alter personality states embodying mutually exclusive responses to a specific situation— for example, opposite reactions to an emotionally charged experience, such as a visit home with abusive parents.

Impaired and Depersonalized Autobiographical Recall

Preliminary data suggest that patients reporting a history of sexual abuse show an impairment in the retrieval of nontraumatic autobiographical memories (Kuyken and Brewin, 1995). Using standard methodology to test autobiographical memory, Kuyken and Brewin found that depressed women reporting a history of physical or sexual child abuse produced more overgeneral memories to standard cues than patients without a history of abuse. Patients who reported trying to avoid memories of childhood abuse in the week prior to testing also produced more overgeneral memories.

As discussed in Chapter Five, MPD patients report extensive gaps in recall of their past. To date, only single-case studies have systematically investigated autobiographical memory in MPD patients (Schacter et al., 1989; Bryant, 1995). Prior to a diagnosis of MPD, Bryant (1995) tested a patient who complained of memory problems. The patient did remember numerous incidents of sexual abuse by multiple perpetrators, but could not recall certain other events from childhood. Approximately 2 years later she presented again, now diagnosed with MPD. Using standard methods, Bryant investigated the autobiographical memories in two alter personalities, the presenting personality and a child alter. Results were compared with thoses for a group of simulating subjects and a group of undergraduate students; Orne's "nonexperiment" procedure was used to control for the demand characteristics of the experimental situation (cited in Bryant, 1995). The patient differed from the controls in having an uneven chronological distribution of memories.

Schacter et al. (1989) studied a 24-year-old woman with MPD. Using standard autobiographical cuing procedures, they found a "striking deficit" in the woman's autobiographical memory for childhood experiences. Specifically, the subject was unable to recall a single memory from before the age of 10 years, and had very limited recall for ages 10–12 years. These findings support clinical reports of unusual gaps in autobiographical recall in dissociative patients.

In Chapter Four, I have discussed the defensive function of a sense of detachment from self and situation that sometimes occurs in people facing imminent death. From a psychological perspective, the subjective distance inherent in depersonalized detachment seems to provide protection for an individual's sense of survival in the face of apparent annihilation. That is, by mentally stepping far back, the individual preserves a sense of self-continuity beyond the events—even in the face of imminent death. It is believed (but has not yet been proven) that repeated experiences of profound depersonalization and detachment lead to feelings of chronic depersonalization, estrangement, and numbing in some traumatized individuals.

Source Amnesias

It appears as if one of the consequences of a chronic sense of depersonalized detachment is that autobiographical recall of past events has a dream-like quality. Such individuals are left feeling uncertain as to whether or not something that they recall as happening actually happened. Several questions on the DES tap into this difficulty (see questions 15 and 24 on the DES-II in Appendix One). We find that patients with dissociative disorders endorse these or similar statements at significantly higher levels, compared with nontraumatic clinical and nonclinical groups.

In many instances, the recalled events did occur. However, dissociative patients report that their recall of verifiable events is often such that it "seems" as if the events happened to someone else or are memories from a dream. In some instances, dissociative patients do elaborate/confabulate information acquired from other sources into "memories" that are recalled as if the events had happened to them. The contribution of source amnesia to susceptibility to pseudomemories is discussed below.

Memory, in all of its complexity, is a critical element of reality testing. The various disturbances of memory associated with pathological dissociation can alter an individual's ability to judge whether an autobiographical "memory" reflects an actual experience that directly involved the individual. In my clinical experience, most dissociative patients are tentative about stating that their "memories" represent actual events.

In a series of experiments (most as yet unpublished), we (Weingartner et al., 1995) have been able to reproduce dissociation-like problems with source amnesias in normals and alcoholics. Using the benzodiazepine triazolam to create a discrete altered state of consciousness, we set up a within- and between-state experiment much like those described above for MPD patients. Subjects were asked to learn a list of words and to generate an association for each word. Later, either within a state (i.e., placebo–placebo or drug–drug) or across states (placebo–drug, drug–placebo), they were asked to recall all of the words (list words and their associations) and to determine whether or not each word was supplied by the experimenter or was their own association. Within state, regardless of whether it was placebo–placebo or drug–drug, subjects were very accurate at recognizing the source of the words. However, across states they made considerably more errors.

Interestingly, the number of errors a subject made was highly correlated with the difference in DES scores between the placebo and drug states: The greater the difference, the more errors the subject made in recognizing the source of the word. These findings further support the theory that states of pathological dissociation such as MPD alter personalities, can be conceptualized as discrete states of consciousness.

PSEUDOMEMORIES

The "false-memory" debate has definitively established one fact: Memory is falsifiable. That is, memory can be changed by experimental manipulations. This has major forensic implications, particularly as it relates to repeated interrogations about alleged maltreatment events (e.g., Loftus, 1979; Ceci et al., 1991). The extent to which this actually happens in clinical settings remains to be established. But data from studies by Loftus (1979) with adults and Ceci et al. (1991) with children serve as a clear warning that memory is malleable and may be altered by misleading postevent questions and other manipulations.

I am skeptical that the creation of false memories in therapy constitutes a widespread clinical problem. Critics act as if it has been scientifically established that thousands of therapists are systematically creating pseudomemories of childhood abuse in essentially normal women. They have yet to demonstrate that this has actually occurred in a single case. I suspect that instances do occur in which memories for actual events are falsified and pseudomemories are created for events that never occurred. But I do not think that this happens nearly as often in therapy as critics allege. Unfortunately, neither side has good data on the question.

An Example of Pseudomemory Creation: Allegations of Satanic Ritual Abuse

From my perspective, the best example of the creation of clinically and legally significant pseudomemories involves allegations of satanic ritual abuse (SRA). Such allegations are defined here as claims that a vast, international, multigenerational conspiracy is practicing religious worship of Satan or the devil through rituals involving sex, death, torture, incest, human sacrifice, cannibalism, and necrophilia (Putnam, 1991c). With the exception of a few isolated "copycat" incidents, there is no credible evidence that actual SRA is occurring or ever has occurred.

As the best examples of pseudomemories, SRA allegations deserve a fuller examination than the sensationalist treatments—pro and con—that they have received in the popular media. To date, sociologists and anthropologists have taken the most careful look. One thing that emerges is that allegations of SRA occur within a much larger social context than just the therapists' offices. In fact, there are plenty of examples where therapists are not involved in the process. SRA allegations are spawned in social networks composed of all manner of individuals, including police officers, journalists, and religious fundamentalists. There is a reverberating rumor circuit that generates, propagates, back-propagates, amplifies, and self-confirms SRA allegations. As I have said elsewhere, the field of child abuse and neglect is particularly prone to this process, because it encompasses so many different disciplines that have little in common except for a focus on child maltreatment (Putnam, 1991c).

Some critics would contend that virtually every therapist who diagnoses MPD proceeds immediately to implant pseudomemories of SRA. In fact, few MPD patients make SRA allegations. For example, Coons (1994b) found that only 8.5% of his MPD patients made SRA allegations. We found that only 4% of dissociative patients in an outpatient treatment sample reported such experiences (Sariganian and Putnam, 1997). Indeed, even the British False Memory Society's own survey found allegations of SRA were rare (Andrews, 1997).

In the course of a general practice, therapists will occasionally encounter individuals who make such claims. This should not be construed as evidence that the therapists are responsible for the patients' raising these claims in therapy. Critics who boldly tell others what is happening in therapists' offices where they have never actually been are guilty of the same fallacy as those few therapists who regale training workshop audiences with gory details of satanic black masses that they have never seen. Both are telling others about something that they believe is going on; however, neither has ever seen it happen, and neither has any hard proof that it has ever happened.

Pathological Dissociation and Pseudomemories

Several effects of pathological dissociation on memory serve to increase individuals' vulnerability to incorporation of pseudomemories into their life stories. Dissociative compartmentalization and amnesias create gaps in the continuity of autobiographical memory. For example, the Adolescent Dissociative Experiences Scale (A-DES; see Appendix Three) includes the item "I feel like my past is a puzzle and some of the pieces are missing." Feeling such an autobiographical void is a painful psychological experience.

People naturally attempt to fill these gaps with whatever is available or plausible. Depersonalized recall of actual memories may be such that memories for past experiences and events have a dream-like quality, undermining a dissociative person's certainty as to what happened and what did not. Other autobiographical memories may be recalled in a detached fashion, as if they were observed happening to someone else, rather than as direct personal experiences. Finally, source amnesias impair recognition of the origin of information. Dissociative patients may know something, but they do not know how or why they know that information. They cannot be certain whether that information comes from direct personal experience or whether it was acquired in another fashion (e.g., from being told about it).

Synergistically, these disturbances of memory make it difficult for individuals with MPD or other forms of pathological dissociation to be certain of what has happened to them. Thus, it is more difficult for them confidently to reject mistaken information that others offer about their life histories. Clinicians should be attuned to this vulnerability; they should not attempt to fill the voids or gaps in patients' recall with suppositions. In other words, clinicians must be aware that dissociative patients are at increased risk for incorporating extraneous material into their life narratives, and that they may relate this material with the same degree of conviction that they have for experiential memories.

SUMMARY

For more than a century, the effects of pathological dissociation on memory have intrigued clinicians. Modern studies demonstrate that memory is composed of multiple systems, acting independently and synergistically. These systems can be separated by clever laboratory experiments, or as the result of conditions such as Alzheimer's dementia or alcoholism. The two major systems are explicit memory, which requires an effortful awareness of the information and its source; and implicit memory, which influences behavior largely out of awareness.

Although often portrayed as having poor memories, children are now known to have good memories—but ones that differ from those of adults in terms of association patterns and retrieval strategies. By the age of 6 years, children are competent to distinguish between fact and fantasy, are and able to give accurate accounts of salient experiences and observations. Both adults and children are susceptible to postevent suggestions. Pseudomemories may be created in susceptible individuals.

As a group, severely traumatized individuals show significant memory and cognitive impairments on standard tests, and therefore cannot be assumed to have normal memory systems. Traumatic memories appear to differ from normal memories in terms of vividness, intrusiveness, and amnesias. Although many traumatic memories are especially vivid, some may be blurred and difficult to recall. There is ample clinical documentation of amnesias for a variety of traumatic experiences. Research on stressful (but not traumatic) memories indicates that they are more resistant to suggestion effects, but often have a narrower attentional focus with loss of peripheral detail. A number of well-described neurobiological mechanisms are thought to be relevant to traumatic memories.

The effects of pathological dissociation on memory have been primarily studied in MPD patients. These studies indicate that MPD alter personality states may act to compartmentalize information more tightly than in normal individuals. Certain kinds of information (e.g., very ambiguous information or implicit information) show greater alter-personality-state-dependent recall in laboratory studies. MPD patients also exhibit unusual gaps in autobiographical recall, which differ from the normal decline with increasing time. Dissociation-like source amnesias can also be produced in normal individuals by using psychotropic medications such as benzodiazepines. By and large, these experimental and clinical data support the conceptualization of pathological dissociation as discrete states of consciousness.

Pseudomemories do occur, and the best examples are allegations of SRA. However, pseudomemories are not all that common, and it should not be assumed that they were implanted in therapy. A sociological examination of SRA allegations reveals that social networks are often involved in this process—as they are in most contagious phenomena. The cruel paradox, with respect to the "false-memory" debate, is that a person must have been severely traumatized to have the kinds of the dissociative memory dysfunctions that increase susceptibility to acquisition of pseudomemories.

Chapter Seven

Toward a Model of Pathological Dissociation

My intent in this chapter is twofold. In the first half, I examine various aspects of the psychobiology of trauma and dissociation, with an emphasis on setting the stage for the model of pathological dissociation I describe in Chapter Eight. General principles involved in posttraumatic biological functioning are derived; the results of psychophysiological studies of MPD are discussed in some detail, and interpreted as suggesting that alter personalities may best be regarded as discrete states of consciousness; and preliminary research on the neurobiology and neuroanatomy of dissociation is briefly mentioned. In the second half of the chapter, I provide further background for Chapter Eight by critiquing traditional models of MPD.

PSYCHOBIOLOGY OF TRAUMA AND DISSOCIATION

Psychobiological Effects of Trauma: A Mapping of Symptoms and a Set of Principles

In Chapter Two, I briefly cite findings from the growing research on the psychobiological effects of trauma and maltreatment. At this point, my aim is to provide a more generalized integration of the meaning of such findings from a developmental-psychopathological perspective. One way to begin is to examine the ways in which behavioral symptoms map onto biological systems known to be affected by traumatic experiences. Table 7.1 outlines such a mapping. Table 7.1 is based on an extensive review of the biological correlates for these symptoms in general psychiatric samples. This is not to say that in each instance it has been *proven*

TABLE 7.1. Mapping of Trauma-Related Symptoms onto Known or Postulated Stress Response Systems

Symptoms	Systems
Somatization	Immune system Hyptothalamic–pituitary–adrenal (HPA) axis Serotonin
Affect regulation	Catecholamines HPA axis Serotonin Gamma-aminobutyric acid (GABA)*
Suicide/aggression	Serotonin Catecholamines
Anxiety	HPA axis Serotonin Catecholamines
Pain	Endorphins Serotonin Assorted kinins* Catecholamine potentiation
Stress reactivity	HPA axis Endorphins Catecholamines Serotonin Immune system
Dissociation	GABA* Endorphins* Catecholamines* Serotonin* N-Methyl-D-aspartate Glutamate* Glucocorticoids*

Note. Asterisks (*) indicate postulated stress response systems.

that trauma-induced dysregulation of the listed biological systems is directly related to the corresponding symptoms in this table. Rather, the table reflects data-driven hypotheses about possible causal relationships, based on recent research with psychiatric patients.

From this mapping, I move on to sketch out a set of principles concerning the role of various factors in posttraumatic biological functioning. These factors include the disturbances in within-system feedback regulation resulting from trauma-induced changes; the individual's past traumatic history (as opposed to the current stressor); general psychosocial factors; and disturbances in feedback regulation among systems. I also consider the question of the reversibility of trauma-induced biological changes, and hazard some general clinical predicitions.

Disturbances in Feedback Regulation within Biological Systems

Each of the biological systems listed in Table 7.1 is complex and composed of subsystems, some of which are known in detail and many of which are as yet only physiologically and anatomically sketched out. In general, we understand each of these systems as "systems," that is, physiological circuits composed of elements (neurons, brain nuclei, endocrine glands, visceral organs, etc.) that are connected together in feedback loops, so that they turn one another on and off or otherwise reciprocally modulate one another. It is the synergistic and cyclic interaction of these elements as a system that underlies their bodily biology.

Extrapolating from research on systems that we know reasonably well—for example, the hypothalamic–pituitary–adrenal (HPA) axis—I infer that one of the basic principles of trauma-related biological dysregulation involves alterations in feedback and other ways in which system elements interactively modulate one another. Trauma changes the transfer functions among elements within a system, and alters the coupling relations between external and internal milieu changes and biological responses. For example, chronic PTSD is associated with increased negative feedback regulation of the HPA axis and hypocortisolism (Yehuda and McFarlane, 1995). This is markedly different from the hypercortisolism found in depression or anorexia nervosa. In many respects, the end result of traumatic biological alterations appears to be of a "type" nature; in other words, individuals with PTSD show significantly different responses from individuals without PTSD (Yehuda and McFarlane, 1995).

The Role of Past Experience

Past traumatic history appears to play a critical role in an individual's biological response to a current stressor. Many of us have long believed this to be true psychologically, and it is reinforcing to find this principle operating at the biological level. For example, Resnick et al. (1995) studied the cortisol responses of rape victims. Victims with no history of past trauma had increased levels of cortisol that were correlated with severity of sexual assault; conversely, women with a history of past trauma had decreased cortisol levels following a rape. These findings are congruent with animal studies that find an attenuation of HPA axis responses to repeated stress. Yet women with a history of past trauma were more likely to develop PTSD following the rape. This susceptibility is congruent with data indicating that histories of prior trauma—particularly childhood maltreatment—appear to increase vulnerability to developing PTSD to new trauma (Bremner, Southwick, Johnson, Yehuda, and Charney, 1993b; Engel et al., 1993; Resnick et al., 1995).

The principle that prior trauma influences the biological and psychological outcomes of current trauma is very relevant to child maltreatment, with its typical course of multiple traumas spanning years. There is reason to believe that there are critical periods in early child development during which aversive or traumatic experiences may have disproportionate influences (compared with their influences during other developmental periods) on the subsequent regulation of biological systems and psychological functions. At present, this has not been definitively demonstrated in humans, but animal studies offer ample support for this hypothesis (Escorihuela, Tobena, and Fernandez-Teruel, 1994).

Psychosocial Effects

Animal studies demonstrate that general social factors can also have strong effects on stress responses. For example, the elegant and arduous research conducted by Robert Sapolsky (1996) with free-living baboons on the Serengeti plain of East Africa documents the complex interaction of social status (dominance hierarchy) and biological stress response systems. Dominant males had lower basal cortisol levels, bigger and faster stress cortisol responses, faster recoveries, and greater sensitivity to HPA axis negative feedback inhibition. They were more resistant to stress effects on testosterone levels, had higher levels of high-density-lipoprotein cholesterol, and were more sensitive to catecholamines. Finally, they had lower resting blood pressures, but faster increases in heart rate and blood pressure to stress.

In many respects, humans are biologically similar to these Serengeti baboons. Human stress responses are also likely to be powerfully affected by social factors. I sometimes wonder whether the profound effects that we see in biological father–daughter incest (compared with sexual abuse in which nonbiological father figures are the perpetrators) reflects some basic psychosocial endocrine response.

Feedback Interactions among Biological Systems

We know that stress-sensitive biological systems are densely interconnected at multiple levels. Major changes in one system reverberate through related systems. General research is providing us with important information about the nature of these interconnections; for instance, a mechanism by which HPA axis glucocorticoids suppress the immune system was recently discovered (Marx, 1995). These interconnections should be understood as another level or layer of feedback.

When one begins to model complex feedback interactions among a set of interconnected biological systems (e.g., McAdams and Shapiro, 1995) it rapidly becomes apparent that all sorts of unexpected phenomena can occur. The complex tangle of interconnections among these systems and their circuits—each feeding back on itself and interactively modulating other systems and their circuits—sets off a biological horse race. (Digital engineers call such competing feedback in computer circuits a "logic race.") The eventual outcome is hard to predict, particularly since past history and general social factors play key roles.

Reversibility of Trauma-Induced Biological Alterations

One of the most troubling questions raised by the research findings of trauma-induced biological dysregulation is the question of permanence. PTSD research with combat veterans and Holocaust survivors indicates that biological changes endure over extended periods. However, research with children who present with "psychosocial dwarfism" (also called "nonorganic failure to thrive" or NOFTT) indicates that at least some maltreatment-related biological changes may be reversible if a child's environment can be changed. NOFTT children are often neglected or abused (De Bellis and Putnam, 1994; Skuse, Albanese, Stanhope, Gilmour, and Voss, 1996).

Skuse et al. (1996) have identified a subgroup of NOFTT children, characterized by growth failure, hyperphagia, excess thirst, and a high likelihood of abuse, who show rapid reversal of growth retardation and normalization of nocturnal growth hormone secretion profiles. This demonstrates that profound biological responses to maltreatment and stress can nonetheless be rapidly reversed by general interventions aimed at changing a child's life circumstances. Our research (De Bellis et al., 1994a, 1994b) has also raised the possibility that certain biological dysregulations, such as HPA axis changes and increased urinary catecholamines, may be improved or exacerbated by medication. Questions of the permanence and reversibility of trauma-induced biological changes must be added to the field's research agenda immediately.

Clinical Predictions

Given these general principles, it is not surprising that we find an array of different psychological and biological outcomes to nominally the "same" traumatic experience (e.g., rape or incest). Nor should it be unexpected that a given stressor produces very different responses in the same individual at different points in time. What we can anticipate is that traumatized individuals are going to be very sensitive to future trauma and stressors. Trauma victims have lost some "buffering" capacity, because their stress response systems have been driven farther from normal homeostatic ranges by posttraumatic compensatory feedback processes—for example, the increased negative HPA feedback phenomena seen in PTSD (De Bellis and Putnam, 1994; Yehuda and McFarlane, 1995). We can anticipate that apparently small changes in stress, or in medications that interact with one or more stress response systems, may lead to disproportionately large responses in a traumatized individual. Experienced clinicians intuitively understand this sensitivity and have learned to proceed slowly and gently with trauma victims, both psychologically and psychopharmacologically.

The Psychopathology of MPD

Alter Personality State Differences

"Is it real?" is the perennial question raised about MPD. Many have wondered whether psychophysiological studies might hold the answer. Prince and Peterson's (1908) crude EDA study marked the first attempt to find physiological traces of alter personality states. Thigpen and Cleckley (1954) sought to document the three personalities of the famous patient Eve with EEG recordings. They reported differences in muscle tension and a 1.5-Hz shift in alpha frequency. Morselli (1953) described similar results with another patient. In a curious but interesting study, Condon, Ogston, and Pacoe (1969) performed a frame-by-frame analysis of eye movement patterns from a movie of Eve's personalities. They reported differences in three types of divergent eye movements. (For a discussion of all of these studies, see Putnam, 1984.)

The quest for physiological proof was continued by Ludwig and colleagues in the 1970s (Ludwig et al., 1972; Larmore, Ludwig, and Cain, 1977). Their EDA studies have been described in Chapter Six; in addition, they reported changes in modal EEG alpha frequency and muscle tension (Ludwig et al., 1972). In a later study of another patient, they reported differences in visual evoked potential (VEP) components across alter personalities (Larmore et al., 1977).

Coons, Milstein, and Marley (1982) examined EEG frequency power spectra in two MPD patients and a simulating control (played by Coons). There was no difference between the patients and the control in the total number of "significant differences" among alter personality states, but there were interesting differences in the frequency bands in which patient and control differences occurred. Specifically, the significant differences in the patients were in the high-frequency beta 2 band (18.25–24.75 Hz), whereas the control's differences were greatest in the delta band (1–3.75 Hz).

At about the same time, we studied a group of MPD patients and age- and gender-matched simulating controls in the NIMH intramural research program. Some of these studies were published (Silberman et al., 1985; Putnam et al., 1990), but the EEG and VEP data were only presented (Putnam, Buchsbaum, Howland, and Post, 1982). The reason for this is a long story, the gist of which is that the principal collaborators ended up in new jobs on different coasts and never got together to write up the data until much, much later—at which time the technology used for brain mapping was regarded as obsolete by journal reviewers. For the record, I briefly describe the study and results below.

A total of 11 MPD patients (8 women and 3 men) and 10 age- and gender-matched controls participated in the study. Each of the control subjects created a simulated alter personality state, which we called the "imaginary personality" (IP). Each IP had a name, gender, race, height, weight, hair and eye color, occupation, annual income, place of residence, marital status, number of children, hobbies, interests, and any other identifying characteristics or attributes that the creator felt were important. MPD subjects identified alter personality states that they felt could meet the requirements for participation. In each testing session, controls were tested three times as themselves and once in their IP states in a randomized order. Four alter personality states from each patient were tested in a randomized order.

The MPD and control subjects received four VEP trials per day (i.e., one trial for each personality state) for 4 or 5 days in a row. VEPs were stimulated by four different intensities of light. The amplitudes and latencies of the P100, N120, and P200 VEP peaks were measured in a standard fashion. The MPD and control subjects were also each tested four times (in randomized order of personalities) with a 16-channel EEG. Unfortunately, because of the limited number of channels on this early computerized EEG system, only the left hemisphere was wired. A standard fast Fourier transform procedure was used to yield computerized power spectrum estimates that were color-intensity-mapped onto a cortical outline.

Statistically, we asked this question: Was there a greater difference between a given pair of MPD alter personality states than between a matched control and his or her IP? The answer to this question was averaged across cases. To compute the degree of similarity–difference between a pair of alter personality states, or a control and his or her IP, we calculated intraclass correlation coefficients. The magnitudes of these coefficients were compared between MPD patients and simulating controls for each of the variables. Examples of variables included the amplitudes and latencies of the VEP peaks for the different electrode locations, and the relative power in the standard EEG bands (i.e., delta, theta, alpha, beta) for each electrode location.

In every case, MPD subjects had significantly lower correlations for a substantial number of variables. In no case did the controls show larger differences than the MPD patients, and in most cases the controls were very highly correlated with their IPs (i.e., intraclass correlation coefficients of .87–.98). That is, the controls' simulations had little or no effect on their VEPs or EEGs. For the MPD patients, the greatest VEP differences were in the earlier components (P100, N120), for both amplitude and latency variables. In the EEG study, the greatest differences were in total power and the beta 2 frequency band.

When the paper was submitted, reviewers complained that the technology was too old and that the failure to wire the right hemisphere made the EEG findings incomplete. My colleagues and I learned that technology can rapidly pass investigators by if they sit on their data too long (Putnam, Buchsbaum, and Post, 1993a; a copy of this paper is available on request).

Additional studies continued to document apparent physiological differences across alter personalities of MPD patients. Mathew, Jack, and West (1985) reported hemispheric differences in cerebral blood flow across alter personalities, which they attributed to activation of the right temporal lobe. Our study of differential autonomic nervous system activity in nine MPD subjects and five simulating controls found that eight of the nine MPD patients consistently manifested physiologically distinct alter personality states across repeated trials (Putnam et al., 1990). Three of the five controls were also able to produce distinct states (two through hypnosis and one through simulation), but these differed significantly from the alter personality states.

In a pair of studies, Miller and colleagues described optical differences in MPD subjects that were not duplicated by simulating control subjects (Miller, 1989; Miller, Blackburn, Scholes, White, and Mamalis, 1991). These authors found that MPD subjects showed significantly more variability across alter personalities than did controls who based their simulations on videotapes of MPD patients. MPD subjects showed greater differences in visual acuity, visual fields, manifest refraction, and eye muscle balance (Miller, 1989). These results were largely replicated in a second study with 20 MPD patients and 20 simulating controls (Miller et al., 1991). There were, however, some differences across the two studies. The authors observed that "psychophysiological differences between personalities may be more labile than previously thought" (Miller et al., 1991, p. 135).

The trickle of psychophysiological studies has continued in the 1990s. A single-case study by Hughes, Kuhlman, Fichtner, and Gruenfeld (1990) found replicable alter personality differences with EEG brain mapping. Their control, a professional actress familiar with the patient's alter personalities, was unable to produce equivalent changes by simulation. The EEG differences were especially significant in the beta 2 band (18–30 Hz)—the same frequency band associated with significant personality state differences in the Coons et al. (1982) study and our data (Putnam, Buchsbaum, and Post, 1993). The beta 2 band is involved in behavioral state differences in other psychiatric disorders (Hughes et al., 1990). Flor-Henry, Tomer, Kumpula, Koles, and Yeudall (1990) compared the EEGs of two MPD patients with a group of women with "chronic hysteria." They did not examine individual alter personality states, but reported unusual levels of left-hemisphere activation.

Using single-photon emission computerized tomography (SPECT) imaging to examine regional cerebral blood flow in four alter personality states of a single MPD patient, Saxe, Vasile, Hill, Bloomingdale, and van der Kolk (1992) found significant differences in the left temporal lobe. This region showed a 10.7% mean blood flow change, compared with control brain areas, which showed changes of 2.5%. This finding led the authors to postulate that temporal lobe mechanisms may be involved in MPD (see the discussion of neurobiological models of MPD, below). An EEG study of the alter personalities of two MPD patients— including hypnosis and nonhypnosis conditions—found significant differences in the delta, theta, alpha, and beta frequency bands across alter personality states for one or more comparisons (Cocker, Edwards, Anderson, and Meares, 1994).

Switching

Switching, or the transition between two discrete states of consciousness, has been studied in a number of psychiatric conditions—for instance, rapid-cycling bipolar illness (Bunney et al., 1977) and periodic catatonia (Gjessing, 1974). State transitions have also been studied in meditators and in subjects who got stoned on marijuana or drunk on alcohol (Putnam, 1988). One common feature that emerges across these different examples is that subjects rarely recognize the state transition process as it is occurring. Rather, they can only identify a switch some time after it has been completed. It is as if the "self" that observes and remembers is state-dependent and is somehow suspended during the transition between two different states of consciousness.

I have studied switches between alter personality states in MPD patients (Putnam, 1988). By and large, these resemble state transitions described in other psychiatric disorders. Switches typically occur in seconds to a few minutes and are manifested by changes in facial expression, quality and quantity of speech, attentional focus, cognitive capacities, and affect. There are often abrupt changes in heart rate (typically, differences of about 8–10 beats per minute). The period of transition between alter personality states is typically marked by behavioral, cognitive, and physiological disorganization. As the new alter personality state organizes itself, the individual reenters into social interactions, and physiological systems restabilize at new activity levels.

In the laboratory, we can get many MPD patients to switch personality states on demand—although this is not always under their control. Sometimes we get a different alter personality state than the one that we asked for, or the desired alter personality state is not able to stabilize and is replaced by another. There are also "order effects." Long observed clinically, order effects are manifested in the need to access certain personality states by first going through intermediate personality states. All of these phenomena are congruent with the notion that MPD alter personalities represent discrete states of consciousness, and that clinical phenomena such as switching are similar to or the same as state transitions reported for altered and alternative states of consciousness.

Implications of the Psychophysiological Research to Date

The results from psychophysiological studies are intriguing. As yet, no clear-cut physiological "signature" has been found that would aid in diagnosis. (There are clinical abnormalities of the EEG associated with MPD, as discussed below in connection with the epilepsy temporal lobe dysfunction model of MPD.) Experimental studies most consistently find EEG differences in the beta frequencies, which are consonant with research on changes in anxiety and affect states and on the effects of deep relaxation. However, there has been little replication across studies to date, in large part because each study has used different methodology.

In several studies, simulating controls were not able to produce changes equivalent to those of MPD patients. Some controls can produce reliable and significant differences on different variables (Coons et al., 1982; Silberman et al., 1985; Miller, 1989; Hughes et al., 1990; Putnam et al., 1990; Miller et al., 1991). This suggests that controls can produce discrete states of consciousness on demand, but that these states differ from the dissociative personality states of the patients.

This is all very interesting and should stimulate additional studies. Unfortunately, progress has been slow for a number of reasons. To study alter personality states, one must do repeated scans under con-

trolled conditions, so each patient costs more; also, in the case of iso-
tope-based brain imaging (e.g., positron emission tomography [PET]),
the subject is exposed to higher doses of radiation. Fortunately, PTSD
researchers with Department of Veterans Affairs backing are becoming
interested in dissociation and are able to bring to bear their more sophisticated research programs on these problems. Newly emerging technologies for functional brain imaging (e.g., PET, SPECT) hold considerable promise for moving MPD research beyond its current case study
nature.

My interpretation of the physiological data is that they are most
parsimoniously explained by regarding the alter personalities as discrete
states of consciousness. What are being found are differences in the psychophysiological variables associated with changes in discrete states of
consciousness. The relationships of the measures (e.g., EEG and EDA)
to the specific states and state transition phenomena are probably more
correlational than causal, and therefore lack the specificity of "signature" variables. The types of differences found across the different personalities of MPD patients resemble those reported across changes in
other discrete states of consciousness.

In my opinion, one of the best ways to study these questions is to
focus on transition events. Systematic efforts should also be made to
compare transition events within a variety of clinical phenomena, such
as normal sleep, panic attacks, flashbacks, catatonic reactions, explosive
dyscontrol, hypnosis, substance abuse, premenstrual syndrome, and
rapid-cycling bipolar illness. Knowledge about the neural mechanisms
involved in transitions of behavioral states would have widespread applications in psychiatry.

Another promising area is the integration of cognitive tasks with
psychophysiological measures. Functional brain imaging approaches are
important, but psychoendocrine and psychoimmune measures will also
advance our understanding of the mind–body linkages between psychological and physiological states of being.

Neurobiology and Neuroanatomy of Dissociation

Research on the neurobiological and neuroanatomical mechanisms of
dissociation is in a fledgling state. There appear to be some interesting
tie-ins between clinical phenomena such as flashbacks, and responses to
pharmacological probes such as yohimbine and ketamine. Flashbacks—
the multimodal reexperiencing of past traumatic events—are widely regarded as a core posttraumatic symptom. (Many regard flashbacks as a
dissociative symptom of PTSD; see, e.g., American Psychiatric Association, 1994, and Krystal et al., 1995.) Infusion of yohimbine, which acti-

vates central noradrenergic neurons through blockade of their inhibitory alpha-2 receptors, produces flashbacks and increased recall of traumatic memories in a substantial number of PTSD patients (Krystal et al., 1995).

A number of medications and illicit drugs produce dissociation-like states in normal individuals (Good, 1989; Krystal et al., 1995). Perhaps the best studied is ketamine, an anesthetic commonly used by veterinarians (Krystal et al., 1995). Ketamine and its illicit cousin, phencyclidine, produce a constricted field of attention associated with a feeling of mental fogginess, often accompanied by a sense of depersonalization/derealization and sometimes by a sense of identity alteration. Marijuana (cannabinoids) and serotonergic hallucinogens such as LSD also produce dissociation-like states in some individuals. An experimental drug, M-chlorophenylpiperazine (MCPP), produces depersonalization in some normal individuals and flashbacks in some PTSD patients. Interestingly, PTSD patients who get flashbacks with MCPP usually do not have flashbacks with yohimbine, and vice versa (Krystal et al., 1995).

None of these drugs produce clear-cut dissociative disorders, but the similarities of these drug states with dissociative symptoms suggest possible common neurobiological mechanisms. If this is true, this would implicate a number of transmitter systems in pathological dissociation, including central noradrenergic systems, serotonin systems, N-methyl-D-aspartate and glutamate receptors, and perhaps brain glucocorticoid receptors (Krystal et al., 1995). As yet, only one study has measured cerebrospinal fluid (CSF) levels of neurotransmitters. We found significant correlations between DES scores and several neurotransmitters or their metabolites in the CSF of eating disorder patients (Demitrack et al., 1993). Most intriguing was a strong negative correlation ($r = -.63$, $p <$ .05) between CSF beta-endorphins and DES scores in 16 bulimic patients.

The neuroanatomy of dissociative states has been the subject of considerable speculation, dating to Benjamin Rush's 18th-century notions about shifts in hemispheric dominance (Putnam, 1991b). Hemispheric laterality models continue to be offered (see the discussion of neurological models of MPD, below). The limbic system (hippocampus, hypothalamus, cingulate gyrus, amygdala, and septum) and the thalamus have been implicated by recent functional imaging and pharmacological challenge studies (Krystal et al., 1995; van der Kolk and Fisler, 1995; Rauch et al., 1996). Krystal et al. (1995) make a persuasive argument that the thalamus—which functions as a major sensory filter—plays a critical role in dissociation by altering sensory input to cortical and limbic structures. Functional brain imaging should allow for testing of these theories during the next decade.

TRADITIONAL MODELS OF
MULTIPLE PERSONALITY DISORDER

What Should a Good Model of MPD Account For?

As much as I love to play on my computer with mathematical models of neurobiological processes, I must admit that their purpose is largely heuristic. Theoretical models, be they quantitative or qualitative, are almost impossible to validate. Their primary function is to organize our thinking about the processes they seek to represent. A good model will provide testable hypotheses, and perhaps even an opportunity to simulate the behavior of the process under a variety of conditions. But a model, no matter how closely it simulates an aspect of a process, is not the process itself.

Dissociation and MPD served as a stimulus for many of the early polypsychic theories of human consciousness and were instrumental in the development of dynamic psychiatry (Ellenberger, 1970). Yet the models put forth to explain MPD and dissociation have been surprisingly narrow. Most focus exclusively on MPD and ignore the larger questions of pathological dissociation.

Traditional models of MPD begin with a process known from another context—for example, hypnosis, epilepsy, cerebral hemispheric laterality, or social role theory. This process is then invoked to explain a few specific features, such as trance-like states (hypnosis), unremembered behavior (epilepsy), differential handedness of alter personality states (hemispheric laterality), or creation of alter personalities (social role theory). Consequentially, historical models and their modern descendants are extremely limited. Most offer little guidance with regard to the clinical approaches to pathological dissociation.

In order to evaluate theories and models of MPD, it is worth thinking about which features of the disorder should be accounted for by a reasonable model. My short list includes the nature of the functional amnesias; the basis of dissociative identity disturbances (particularly the alter personalities); and the relation between trauma and pathological dissociation. Ideally, a good model will also help conceptualize the differences between normal and pathological dissociation, and inform us about treatment.

From this vantage, I briefly critique the traditional models offered to "explain" MPD. These include (1) the autohypnotic model of MPD, currently the most widely held theory; (2) two neurological models, the epilepsy/temporal lobe dysfunction and cerebral hemispheric laterality models; (3) social role/simulation/malingering models; (4) animal models; and (5) computer metaphors and neural network models. Each explains a little, but all fall considerably short of providing a larger picture, particularly with regard to guiding clinical interventions. To address this deficit, in Chapter Eight I offer what I call the "discrete behavioral states" (DBS) model of pathological dissociation and MPD.

The Autohypnotic Model

The autohypnotic model of MPD is the most widely accepted theory of the disorder (Putnam and Carlson, in press). It is rooted in the historical equation of hypnosis with dissociation. Its basic assumptions can be dated back to Eberhard Gmelin in 1789 (see Bliss, 1983). In brief, the modern form of the autohypnotic model of MPD postulates that a traumatized individual—usually a chronically abused child—uses his or her innate hypnotic capacity to induce "self-hypnosis" as a defensive response to repeated traumatic events. With repetitive use, the autohypnotic state is transformed into an alter personality, giving rise to MPD.

Supporting Arguments

Five lines of argument are invoked to support the model. The first is that MPD patients are significantly more hypnotizable than are other psychiatric patients or normals. The second is that analogues of dissociative symptoms (e.g., auditory hallucinations, age regression, motor paralyses, and amnesias) can be produced by hypnosis. The third is that hypnosis is beneficial for MPD; therefore, it must be acting through a common mechanism. The fourth is that childhood trauma increases hypnotizability. The final argument is that alter-personality-like entities can be created under hypnosis.

Each of these arguments should be interpreted in the light of experimental data. The first argument is an overgeneralization from two small-sample studies, which found that hypnotizability scores of MPD patients were higher on average than those of comparison groups; however, most of the MPD subjects were not "highly" hypnotizable (Putnam and Carlson, in press). For example, Frischholz, Lipman, Braun, and Sachs (1992) reported a mean Stanford Hypnotic Susceptibility Scale, Form C score of 8.9 for MPD subjects, which is below the accepted threshold (9–10) set for "high hypnotizability."

However, I agree that the widespread clinical impression that MPD patients are highly hypnotizable probably reflects an above-average hypnotic capacity in a substantial percentage of patients. Whether or not increased hypnotizability is integral to the pathology of MPD, as believed by many, remains to be seen (see "Empirical Studies of Hypnosis and Dissociation," below).

The second line of argument—the creation of analogues of dissociative symptoms through hypnosis—does not constitute proof of a common mechanism. As noted earlier, dissociation-like phenomena can be produced by certain drugs, such as marijuana, phencyclidine, and some benzodiazepines (Good, 1989; Krystal et al., 1994; Weingartner et al., 1995). As far as we can tell, these psychoactive substances target different neurotransmitter systems, implying different mechanisms of action. Thus, the similarity of phenomena does not necessarily establish a common neurobiological mechanism.

There is no question that the judicious use of hypnosis is an important therapeutic adjunct to psychotherapy with adult MPD patients (Putnam and Loewenstein, 1993). However, the third line of argument—that the therapeutic effects of hypnosis imply a common psychobiological process—risks the same fallacy as the second (above). Indeed, hypnosis is also an important adjunct to psychotherapy for a number of disorders that are not considered dissociative (e.g., Kirsch, Montgomery, and Sapirstein, 1995). Two studies of the clinical phenomenology of MPD patients treated with and without hypnosis did not find any significant effects of the use of hypnosis on symptom patterns (Putnam and Carlson, in press). Beneficial effects do not prove that the disorder and treatment involve a common mechanism.

The fourth line of argument—that childhood trauma increases hypnotizability—has been demonstrated to be false in at least a half dozen clinical studies. Elsewhere, we review this research in detail (Putnam and Carlson, in press). In summary, neither adult nor child trauma samples have higher hypnotizability than nontraumatized comparison subjects. For example, our longitudinal study of sexually abused girls found no effects of short- or long-term abuse on hypnotizability scores (Putnam, Helmers, Horowitz, and Trickett, 1994). Nor were there any "dose–effect" relationships between trauma variables (e.g., age of onset, number of types of abuse) and any component of hypnotizability scores (Putnam et al., 1994). There were significant relationships between trauma variables and dissociation scores. However, we did find a subgroup of traumatized girls who scored high on both dissociation and hypnotizability scales; this finding is discussed below.

Finally, the argument that MPD-like alter personality states can be created under hypnosis is an exaggeration of old, uncontrolled reports. Reanalyses conclude that these hypnotically induced entities do not resemble MPD alter personalities on clinical variables. They are better understood as examples of transient ego state phenomena (Putnam and

Carlson, in press). One such hypnotic alter entity, the "hidden observer," has sometimes been compared to an MPD alter personality. Commenting on these comparisons, the distinguished hypnosis researcher Ernest Hilgard (1984) notes that although certain aspects of the hidden observer "bear some resemblance to those of multiple personality . . . it is a mistake to extrapolate too quickly to the more profound and enduring changes found in clinical cases of multiple personality" (p. 252).

Empirical Studies of Hypnosis and Dissociation

Examining the relationship between measures of hypnotizability and measures of dissociation, we find strikingly low correlations. For example, we (Putnam and Carlson, in press) reviewed 13 published and unpublished studies with a total of over 2,000 subjects, and found that the sample size weighted mean correlation was very low (Pearson $r = .12$). This explains less than 2% of the variance. Faith and Ray (1994) report a similar low correlation for a total of 866 subjects ($r = .09$, n.s.), which explains 1% of their variance (Faith and Ray, 1994). In short, in both general population and trauma samples, there is little statistical relationship between an individual's dissociativity and hypnotizability (Putnam and Carlson, in press).

"Double Dissociators"

However, within a trauma sample there may be a relatively small subgroup of subjects who score high on both dissociativity and hypnotizability measures. We label such individuals "double dissociators." In our study of sexually abused girls, the trauma histories of double dissociators were significantly different from those of other abuse victims (Putnam et al., 1994). Specifically, they had a much earlier onset of incest and many more perpetrators.

One implication of a "double dissociator" subgroup is that the higher mean levels of hypnotizability reported in MPD patients reflect the higher percentage of these individuals in that population. Thus, the hypnotizability–dissociation relationship is not true for the general population, but may hold for a subgroup of highly traumatized individuals. A number of investigators have raised the possibility that the relationship between hypnotizability and trauma is "nonlinear" (Nash, Hulsey, Sexton, Harralson, and Lambert, 1993; Faith and Ray, 1994; Putnam et al., 1994). These data would be consonant with the taxonic model of pathological dissociation.

Current Status of the Model

In summary, the current evidence for the autohypnotic model of MPD consists primarily of metaphorical arguments based on analogies between experimental hypnotic phenomena and clinical dissociative symptoms (Putnam and Carlson, in press). Such similarities, although descriptively compelling, do not constitute proof of a common hypnotic mechanism. Dissociative phenomena can also be produced by certain experimental processes, such as mirror gazing (Miller, Brown, DiNardo, and Barlow, 1994), drugs (Good, 1989; Weingartner et al., 1995), and meditation (Castillo, 1990).

To date, empirical studies find little relationship between hypnosis and dissociation. Histories of antecedent trauma do not appear to increase hypnotizability in the majority of subjects studied. However, a minority of traumatized individuals are both highly hypnotizable and pathologically dissociative. These "double dissociators" have experienced trauma at significantly earlier ages and at the hands of more perpetrators. There is the possibility that such differences in trauma history interact developmentally, perhaps during critical developmental periods, to increase both hypnotizability and dissociativity in some fashion. Alternatively, Judith Armstrong (personal communication, January 1996) suggests that the low correlations between dissociation and hypnosis scales may reflect differences between heterohypnosis, which is measured by standard hypnosis scales, and autohypnosis, which is not.

Neurological Models

The Epilepsy/Temporal Lobe Dysfunction Model

The epilepsy/temporal lobe dysfunction model of MPD was first offered by Charcot in 1892 (see Putnam, 1986a). Two lines of evidence underpin this model. First, the prevalence of seizure disorders is said to be much higher in MPD patients (Mesulam, 1981; Schenk and Bear, 1981; Benson, 1986; Perrine, 1991). Second, dissociation-like symptoms are sometimes reported, ictally and periictally, by seizure patients. In epileptics, dissociation-like symptoms include depersonalization, fugues, amnesias, and autoscopy (i.e., seeing an externalized image of oneself).

A neurobiological mechanism, kindling, can potentially explain how epileptic-like phenomena might arise from repeated trauma such as incest. Kindling is a behavioral sensitization and convulsive response that occurs when an animal is subjected to a repeated noxious stimulus over a period of time (Post et al., 1995; see Chapter Six for a fuller discussion).

Attempts to test the epilepsy/temporal lobe dysfunction model of dissociation have taken two forms: (1) studies of epileptic phenomena in dissociative patients, and (2) the search for dissociative phenomena in epileptic patients. So far, the data are equivocal. Although some neurological case series describe epilepsy in dissociative patients, there are questions about the validity of the dissociative disorder diagnoses (i.e., many cases do not fulfill standard criteria). Two widely cited, and supposedly independent, case series (Mesulam, 1981; Schenk and Bear, 1981) actually discrepantly report on the same set of patients (see review in Loewenstein and Putnam, 1988). Pseudoseizures, void-like trance and catatonic states, and other weird clinical phenomena in MPD patients may sometimes be mistaken for seizures, leading to the misdiagnosis of these patients as epileptic (Devinsky et al., 1989).

My reading of the current data is that neurological abnormalities, especially abnormal EEGs, are more prevalent in MPD patients than in normal or general psychiatric populations. However, few of these abnormalities are epileptoid. In the most definitive study to date, Devinsky et al. (1989) conducted lengthy video EEG monitoring of MPD patients diagnosed as having epilepsy. Although they found plenty of EEG abnormalities, dissociative phenomena were not correlated with epileptiform EEG activity.

Devinsky et al. (1989) also compared the DES scores of normal controls, MPD patients, and epileptic patients with documented epileptic foci. Epileptic patients' scores were higher than those of normals, but were significantly lower than those of dissociative patients. Similar DES findings for epilepsy have been reported in other studies (Loewenstein and Putnam, 1988; Ross, Heber, and Norton, 1989a). Interestingly, seizure patients with dominant-hemisphere foci had higher DES Depersonalization subscale scores than seizure patients with non-dominant-hemisphere foci (Devinsky et al., 1989). Hollander et al. (1992) have reported left-hemisphere activation in patients with depersonalization disorder.

Thus, clinical data raise the possibility that temporal lobe abnormalities play a role in pathological dissociation. Typical EEG abnormalities found in dissociative patients involve temporal or frontal slow-wave activity. Recent studies by Teicher, Glod, Surrey and Swett (1993) and Ito et al. (1993) have found frequent and unusual EEG abnormalities in victims of child abuse. Several brain imaging studies describe hippocampal abnormalities in trauma patients (Bremner et al., 1995a, 1995b). Persinger (1993) has linked psychometric indices of temporal lobe dysfunction to dissociative states. In the aggregate, these data suggest that trauma may produce detectable alterations in brain function and anatomy, particularly in the temporal lobe and paralimbic brain areas. The epilepsy/temporal lobe dysfunction model of pathological dissociation clearly deserves further investigation, but current data do not support a simple, direct connection between epilepsy and dissociation.

The Cerebral Hemispheric Laterality Model

The discovery of the left-hemispheric lateralization of language function in the brain by Pierre Paul Broca, a mid-19th-century surgeon, set the conceptual stage for the cerebral hemispheric laterality model of MPD. During the period from 1880 to 1920, the theory that either an anatomical or a functional disconnection between the two hemispheres of the brain was the source of "double personality" was a popular notion (Ellenberger, 1970; Quen, 1986; Putnam, 1989a).

The laterality model is bolstered by repeated clinical observations of changes in dominant handedness described in both early and modern case reports and surveys of clinicians (e.g., Brende, 1984; Gott, Everett, and Whipple, 1984; Putnam, 1986a; Henninger, 1992). Recent single-case studies document laterality differences across alter personalities in MPD patients (e.g., Brende, 1984; Henninger, 1992; LePage, Schafer, and Miller, 1992; Ahern et al., 1993). In an especially intriguing study, Ahern et al. (1993) used an intracarotid injection of amobarbital (the Wada test) to anesthetize each cerebral hemisphere individually in two MPD patients with epilepsy. This reproduced the alter personality changes associated with seizure activity in these two patients.

The cerebral hemispheric laterality model of dissociation becomes more difficult to support when one considers that most MPD patients have more than two discrete alter personality states. To handle this problem within the model, one has to postulate that activation or dominance of smaller brain regions is responsible for each alter personality state. The only controlled test of the laterality model did not find evidence of shifts in lateralization in galvanic skin response across repeated, randomized testing of alter-personality states (Putnam et al., 1990). Studies of epileptic patients who had commissurotomies for intractable epilepsy do not find evidence of the alter-personality-like phenomena induced by cutting the corpus callosum (Sidis, 1986). In short, intriguing as the shifts in dominant handedness reported in single-case studies are, global differences in hemispheric activation/functioning do not account for many of the clinical features of MPD.

Social Role/Simulation/Malingering Models

The social role model of MPD can be dated back to Pierre Janet, among others (Putnam, 1995). Although Janet clearly did not believe that dissociative disorders are created by simulation or malingering, he did believe that dissociative symptoms could be shaped by social contingencies or by displays of fascination from authority figures such as physicians. Social role theories of MPD are favored by critics who believe that MPD is iatrogenically created (e.g., Merskey, 1992, 1993; Piper, 1994).

The late Nicholas Spanos (1986) is sometimes credited with experimentally producing MPD by asking psychology undergraduate students to simulate an accused murderer's being interrogated in the fashion of the Los Angleles "Hillside Strangler" case. Critics point out that any psychiatric disorder can be simulated with sufficient cuing of motivated subjects. Spanos's undergraduates did not have any of the clinical features of MPD, nor did they fool clinicians.

When simulating controls are compared with actual MPD patients in psychophysiological and cognitive studies, patients produce changes that the controls cannot duplicate (e.g., Silberman et al., 1985; Miller, 1989; Putnam et al., 1990; Miller et al., 1991). For social role/simulation/malingering models to be convincing, experimentalists must produce examples that closely mimic symptoms, psychophysiology, cognitive features, and clinical course. Until then, little credence should be given to Spanos's transparent fabrications.

Animal Models

Ethologically oriented theorists point out that a number of predator-activated behaviors in prey species, particularly freezing behaviors, appear analogous to dissociative behaviors in humans. Ludwig (1983) was the first to discuss this; others have subsequently raised this possibility. Two sources of data inform this theory. The first comes from field-based observations of prey–predator interactions, and the second comes from laboratory studies of inescapable shock (IES).

In the field, prey animals such as rodents respond to the presence of a predator with a series of discrete behavioral states separated by abrupt behavioral shifts. Regardless of the predator's distance, freezing is the dominant first response (Brain, Parmigiani, Blanchard, and Mainardi, 1990; Henning, Dunlap, and Gallup, 1976). All ongoing behavior is suppressed, and the prey remains motionless until it is clear that an attack is imminent. At this point, the prey animal bursts into escape activity and attempts to flee as rapidly as possible. If caught, the prey animal will struggle violently, but only briefly if it is apparent that it cannot escape (Rovee, Kaufman, Collier, and Kent, 1976). When escape is not possible, the captured prey becomes limp and suppresses distress and emotional behaviors (e.g., it ceases movement and vocalization). On occasion, this "playing possum" strategy may ultimately allow the prey to effect an escape. It is believed that stress-activated biological responses, such as the release of endorphins, enable prey animals to endure the terror and pain of being mauled and eaten.

IES studies involve placing animals in situations where they are exposed to noxious stimuli, typically electric shocks to the feet. A number of other stressors (e.g., rapid rotation, vaginal stimulation, tail pinching, or immersion in hot water) can elicit similar behaviors. (Many of the same stressors produce kindling.) Once conditioned by IES, animals subjected to further painful shocks will fail to avail themselves of opportunities to escape, even when the means to do so are immediate and obvious. Responses to IES are a function of the intensity of the pain and the uncontrollability and unpredictability of the experimental situation. Controllability (or the lack thereof) of the stressor appears to be an especially important variable (Maier, 1986). Of considerable interest is the widely replicated finding that IES procedures produce significant analgesia in experimental animals (Kelly, 1986). This analgesia appears to involve both opioid and nonopioid mechanisms (Maier, 1986).

These studies are intriguing. They demonstrate that life threat and uncontrollable trauma produce discrete, highly change-resistant behavioral states with significant neurobiological alterations. Originally interpreted in the framework of "learned helplessness" theories of depression, trauma researchers have subsequently reinterpreted these experiments as responses to uncontrollable trauma and stress (e.g., van der Kolk, Greenberg, Boyd, and Krystal, 1985; Foa, Steketee, and Rothbaum, 1989). The DBS model of dissociative disorders, discussed in the next chapter, is compatible with many of the animal data.

Computer Metaphors and Neural Network Models

From clockwork men, to Freud's steam engine metaphors, to telegraph and telephone wiring diagrams of the nervous system, every age turns to its technology for descriptions of the mind. Not surprisingly, computer-based models of MPD have surfaced. These range from simplistic metaphors of the brain as a "microprocessor" and alter personalities as "programs" (e.g., Andorfer, 1985) to more sophisticated neural network models of dissociated mental processes (e.g., Farah, O'Reilly, and Vecera, 1993).

Neural networks have considerable potential for modeling dissociative cognitive phenomena, but models that replicate important clinical features have not yet been presented. I would point to the neural network modeling of schizophrenic thought processes by Hoffman and McGlashan (1994) as a good example of the power of this approach to illuminate abnormal cognitive processes. The chaos models of switching and state changes discussed at the end of the next chapter provide another exciting area of computer exploration.

SUMMARY

Recent research establishes that trauma can produce significant biological sequelae. Major stress response systems, such as the HPA axis, the sympathetic nervous system, and the immune system, become dysregulated in traumatized children and adults. The disturbances in these densely interconnected systems appear to reflect alterations in feedback mechanisms that disrupt homeostasis and make an individual less able to compensate for new or additional stress.

Psychophysiological studies of MPD patients have often demonstrated significant differences in alter personality states that cannot be duplicated by simulating controls. A number of promising leads have also appeared in the neurobiology of dissociation, including studying neurotransmitter systems affected by "dissociative" drugs such as ketamine. Theories that implicate such brain regions as the thalamus and hippocampus are likewise generating new studies, particularly at PTSD research centers.

More studies are needed, but unfortunately sometimes the acrimonious criticism of the validity of the MPD diagnosis generates a reluctance on the part of grant review groups to support studies of MPD patients. Nonetheless, a trickle of research continues because there is something happening here that demands a scientific explanation. (One would think that skeptics would welcome scientific studies as the quickest route to disproving the disorder, but some use their influence to block funding and publication of MPD research.)

Theoretical modeling is an important task of science. It organizes our thinking and highlights discrepancies in the data (i.e., what fits and what does not fit). Modeling should lead to testable hypotheses—and thus to prediction, a central goal of the scientific method. A good model of MPD and pathological dissociation should account for core features including functional amnesias, identity disturbances, the relationship with trauma, and differences between normal and pathological dissociation.

Various traditional models have been offered as explanations of MPD. These include autohypnosis, epilepsy/temporal lobe dysfunction, cerebral hemispheric laterality, social role theory, fear-conditioned responses, and computers. All are invoked to explain specific features of MPD, but none provide very comprehensive explanations.

Chapter Eight

The "Discrete Behavioral States" Model

The concept of "state"—from the Latin *status*, meaning a condition of being—is ubiquitously invoked to describe mental and emotional conditions. The notion of a mental state as a transient but important determinant of behavior was common by the early 18th century, and continues to be used in much the same fashion today. Curious about the modern psychiatric usage of "mental state," I phoned Robert Spitzer, chair of the DSM-III-R work groups, and asked to borrow a copy of the DSM-III-R text on floppy disks so that I could search for references to this term. "State! We don't mention state in the DSM," Bob protested. I did not have my copy on hand to provide an example, so I said that I would call back shortly. Bob called me a few minutes later to say that the disks were on their way. "I guess you caught me in the wrong state," he laughed. Searching Bob's disks, I found over 100 references to "mental state" in the DSM-III-R.

The ubiquity of the notion of a mental state has worked against its acceptance as a scientific concept. Although researchers recognize the importance of this concept, the bulk of investigational effort remains focused on its supposed antithesis, the "trait." Traits—technically, distinguishing qualities in the personality of an individual—are generally viewed as the true foci of scientific psychiatry and psychology. Traits are considered to be genetically based and to serve as markers for underlying biological processes. In contrast, states are widely viewed as mere behavioral noise, cluttering our efforts to find the root and cause of mental disturbances.

I argue that mental states are core components of consciousness, behavior, and personality. Many of the mental and behavioral phenomena associated with pathological dissociation—as well as certain other psychiatric disorders—can be best understood by focusing on their state-related properties. MPD in particular can be understood as arising from a traumatic disruption in the early developmental acquisition of control and integration of basic behavioral states coupled with the creation of highly discrete dissociated states organized around differences in sense of self. This conceptual framework provides an interesting perspective on the genesis, evolution, and nature of MPD. In this chapter, I outline the "discrete behavioral states" (DBS) model of MPD and pathological dissociation.

DEFINING AND CONCEPTUALIZING MENTAL STATES AT DIFFERENT LEVELS OF ANALYSIS

There are numerous literatures on states of mind, ranging from rigorous scientific research through pop psychology and out into the great flaky beyond. This breadth of interest attests to the universality of the notion of states of consciousness as critical determinants of mental experience. A review of these diverse literatures is beyond the scope of this book. (I hope one day to have an opportunity to write an expanded explication of the DBS model.) Among the scientific literatures on mental states that one can explore are studies of the following: meditation and deep relaxation; sleep and dreaming; hypnosis; drug-altered states of consciousness; pathological states (e.g., depression, mania, panic attacks, abreactions, and catatonia); and normal infant behavior. The last of these—research on behavioral states in infancy—is an excellent place to begin the present discussion of the DBS model.

Mental states are unique organizations or structures of consciousness and behavior. A given mental state is recognizable by its distinctive pattern of psychological and physiological variables. Charles Tart (1972, 1975), one of the important investigators of the science of states of consciousness, says that it is more precise to speak of "discrete states of consciousness." To reduce the monotony, I vary my terminology a bit in this chapter. I speak of "discrete states of consciousness" after the fashion of Tart, and "behavioral states" after the fashion of Peter Wolff (1987); I also occasionally throw in plain old "states of consciousness" and "mental states." In each instance, I am referring to the concept of a discrete state of consciousness as a specific and unique configuration of a set of psychological, physiological, and behavioral variables. This is the essence of the various definitions arrived at by investigators studying examples of such states.

The "levels of analysis" problem plagues the neurosciences, particularly as it relates to understanding the nature of consciousness. Is consciousness best studied at a cellular level, at the level of brain nuclei and circuits, or at a hemispheric level? Of course, the answer is all three and more. But how can we make sense of data across different levels? How do we integrate what is known about intracellular ion currents with what is known about differential hemispheric EEG patterns? What we need are isomorphic constructs that permit patterns at one level of analysis to be mapped onto patterns at another level. An example from another biological realm is the mapping of primary amino acid sequences onto secondary structures, and, in turn, the mapping of secondary structures onto tertiary protein structures. The first level of mapping (primary to secondary structures) is already well underway, thanks to computational approaches (e.g., Lapedes, 1994). It is likely that similar mappings can be constructed for brain–mind, although the readily apparent complexity of this puts the brain–mind problem in larger perspective.

The concept of "state" is encountered at all levels of brain–mind analysis. From the resting and hyperpolarized states of individual neurons to the global behavioral pattern of a manic patient, neuroscientists invoke the concept to organize and classify behavior that they are interested in. Physiologists have long recognized the ubiquity of behavioral state dependency in physiological regulation (e.g., Lydic, 1987). Missing, however, are the mappings of states across levels of analysis. How do specific firing patterns of certain neurons relate to a state of resting alert attention? Attention to the correspondences of states at different levels of analysis may help to integrate neuroscientific approaches to the really big problems, such as consciousness.

INFANT BEHAVIORAL STATES AND STATE-DEPENDENT STIMULUS RESPONSIVENESS

Each and every discrete state of consciousness may be defined in terms of a specific configuration of the system of variables used to define states of consciousness in general. In many respects, researchers of infant behavioral states—notably Heinz Prechtl, Robert Emde, Robert Harmon, and Peter Wolff—have done the best job of specifying and empirically testing classification systems of state-defining variables. In particular, much of the present discussion of infant behavioral states is based on the seminal work of Wolff and described in his important book, *The Development of Behavioral States and the Expression of Emotions in Early Infancy* (1987).

Prechtl and his colleagues formulated a logically consistent and operationally defined classification system for infant states. Prechtl's taxonomy was subsequently adapted by Wolff (1987) and others. Generally, four or five independent variables are sufficient to classify the discrete behavioral states of healthy, normal infants. Each additional variable increases the degrees of freedom, but adds to operational complexity.

State-defining variables may be continuous or dichotomous. For example, respiratory rate is a continuous variable, whereas eyes open or closed is a dichotomous variable. In practice, continuous or quasi-continuous variables provide more classificatory power than binary variables. Wolff's classification system uses easily observed or measured variables (e.g., respiratory rate, extremity motor tone, activity level, vocalization, facial expression, and eye movement patterns) to classify the confusing range of infant behaviors into a set of discrete states. When viewed from within this classification framework, complex and shifting infant behavior resolves itself into a series of orderly transitions among a limited set of discrete behavioral states.

Healthy children are born with a basic set of behavioral states. Indeed, there is evidence for the existence of a basic set of behavioral states *in utero* (de Vries, Visser, and Prechtl, 1988). Newborns exhibit five basic behavioral states, which are distinguishable by unique configurations of the state variables discussed above (Wolff, 1987). For example, in State I (regular, quiet, synchronous, or non-rapid-eye-movement [non-REM] sleep), the infant is at rest. Motor tone is low, with little resistance to passive movement of the limbs. Motor activity is infrequent, except for periodic bursts of rhythmic mouthing and occasional clonic jerks. The eyes are closed, with rare spontaneous movements. The face is relaxed and symmetrical. Breathing is regular in rhythm and amplitude, with a mean frequency of 36 breaths per minute (Wolff, 1987).

In contrast, State II (irregular or REM sleep) is characterized by periodic movements of the limbs and truck and generalized stirring. Motor tone is increased. The baby's face alternates between periods of relaxation and intermittent grimaces, frowns, smiles, or precrying expressions. Mouth movements are grosser and less regular, without the rhythmic quality of State I. The eyes are closed, but intermittent movements in both horizontal and vertical directions are visible through the eyelids. Respiratory rate is much faster, averaging about 48 breaths per minute, and is irregular in amplitude and rhythm (Wolff, 1987).

In State I, infants can be picked up, carried about, and dressed or changed without waking them. In State II, they are easily awakened by noise or movement. In State II, but not in State I, certain high-pitched sounds will elicit smiling expressions (Wolff, 1987). A small stimulus, such as a slight bump to the crib, will produce a massive startle response in State I, but not in State II or in awake states (Wolff, 1987). These are early examples of different state-dependent behaviors in response to the same stimulus. Such differences in state-dependent behaviors to a given stimulus are fundamental features of a system of discrete states of consciousness. With maturation, metacognitive mechanisms increase the generalization of state-specific adaptive responses to other discrete behavioral states—and thus the generalization of overall stimulus responsiveness.

State-dependent stimulus responsiveness produces differential responses to the same stimulus, depending upon the state the individual is in at the time. In adults, this type of differential responsiveness is most apparent in such disorders as bipolar illness and MPD. Differential VEP responses across MPD alter personality states, described in Chapter Seven, constitute a good example of this phenomenon.

Differential responsiveness demonstrates that the observable differences between two discrete states are not a simple function of moving up or down a linear response gradient. Wolff (1987) highlights differential responsiveness as an example of the nonlinearity of input–output relations in different states of consciousness. Nonlinear dynamic features of the DBS model are discussed at the end of this chapter.

The set of newborn waking states also includes State III (alert inactivity), State IV (waking activity or precrying), and State V (crying). The newborn's general behavior consists of an orderly cycle of transitions among these five states, as illustrated in Figure 8.1a. An infant alternates among several behavioral loops. Infant sleep is characterized by periodic oscillation between regular (State I) and irregular (State II) sleep until the infant passes from State II through a drowsy state and then into State IV (waking activity). State IV—often referred to as "fussy"—is characterized by frequent bursts of generalized motor activity and periodic moans, grunts, or whimpering, but not sustained crying. The infant is active and periodically verges on crying with pinched, precrying facies, irregular respiration, and flushing of the skin. Eyes are open and scan the surroundings during periods of inactivity (Wolff, 1987). The infant typically moves from State IV into State V, full-fledged crying—a state well known to parents.

Transitions from "fussy" into "crying" can sometimes be averted by timely interventions from a caretaker—for instance, feeding, picking up, or playing with the infant, or attending to an area of discomfort. As the result of such an intervention, the infant may bypass State V (crying) for this cycle, and move instead into State III (alert inactivity). State III (also known as "bright and shiny eyes") is characterized by an alert, focused gaze, regular respirations, and little spontaneous movement beyond occasional postural shifts. The infant scans the surroundings with directed eye movements and appears to be processing his or her environment. No one knows what is going on in the mind of an infant, but adults observing the "bright and shiny eyes" state are frequently moved to comment on what they think the infant "sees" or "thinks."

BEHAVIORAL STATE SPACE AND STATE TRANSITIONS (SWITCHING)

Figure 8.1 also illustrates the concept of "behavioral state space." This term refers to the idea that individual behavioral states exist within a larger multidimensional framework or space defined by a chosen set of variables. Individual behavioral states occupy discrete volumes of state

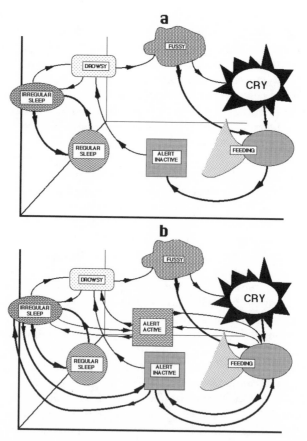

Figure 8.1. An infant's state space architecture at the ages of 1 month (a) and 3 months (b). Based on data from Wolff (1987).

space, centered around the intersections of the state-defining variables. An individual's behavior traverses state space in a series of discontinuous jumps or "switches" from one state to another. Theoretically, state space may be vast, but one can only regularly visit those regions in which one has created stable, discrete states. Discrete states are linked together by directional pathways forming a behavioral architecture (see Figure 8.2). Movement along these pathways occurs in a probabilistic fashion, which lends some degree of predictability to human behavior.

In total, this behavioral architecture defines an individual's personality by encompassing both the range of the behavioral states available to the individual and the sum of prior experiences that have created distinct, stable states of mind. This architecture can be traversed in multiple ways, but individuals tend to follow roughly predictable sequences. The phenomenon of "order effects" described in Chapter Seven probably reflects the directionality of state space pathways. An individual may spend considerably more time in certain regions of state space than in others. Some discrete behavioral states are only activated by highly unusual circumstances or in response to distinctive cues, and thus may only be seen in very specific circumstances.

Discrete states are transitory behavioral structures. Within time limits, states are self-organizing and self-stabilizing (Wolff, 1987). When a state is newly activated—for instance, when a sleeping infant wakes up (technically a transition from State II [irregular sleep] to State IV [alert activity])—the newly activated state progressively organizes and stabilizes itself. However, even when conditions are highly favorable for a given state, it is only sustained for a finite length of time. Eventually a

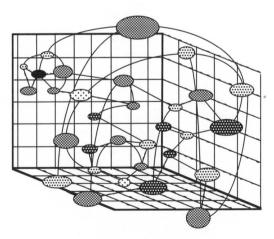

Figure 8.2. Discrete behavioral state system as "personality."

state is destabilized in some fashion, and the locus of organization for cognition and behavior shifts to another region of state space.

States vary in their capacities for self-stabilization and resistance to destabilization. Resistance to destabilization for a given state will also vary over the course of its activation. In other words, it may be easily disrupted as it first consolidates and again later after a period of time has elapsed, but during the intervening time it will take a major event to disrupt the continuity of the individual's mental state and behavior. Eventually each and every state is replaced by another, and so forth.

Transitions between behavioral states are often referred to as "switches" (Putnam, 1988). A switch is manifested by an abrupt change in the values of the constellation of state-defining variables. Examples include the transitions from waking to sleeping and from sleeping to waking (which appear to traverse different pathways); the switches in bipolar illness from mania to depression and from depression to mania (which also traverse nonreciprocal pathways); and the switches in panic disorder from euthymia to panic attacks and vice versa. Switches among alter personality states in MPD patients (discussed in Chapters Five and Seven) are excellent examples and are especially suitable for laboratory investigation. The relative ease with which they are elicited, and their behavioral distinctness, lend themselves to scientific investigation.

Figure 8.3 is a schematic depiction of different types of switching behavior. Pathway A. represents a significant leap across state space between two widely separated states, 1 and 2. This is manifested by a marked change in the values in many or all of the state-defining variables (e.g., a switch from depression to mania). Pathway B represents an oscillatory pattern, such as the periodic alternation that occurs between States I and II in the sleep of 1-month-old infants. In this schema, two states (here called 4 and 5) lie close in state space. They almost blend into each other as they cycle back and forth. Reciprocally alternating states are common at global boundaries, such as the one between sleeping and waking.

Pathway C demonstrates a nonreciprocal return route from state 2 back to state 1, requiring passage through state 3. The switch from mania to depression often passes through an unstable, intermediate state that contains both manic and depressive features, whereas the transition from depression to mania can be a direct switch (e.g., this may occur with sleep deprivation). Interestingly, reciprocal transitions between depression and mania may occur following an intervening period of sleep, so that a patient may go to sleep in one affective state and awake in the other. This period of sleep may be very short; we (Rubinow and Putnam, 1981) once studied a rapid-cycling bipolar patient who only re-

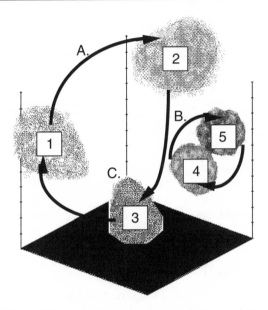

Figure 8.3. Switches among discrete behavioral states.

quired 6–10 seconds of stage II sleep to make the transition from mania to depression.

One feature of switches that helps to define them as transition processes (as opposed to discrete states) is that the time spent in the switch is considerably less than the time spent in either the initial or final state. If one chooses a sufficiently dense multivariate system of state definition, it may be possible to resolve switch pathways into rapid sequences of unstable transition states. It is a question of time scaling.

BEHAVIORAL-STATE-RELATED DEVELOPMENTAL TASKS

Creation of New States and Development of New Pathways

As children grow older, additional states appear and more complicated interconnecting pathways develop. Figure 8.1b shows the state system architecture of a 3-month-old infant. A new state, State VI (alert activity), emerges at about this age (Wolff, 1987). Additional pathways between states have also developed. Now it becomes possible for the infant to make the transition from irregular sleep (State II) to alert inactivity (State III) without passing through the drowsy and fussy states. Branching of pathways has begun to occur as well, yielding new behavioral loops. For example, at this age either the alert active or alert inactive state may follow a caretaker's intervention, such as feeding or changing a dirty diaper.

The creation of new discrete states, together with the evolution and elaboration of existing states, contributes to the increasingly complex behavioral repertoire of the growing child. The development of new pathways between existing states, and the incorporation of new and existing states into branching behavioral loops, contributes further to the growing richness and flexibility of the child's overall behavior. These two interconnected processes of state creation and pathway development are ways in which the developmental web continues to expand throughout the life span.

Modulation of Behavioral States

As the infant matures, an additional type of strand in the developmental web becomes apparent—the child's attempts at gaining control over his or her behavioral states. In early infancy, this is evidenced by self-stimulation and self-soothing behaviors (e.g., sucking on pacifiers and rhythmic rocking when stressed). In the beginning, it is the caretaker who primarily modulates the infant's behavioral states with timely interventions to meet the child's needs, both physical and psychological. As I discuss further below, the congruence and reciprocity of shared states, and the interactive modulation between caretaker and child, constitute a fundamental social experience and a core component of the attachment response.

Children gradually learn to acquire control over their own states. In Western society, some of the first states that adults actively teach children to recognize and to regulate involve the elimination of bodily wastes. Children are taught to recognize the impending signs of urination and defecation and to initiate appropriate action, which in some cases involves resisting the emergence of the elimination state until the proper context (a bathroom) is available. We normally think of waste elimination as more of a biological act than a state of mind. In early development, biological acts and states of mind are so closely paired that they are more or less one and the same—a sort of "state/act." Introspection or observation should convince the reader that preparing for, participating in, and cleaning up after a bowel movement are associated with specific states/acts, including unique biological activity (rectal peristalsis) not found in other states of consciousness. For infants, waste elimination is as much a reciprocal social experience as feeding is; indeed, the gastrocolic reflex frequently insures that one follows the other.

Physiological processes can initiate or modify states of consciousness, and specific states can initiate or modify physiological processes. Every individual has a set of states that are associated with specific biological acts, such as eating, sleeping, sex, and waste elimination. These behavioral states are entered into or exited from largely in response to physiological cues. A great deal of social and cognitive overlay accrues with time, particularly as a result of aversive experiences (e.g., embarrassment). By and large, the mental content of these routine biological states/acts is not part of the stream of consciousness during the course of the day. They are partially partioned off from other mental life. In infancy, the physiology (e.g., hunger, rectal peristalsis, fatigue) drives the switch to a given discrete state/act. As self-control is acquired, these states/acts must be entered more volitionally. For some individuals, a ritual may be necessary to prepare mind and body; for others, a good magazine or interesting catalog is sufficient.

Caretakers use a range of techniques for modulating the behavioral states of young children. Distractions, for example, are commonly used to change a child's state (see below). Children also learn the value of distractions, and in the face of discomfort may make their own "spontaneous" attentional shifts to pleasantly distracting stimuli. Indeed, refocusing of attention is a powerful technique used by harried parents and ethereal mystics alike to alter states of consciousness.

Control or modulation of behavioral state involves a number of component processes. These include (1) the ability to sustain a desired state in the face of distractions and destabilizing stimuli; (2) the ability to recover from disruption of a state by reactivating the desired state; and (3) the ability to match the appropriate behavioral state with the contextual demands of the situation. Again, diligent caretakers spend a great deal of time and effort nurturing the development of their children's state-modulating capacities. They focus on increasing the children's attention span (i.e., maintaining alert, attentive states). They provide the children with tools and tricks to recover from disruptions of states. Finally, they explain and model for the children how people "behave" in certain situations.

Modulation of affective behavioral states is a critical aspect of emotion regulation, as well as of social behavior. Children with poor emotional regulation have significant behavior problems. Indeed, researchers find a significant relationship between poor emotional regulation and psychological and behavior problems across all ages, from infancy to adulthood (e.g., Gralinski, Safyer, Hauser, and Allen, 1995; Rubin, Coplan, Fox, and Calkins, 1995).

Socialization of Behavioral States

States are contagious: They can be transmitted from parent to child, and most certainly vice versa. That is not to say that shared states are manifested in exactly the same fashion in two individuals, but rather that they are parallel or complementary in important respects. Such sharing of states—be they positive or negative—is a powerful component of "bonding" between individuals. We know very little about the processes underlying the sharing of parallel or complementary behavioral states by two or more individuals; however, I offer some speculations later in the chapter on the occurrence of these processes within families.

Developmental psychologist Tiffany Field (1985) has shown that powerful synchronizations occur in the physiological processes (e.g., heart rate) of a mother–child dyad when their behavioral states are complementary. Deliberate desynchrony of parent–child behavioral states produces strong disruptive effects, out of proportion to the actual behavioral acts (Field, 1985). Field et al. (1992) have also shown the importance of state-matching behaviors in social relationships with peers.

Metacognitive Integration

Integration of Information and Behavior in General

Still another type of strand in the developmental web, becoming apparent during toddlerhood and early childhood, involves the metacognitive processes of integrating information and behavior across different states. Unfortunately, for a host of reasons, there is little research on the subject of state dependency in children. Observation suggests that young children exhibit strong state and context dependency in their ability to recall learned information. In general, young children must be helped to generalize information acquired in one state or context to others. Very little is known about the development of such integrative metacognitive functions in children. However, varying degrees of disruption in the task of integration of information across behavioral states and contexts probably underlie the larger failures of integration of self and behaviors seen in many victims of childhood trauma (see below).

The development of behavioral-state-integrative metacognitive processes probably overlaps with the acquisition of other metacognitive functions, such as distinguishing between appearance and reality, source monitoring, visual perspective taking, conceptual perspective taking, seriation, and transitivity. Most of these capacities appear between the ages of 1 and 5 years, although they take many additional years to mature (Flavell, 1989).

Gopnik and Slaughter (1991) studied the ability of children to retrieve information about pretenses, images, perceptions, and beliefs across changes in behavioral state. Three-year-olds were able to recall past pretenses, images, and perceptions, but had difficulty with past desires, intentions, and beliefs. Four-year-olds did well on all categories of information except past beliefs. A great deal more could be said about the development of children's theory of mind and associated metacognitive functions, but these examples suffice to illustrate that state-bridging metacognitive capacities begin coming "on line" during early childhood.

As always, parents and other primary caretakers are instrumental in helping children integrate information and behavior across behavioral states and social contexts. The caretakers remind the children of what they have already learned in other states and contexts, and help the children to adapt and apply this previously learned information to new situations. Caretakers also help children generalize what they know from one set of situations or experiences to the ever-enlarging world around them. These connections usually include logical, temporal, historical, and causal components.

Development and Integration of Sense of Self

Early evidence for the differential influence of behavioral state on sense of self and on social interaction comes from studies of infants presented with a familiar face obscured by a clear plastic mask that obscures finer details of facial expression (Kaufman and Kaufman, 1980). In the alert, active state, infants typically respond by stopping all movement and staring with "consternation." In the fussy state, they respond with full gaze aversion and rapid transition to vigorous crying (Wolff, 1993).

Many aspects of self are state-dependent. That is, the particular mental state that one is in at a given moment influences how one feels about and expresses various aspects of oneself, and how one relates to others. Research with drug- and mood-induced behavioral states indicates that an individual's autobiographical recall of events and experiences can be strongly state-dependent (Weingartner et al., 1995). Clinically, this is dramatically manifested in such disorders as rapid-cycling bipolar illness (Weingartner, 1978; Szostak, Lister, Eckardt, and Weingartner, 1994). In the depressed state, bipolar patients have poor self-esteem and feel powerless to affect the world around them. When asked about their past, depressed individuals disproportionately recall negative events. Yet immediately following a switch into mania, the same individuals are inappropriately grandiose, with an exaggerated sense of self-importance and influence. They will recall, inflate, or even confabulate all manner of personal successes. "Personality" markers (e.g., manner of speech, use of gestures, gait, posture, etc.) will be strikingly different from those in the depressed state.

In normal individuals, mood state has a lesser but still noticeable impact on how an individual perceives and represents himself or herself. In this sense, everyone manifests a range of "selves" that are to some extent state-dependent (Bower, 1994). However, in a normal individual, specific state-dependent senses of self are sufficiently integrated with one another that the individual maintains a sense of continuity of self across state and context. This is one of the critical differences between the contextual "selves" of normal individuals and the dissociated "selves" of MPD patients.

State dependency of senses of self appears to be especially true for young children. Investigators studying the development of self note that young children have multiple senses of self, depending on their internal states and environmental contexts (Wolf, 1990). With maturation, children develop "selves" that bridge contexts and can be volitionally activated as necessary. For example, during the period roughly between the ages of 2 and 4 years, children develop an "authorial self." The authorial self is sufficiently independent of context or state to enable a child to begin selecting modes and aspects of self to emphasize in given situations. As developmental researcher Dennie Palmer Wolf (1990) notes, "It [the authorial self] is a new kind of self, one who can speak as object or subject, as observer or participant" (p. 185).

The authorial self represents a preliminary metacognitive integration of the child's state-dependent aspects of self. The authorial self permits the child to emphasize different aspects of self volitionally, according to his or her wishes and needs. Beginning at about 2½ to 3 years or age, this developing capacity is beautifully expressed by the appearance of fantasy play. As children pretend to be different selves—often socially coordinating their roles with playmates—they begin the larger process of uncoupling sense of self from the immediate situation.

PARENT–CHILD BEHAVIORAL STATE INTERACTIONS

Parents and children recurrently alter each other's states of consciousness—often deliberately! Parents are biologically "wired" to respond to their children's states. To interact with these states, they use sets of child-rearing techniques that are passed on from generation to generation by example. The transgenerational and cultural transmission of parenting behaviors is an extraordinary example of the interaction of powerful biological and cultural forces on human behavior.

For their part, children are equally attentive to parental states and rapidly learn what works best to meet their own needs. They also augment their experience with examples from siblings and peers. Indeed, below I argue that the interplay of discrete states of consciousness is a major vehicle for family interactions. Surprisingly little attention has been paid to this phenomenon, which constitutes one of the major modalities of child–parent interactions in daily life. One manifestation of this process in action is the ubiquitous family battle of whose mood state is going to prevail.

Parental State-Altering Behaviors

An infant communicates his or her needs primarily through alterations of behavioral state. Crying (Wolfe's [1987] state V) is a common behavioral state that infants and preschoolers enter when stressed. Crying usually captures caretakers' attention, and most respond—at least initially. In many parents, crying induces a vigorous attempt to switch their infants into a less noxious behavioral state (e.g., sleep). These first interactions are the beginning of a complex dance between the parents and children around the modulation of each other's states of mind.

Caretakers, especially mothers, intuitively learn to read their children's current states and to anticipate the children's future states (based on their intimate knowledge of their children's cyclic behavioral state architecture). They use this information to plan daily activities. For instance, a caretaker who anticipates that a child may be situationally stressed later in the day may try to time a nap or feeding to maximize the likelihood of a cooperative state during the stressful period. The success of these interventions depends on the caretaker's ability to read the child's state, familiarity with the child's behavioral state cycle, and ability to make effective interventions in the child's state cycle. This is one of the areas in which good parents/caretakers differ significantly from not-so-good ones.

When a child's crying or distress is not due to directly remediable causes (e.g., hunger or a wet diaper), a parent often uses distraction and other techniques to alter the child's state. Distraction works best with infants and young children, but it continues to be effective under special circumstances throughout the life span. In older individuals, distraction is often achieved by a voluntary concentration of attention. When coupled with suggestion, distraction can block significant pain and other noxious perceptions by altering state of consciousness. À la James, one can postulate two basic types of distraction, voluntary and involuntary. In voluntary distraction, individuals consciously focus their cognitive resources in order to distract themselves from something, usually a noxious situation.

Involuntary distraction, such as that practiced by parents seeking to alter a child's behavior, occurs when an individual's attention is caught and held by an external stimulus. Capturing the attention of a crying toddler often breaks the crying state, which dissipates in a scattering of sobs and shudders, to be replaced by smiles and laughter. During the transition period, it is not uncommon to see a mixture of tears and laughter. Every parent knows that there is often a critical moment when the balance can tip back toward tears if another disruption intrudes. Susceptibility to involuntary distraction declines with age, perhaps reflecting increased self-monitoring of attentional resources.

Parents sometimes attempt to break a noxious state in a child by attempting to elicit a psychophysiological response associated with a more desirable state ("Come on, Billy, give me a smile"). By jollying their child into the act of smiling, parents may be destabilizing the negative state by modifying the child's physiological organization. Ekman, Levenson, and Friesen (1983) have shown that significant physiological changes occur when facial muscles are arranged in certain configurations. Children, sensitive to the disruptive effects of smiling on their angry demeanor, may sometimes refuse to comply—yet another round in the family "war between the states."

Parental Lessons in Monitoring Others' States of Mind

The social monitoring of discrete behavioral states in others, and the adjustment of one's own states in accordance or opposition to the states of others, constitute a basic social skill. The acquisition of this skill—which is a dimension of social intelligence—is probably dependent on a complex set of genetic and environmental factors interacting with the cognitive capacities and learned behaviors of the individual. Some people excel at this art, whereas others are social morons. Although there are clearly universal states (e.g., anger and terror), many social states have features that are unique to each culture. Even socially perceptive individuals have difficulty detecting differences in social-emotional states in people from a different culture.

By word and deed, parents and significant others teach children how to recognize social states. Ideally, they identify for the children salient states in themselves and others ("She is feeling sad because her dog died"). They also help the children to understand when and how to initiate an appropriate response to a prominent state in another ("Tell her that it makes you feel sad too"). Parents help the child to assume an appropriate state in response to specific contexts—for instance, a solemn state of mind in church, or good humor in response to friendly teasing. Finally, parents teach children to recognize and respond to dangerous states in others ("Jimmy, don't stare at that man! He's acting strange").

Children generally catch on fast, and by the age of 18 months they are capable of articulating their perceptions of basic emotional states (e.g., anger, fear, amusement, etc.) in others. Refinement of this capacity is an evolving developmental thread spanning the life cycle. With time, an exquisite degree of sensitivity—for better or for worse—can develop in parent–child and spousal relationships.

States of Mind as a Modality of Family Transactions

Discrete states of consciousness, especially mood states, are a basic modality of family transactions. We all react, consciously and unconsciously, to the emotional and behavioral states of our significant others. Struggles around issues of control often revolve around the question of whose state is going to dominate the family scene. Children are formidable competitors, equipped with an armamentarium of emotional states capable of pushing biological buttons in their elders. Parents react to their children's given states in voluntary and involuntary ways. Sometimes they have to catch themselves and substitute a deliberately adopted state/behavior for a child's reflexive emotional response ("Remember! We agreed that you and I would count to 10 together when you feel like hitting your brother").

An extended look at the "state" expressions of family dynamics is beyond the scope of this book. Here I simply highlight a few examples of what I think is going on. The family state game is about power, influence, and control (i.e., the usual human stakes). It is played differently in different families—sometimes playfully, sometimes vengefully.

Family dynamics, viewed from a clinical perspective, are influenced by a myriad of factors: demographics; family history at many levels; economic, social, and cultural factors; current and past stressors; existent pathology; and many others. The point is that every family reflects a unique and dynamic blend of factors that must be considered. (As Tolstoy observed in *Anna Karenina*, every unhappy family is unhappy in its own way.) Family psychopathology, both as manifested in discrete disorders within family members (e.g., schizophrenia, social phobia) and as expressed within family interactional patterns (e.g., the setting up of double binds), influences and is expressed in the language of affective and behavioral states.

The goals of the family state game involve influence and control over interactions within the family. There are many reasons why individuals want to influence the states of mind of their family members. In addition to the issues of power and authority, there are more subtle positive human needs, such as feeling understood. Struggles to set a dominant affective tonal state for family interactions may revolve around the need for congruency of affect and emotional perspective. Sometimes this is driven by a very specific family issue ("We all feel the same way about what Uncle Jack did").

Because of their lower-power position in the family hierarchy, children often play the family state game by activating specific behavioral states that passively impede or negatively tinge the state/mood/contextual behavior that the parents are trying to envoke—for example, by "becoming" oppositional to parental wishes. When they are unable to dominate the family scene directly, children may snipe away from the periphery by adopting a quasi-acceptable state/demeanor that still communicates their feelings and exerts their influence on family socialization (e.g., sulking). Adolescent negative states (e.g., sullen silence) are common forms of "payback" against parents. Indeed, adolescents become adept at maintaining such emotional states for protracted periods.

Children quickly come to recognize which states can be expressed under what circumstances. Certain states that are appropriate when a child is alone with one or the other parent are not acceptable in the presence of both parents or another party. Siblings play off each other's states in complex ways. At least a few children have learned to exert indirect influence on the family affective environment by cranking up a noxious state in a sibling ("Johnny, stop teasing your sister this instant!"). Extended family, friends, and others periodically enter the arena and sway the process in ways that are unique for every family.

Tolerance for one another's states is an important socialization process within the family. The experience of problematic states in other family members is leavened by a knowledge of their prior history and by the recognition that they will pass with time or a change of context. Recognition of the role of context is a particularly important factor in defusing the provocative nature of noxious states in family members ("Oh, your father doesn't really mean what he said. He always gets like that when he's paying the bills"). Time outs, restriction to one room, or mandated changes in setting or activity are often used by parents to interrupt or isolate negative states in their children. Likewise, children come to know when to leave a parent alone or to save a delicate question for another time.

THE EFFECTS OF MALTREATMENT ON THE
DEVELOPMENT OF BEHAVIORAL STATES

For better or for worse, therefore, parents have an array of techniques and processes with which they can influence the behavioral states of their children. Maltreatment, particularly early in childhood, has a significant effect on the various state-related developmental tasks discussed above. The terror, despair, torment, helplessness, guilt, self-loathing, and other painful emotions associated with being a maltreated child may stimulate the creation and elaboration of discrete emotional states that the child recurrently reexperiences following a triggering stimulus. Some of these states may be fear-conditioned and may involve amygdaloid/temporal lobe responses to threatening stimuli (Aggleton, 1992; see discussion in Chapter Seven). Other states may be activated in the aftermath of maltreatment, as the child struggles to reconstitute himself or herself after physical and emotional intrusions. Internally focused, reality-altering states of deep fantasy located in magical mental worlds are a common restitutive response of tormented children.

Creation of Traumatic States

Fear-conditioned states—for example a discrete behavioral state activated in response to a stimulus reminiscent of a previous terrifying maltreatment experience—are typically associated with significant physiological arousal. Blood pressure, heart rate, central and peripheral catecholamine levels, and other autonomic indices are markedly elevated in these states in both animals and humans (Aggleton, 1992). Although fear-conditioned states have been part of human experience from the beginning of our species, for most of us they exist outside of the range of daily experience and represent non-normal, altered states of consciousness. They are extremely unpleasant experiences, even when the perception of the threatening stimulus turns out to be mistaken.

Indeed, individuals have developed full-fledged PTSD as a result of exposure to objectively minor stressors that they misperceived as life-threatening. Typically, fear-conditioned states have a rapid, "emergency response" activation pattern and a much slower offset, leaving the individual feeling shaky, enervated, and unable to concentrate. Pitman et al. (1990) speculate that the high arousal levels associated with fear-conditioned states may release increased levels of endogenous opiates, which create a biological "addiction" to trauma and thrill-seeking behaviors.

Traumatic Alterations of the Architecture of Behavioral State Pathways

Maltreatment can interfere with the associative pathways connecting sequences of states. New, trauma-associated pathways are generated, producing abnormal behavioral sequences. Exposure to fear-conditioned stimuli can interrupt normal behavioral loops, sending a child into trauma-related behavioral states; this has a disorganizing effect on the child's overall behavior. Traumatized children are vulnerable to trauma-reminiscent stimuli that activate abnormal state sequences (e.g., flash-backs). These may be manifested in agitated, hyperkinetic, disorganized, and affectively labile behavior. Such a child has a dazed, "out-of-it" quality. Attempts to make contact or otherwise control his or her behavior are frequently unsuccessful. Recovery from such behavioral disruptions can be slow and may require a change of context or other major intervention to break the child's mental set.

Perry, Pollard, Blakely, Baker, and Vigilante (1995) have thoughtfully articulated a theoretical neurobiological model to account for how trauma-induced behavioral states in children ultimately evolve into behavioral/personality "traits." This model revolves around newly emerging research on the "use-dependent" capacities of the developing brain. Repeated activation of specific trauma-related behavioral states and associated pathways (i.e., "use") influences developing neurobiological processes, including synaptic function and second- and third-messenger cellular systems, so that the states/acts become "hard-wired" into the brain. Sensitization of hyperarousal responses to threat stimuli, involving activation of the locus coeruleus and ventral tegmental nucleus norepinephrine systems, plays a central role in the Perry et al. (1995) model.

Data from a number of research areas, particularly the development of cortical representation of motor functions, demonstrate the importance of use-dependent neural development (e.g., see Thelen and Smith, 1994). From animal (and to some extent human) studies, it seems likely that there are "critical periods" during early development in which use-dependent organizational effects are more influential. Research suggests that the critical period for certain types of use-dependent capacities seems to close at about 6 years of age. For example, for players of stringed instruments who begin their musical instruction before age 6, the increase in cortical representation for the left hand is significantly correlated with the age at which they began to play (Elbert, Panev, Wienbruch, Rocksroh, and Taub, 1995).

Disruption of Capacities for Behavioral State Modulation

Continuing maltreatment or other stress can interfere with a child's acquisition of self-control over behavioral states. Feelings of helplessness and lack of control are common characteristics of trauma-associated states of consciousness. These same feelings may be triggered in other situations by stimuli that are reminiscent of the trauma. In many instances, it seems as if traumatized children are not directly aware of the nature of the traumatic stimulus that disrupts their behavior. The experience of having their volitional behavior suddenly derailed for no apparent reason does not foster self-confidence nor reinforce a sense of self-control.

Disturbances in the primary attachment relationship are extremely common in maltreated children (Cicchetti and Lynch, 1995). Attachment is inextricably related to the regulation of psychological and physiological functions (Pipp and Harmon, 1987). Maltreated children typically exhibit "disorganized" attachment (type D). Type D attachment is manifested by a child's first initiating one behavior toward the caretaker, ceasing that behavior, and then initiating another form of attachment behavior (Main and Hesse, 1996). Sometimes the transition between the end of the first attachment behavior and the initiation of the second form of attachment behavior is interrupted by a period of "stilling," in which the child appears to be in a trance-like state (Main and Hesse, 1996). It is tempting to conceptualize this trance-like state as a dissociative state switch, but further research is necessary to determine what is happening here.

Other aspects of inept or malignant parenting in maltreating families also contribute to problems in modulation of state and affect regulation. In many instances, maltreating parents, even when well-meaning and trying to be good parents, simply have grossly deficient parenting skills and are much poorer at nurturing their children's capacity to acquire control over their behavior. Maltreating parents are not as good at recognizing and tracking their children's behavioral states; they are also less able to craft the gentle interventions that reset or sustain appropriate states and dissipate negative or inappropriate states. Moreover, maltreating parents' own state-modulating behaviors are generally poor examples of self-control for their children to introject and identify with.

Maladaptive Attempts at Self-Modulation of Behavioral States

As they grow older, traumatized individuals often seek to compensate for their deficits in state modulation in a variety of ways. Phobic avoidance of traumatic reminders pervades the lives of many. Some use obsessive and ruminative strategies to suppress intrusive thoughts and affects; others use drugs and alcohol as ways of "pharmacologically dissociating," insulating themselves from traumatic material and affects. Such maladaptive attempts at self-modulation of behavioral states add another layer of psychopathology to an already disturbed individual. Treatments aimed only at this highest level of psychopathology are likely to fail, as the individual substitutes other maladaptive state modulation strategies or simply readily relapses under minor stressors.

Disruption of Metacognitive Integrative Functions

Maltreatment interferes with the metacognitive integration of information and knowledge across behavioral states. It does this in a number of ways. As discussed in more detail below, traumatic states of consciousness are widely separated in state space from normal states of consciousness on many psychological and physiological dimensions. This distance, and the powerful and painful emotions associated with traumatic states, make it difficult for a traumatized person to retrieve information learned in other states while he or she is in the traumatic state. In general, investigations of state-dependent learning and retrieval demonstrate that the larger the differences between two states, the greater the dissociations of memory between them (Weingartner et al., 1995). Cognitive deficits and brain damage associated with trauma (discussed in Chapters Two, Six, and Seven) may also interfere with the efficacy of metacognitive processes.

Family environment features commonly associated with maltreatment may also negatively influence a traumatized child's attempts to integrate knowledge and behavior across state and context. Abusive families often maintain significant discrepancies between public and private behavior, so that the child alternates between two dramatically different social contexts. Abusive parents may even actively prohibit the child from generalizing across these two domains, thus creating multiple realities that require differing responses to the "same" situation. Indeed, Richard Loewenstein (personal communication, 1991) has observed that MPD would be more aptly named "multiple reality disorder."

APPLYING THE MODEL TO CORE DISSOCIATIVE PHENOMENA

The DBS model is elaborated in the following chapters. Here, I begin applying the model to the core dissociative phenomena listed in Chapter Seven as demanding explication by a viable model. These include the nature of the functional amnesias; the basis of MPD alter personalities and related identity disturbances; the relation between trauma and pathological dissociation; and the differences between normal and pathological dissociation. First, however, I provide a DBS-based definition of "pathological dissociation" and description of the processes that influence its distance from normal states of consciousness.

Pathological Dissociation versus
Normal States of Consciousness

In the DBS model, "pathological dissociation" is defined as a category of trauma-induced discrete behavioral states that are widely separated in multidimensional state space from normal states of consciousness. This is similar to conventional definitions, which emphasize the separation or segregation of specific ideas or affects from normal mental phenomena (see, e.g., Kaplan and Sadock, 1991). However, the DBS model permits better definitions of the nature and dimensions of this "wide separation." Four main processes intrinsic to the model influence the degree of separation between normal states and dissociative states. When many or all of these processes are significantly different between the two types of states, then the states are separated by a wide gap in state space, and the dissociative states are said to be "pathological." Some of these processes are tapped by current dissociation scales and structured diagnostic interviews.

The first process contributing to the separation of dissociative states from normal states consists of the multidimensional distance, in terms of the variables used to define state space, between the two types of states. That is, a dissociative state (particularly one produced by an acutely terrifying experience) may be very distant from normal states of consciousness along such dimensions as heart rate, respiration, affect, and level of arousal. For example, in the midst of an emergency response state associated with a near-accident on the highway, one's ability to do mental arithmetic or recite memorized poetry is significantly impaired, compared to one's ability in normal states of consciousness. Heart rate, respiration rate and pattern, affect, arousal level, and other state-defining variables are also dramatically different from those in normal states of consciousness.

The second process is the profound state dependency of the accessibility/retrievability of information and knowledge encoded in dissociative versus normal states of consciousness. As discussed in Chapter Six, the mental state present during the encoding of information acts as a sort of address tag for the storage and later retrieval of that information. Information acquired in a specific state is usually more accessible to recall from a state that is the same as or very similar to the encoding state. The same information often becomes significantly less accessible when the retrieval state is markedly different from the encoding state (Weingartner, 1978; Szostak et al., 1994). Trauma-induced dissociative states are markedly different from normal states of consciousness, and these marked differences affect the accessibility of information in both directions. Thus the retrieval of information between dissociative and normal states of consciousness is often inhibited. This bidirectional inhibition in state-dependent retrieval (which is usually somewhat asymmetrical) can account for the personality-state-reciprocal amnesias reported in MPD, and for amnesias in other dissociative disorders. This point is discussed further below.

The third process postulated to influence the degree of separation between the two types of states is the architecture of the pathways connecting the states. Several architectural elements influence the degree of separation. Direct connections are postulated to be closer in state space than pathways that must traverse a series of intervening states. States sharing multiple interconnecting pathways are postulated to lie closer in state space than states sharing only a single connecting pathway. (Recall that behavioral state space is multidimensional.) States lying at the distal ends of infrequently traversed state system pathways are hypothesized to be far apart.

The fourth process considered here resides at the metacognitive level of the integration of knowledge and sense of self. Such integration is hypothesized to be a metacognitive function that exists outside of state space and facilitates a person's observation of his or her own behavior, regardless (more or less) of which state the individual is in. It is postulated that this function facilitates the integration and continuity of identity and behavior across daily fluctuations in behavioral state. To some extent, self-observation and related reflective capacities are state-dependent; however, normal individuals manage to maintain an intact and continuous sense of self, even across marked fluctuations in mental state. Early childhood trauma is postulated to disrupt the development of this important higher-level process, leading to difficulties in integration of self across marked changes in affective, anxiety, and dissociative states. As discussed in Chapter Three, disturbances in identity and sense of self are not confined to the dissociative disorders, but are manifested in one form or another in other trauma-related disorders (e.g., BPD and eating disorders).

Taken together, then, these four processes contribute to the "wide separation" in state space between pathological dissociative states and normal states. The clinical phenomena associated with pathological dissociation can be understood in terms of these processes and this separation.

Dissociative Amnesias

Dissociative amnesias are considered to be "functional," in that the "missing" memories are available (under the right circumstances) but cannot be recalled by the individual in the dissociative state. Dissociative amnesias exhibit many properties consistent with the phenomena of state-dependent learning and memory retrieval (Putnam, 1991b; Szostak et al., 1994, 1997). In the DBS model, dissociative amnesias are postulated to be examples of extreme state dependency in the accessibility of information, caused by the wide separation in state space between the dissociative and normal states.

Dissociative Disturbances in Identity

There are several different manifestations of dissociative disturbances of identity. In dissociative amnesias and dissociative fugue states, the individual typically "forgets" who he or she is. In an acute dissociative state, core personal information such as name, age, and marital status may be temporarily inaccessible to the individual. For example, Hicks (1993) describes the case of a man who could not recall his wife's name or their address after learning that she had just been killed. This profound failure in autobiographical memory retrieval is an extreme form of state-dependent retrieval. Traumatic disruption of metacognitive integrative functions may also be involved. Depersonalization, a common dissociative disturbance in identity, is postulated to result from an alteration of metacognitive self-reflective, self-observing functions. In situations of extreme danger, depersonalization may be part of the identity dimensions of a state of extreme stress. In chronic depersonalization syndrome that occurs without immediate life threat, depersonalization may reflect a basic disturbance in metacognition.

The DBS model hypothesizes that the alter personalities seen in MPD reflect the creation of a set of complex, enduring, identity-based, discrete dissociative states that evolve during childhood and adolescence. Current clinical and research data suggest that alter personalities arise in the context of severe trauma occurring early in childhood. They are hypothesized to begin as trauma-induced states of consciousness. Over time, they become increasingly differentiated as a result of several factors.

The first factor is the repeated induction of a given state as a result of contextual factors associated with a specific, repetitive traumatic experience. Repeated induction leads to easier accessibility from other states, greater differentiation as a result of acquiring a "history," and greater self-organizing/self-stabilizing properties. Many MPD patients describe having alter personalities that "took" specific abusive acts (e.g., one handled fellatio, another absorbed cunnilingus, etc.). An implicit prediction of the DBS model is that autobiographical memories for such traumatic experiences should be strongly alter-personality-state-dependent and not readily retrievable in other states of consciousness. This is amply supported by clinical experience (Putnam, 1989a).

The increasing differentiation and specificity of MPD alter personalitites and other dissociative states also reflect a developmental failure of metacognitive integrative processes. The DBS model postulates that in younger children, metacognitive processes are more rudimentary and therefore more susceptible to disruption. Thus a relationship between earlier trauma and higher levels of dissociation, which has been widely reported, is predicted by the model (see Chapter Nine). The existence of critical periods of vulnerability during early childhood may account for the nonlinearity of this relationship.

The DBS model implies that the identity fragmentation seen in MPD and other disorders associated with childhood trauma is not a "shattering" of a previously intact identity, but rather a developmental failure of consolidation and integration of discrete states of consciousness. In particular, it is a profound developmental failure to coherently bind together the state-dependent aspects of self experienced by all young children that leads to the MPD patient's experience of multiple "selves."

Relationship between Trauma and Dissociation

The relationship between experiences of significant trauma and higher levels of dissociation is also explained by the potent state-generating properties of trauma. Extreme states induced by stress and trauma are robustly different on state-defining variables (i.e., dissociated) from normal states of consciousness. The more severe the trauma, at least on certain indices, the greater the likelihood that an individual will be driven into an altered state of consciousness. Chronic or repetitive trauma leads to a greater number of altered states, which coevolve with time; in a case of MPD, the ultimate result is an alter personality system.

Differences between Normal and Pathological Dissociation

Finally, the DBS model suggests that "pathological dissociation" (i.e., highly discrete dissociative states of consciousness) should differ from "normal dissociation." Recent taxometric analyses suggest that pathological dissociation and normal dissociation may be quite different processes (see Chapter Four). Pathological dissociation is characterized by profound, functional amnesias and significant alterations in identity; normal dissociation is expressed primarily in the form of intense absorption with internal stimuli (e.g., daydreams) or external stimuli (e.g., a fascinating book or television program). Normal dissociation consists of a set of discrete states of consciousness that are characterized by a narrowing of perceptual and attentional focus, but without significant state dependency for memory or identity (i.e., no *wide* separation from normal states of consciousness). In contrast, pathological dissociative states are characterized by significant state dependency of autobiographical memory and identity.

NONLINEAR DYNAMICS AND THE
DISCRETE BEHAVIORAL STATES MODEL

Nonlinear dynamics—popularly termed "chaos theory"—is an interdisciplinary field that draws upon and touches many areas of science, especially mathematics and the physical sciences. Such works for general audiences as Gleick's (1987) *Chaos* are informative and entertaining introductions for readers not familiar with this exciting field. As with any "theory of (almost) everything," cliché overload has dimmed the appeal of chaos theory for some. Nonetheless, nonlinear dynamic approaches inform our understanding of many basic brain processes. In particular, nonlinear phenomena such as self-organization and emergent properties are particularly appealing to neuroscientists attempting to understand how complex behavior emerges from brain systems (Pribram, 1994).

Attempts to apply nonlinear dynamics to psychology have been largely metaphorical, in the sense that analogies are drawn between the phenomena that characterize nonlinear dynamic systems (e.g., sensitive dependency on initial conditions, self-organization, strange attractors, etc.) and psychological phenomena (e.g., Barton, 1994). Although such analogies are descriptively attractive, data to support them have been lacking in most instances. Stronger evidence of the relevance of nonlinear dynamic systems to rapid shifts in mood and behavior has emerged from recent studies (e.g., Gottschalk, Bauer, and Whybrow, 1995).

To my knowledge, Wolff (1987) was the first to point out the relevance of nonlinear dynamic systems theory to discrete behavioral states. In a later publication (Wolff, 1993), he takes the position that behavioral states can be conceptualized as nonlinear systems and that changes in behavioral state (switches) constitute nonlinear transitions in a "qualitatively distinct and multidimensional constellation of nonlinear responses to environmental influences, which from a psychological perspective, can be construed as discontinuous contexts of practical 'meanings' or qualitatively different ways of evaluating the environment through action" (p. 192).

Wolff (1993) presents data from infant studies illustrating that behavioral states are best understood in nonlinear dynamic terms as self-organizing, self-equilibrating systems. A gradual change in one or more variables can drive a state beyond the critical limiting conditions that it can buffer. When a state exceeds the threshold of its self-stabilizing capacities, it disorganizes and reorganizes spontaneously as a qualitatively different pattern (i.e., the person switches to a new state).

Although Wolff does not say this directly, nonlinear dynamic theory would conceptualize discrete behavioral states as "strange attractors" located in state space. Technically, an "attractor" is a stable asymptotic motion, such as a source, sink, saddle, or limit cycle in two dimensions. In three (or more) dimensions, "chaotic systems" (i.e., deterministic systems that exhibit uncorrelated behavior) are "trapped" by strange attractors. To the uninitiated, this probably sounds pretty strange, but nonlinear dynamics provides a sophisticated conceptual language that nicely describes many behavioral state phenomena (Ehlers, 1995).

The study by Gottschalk et al. (1995) of chaotic dynamics in the oscillations of mood states in bipolar patients is evidence that nonlinear dynamic theory may powerfully converge with the DBS model—permitting (among other things) better mathematical modeling of behavior, as well as defining the limits of the predictability of human behavior. Using physiological data from infants learning to walk, Thelen and Smith (1994) provide an elegant synthesis of nonlinear dynamical theory with normal developmental processes. A more comprehensive explication of these ideas would require another book.

SUMMARY

The DBS model is offered as an alternative perspective on the nature of dissociation. Attention is drawn to the ubiquity of the concept of "mental states" in our everyday and clinical thinking. Many forms of mental states are available for study, but the discrete behavioral states of infants provide the best foundation for understanding dissociative states. The discussion draws on work by a number of researchers, exemplified and summarized by the research of Peter Wolff.

Infant behavioral states can be defined by a set of observable continuous and dichotomous variables. When so classified, they reveal that they are arranged in cyclic architectures, which organize infant behaviors into roughly predictable sequences. The number of infant states and their levels of interconnection increase with development and are responsible for the infant's growing behavioral repertoire.

With respect to the self-control of behavioral states, the growing child faces several core developmental tasks. These involve the creation of functional new states and the refinement of existing ones; the creation of new and functional connections/associations between states that increase behavioral flexibility; the acquisition of self-control over behavioral states; the social modulation of states with respect to significant others; and the metacognitive integration of information and behavior (most importantly, a sense of self) across diverse behavioral states.

These developmental tasks are profoundly influenced by early caretaking interactions. Parent–child interactions are discussed first at the infant level, and then again in a more age-ambiguous "parent and child within the family" context, in an attempt to illustrate social influences on behavioral states.

With this background, the effects of maltreatment on behavioral-state-related developmental tasks are considered. Trauma creates specific states that are very different from normal states along many state-defining variables, such as arousal, affect, and physiological milieu. Trauma interferes with associative pathways between states. Trauma also interferes with the acquisition of control over behavioral states, often leading the individual to seek external controls over mental state (e.g., alcohol and drugs). Maltreatment interferes with metacognitive integrative functions. Family environment interacts with maltreatment features in complex ways to exacerbate or mitigate maltreatment's direct effects.

Pathological dissociation, in the DBS model, is defined as a category of trauma-induced discrete behavioral states that are widely separated from more normal states of consciousness in multidimensional state space. The degree of this separation is influenced by four processes: differences in physiological arousal and other state-defining variables; state dependency of the accessibility of specific information, particularly autobiographical information; architecture of the pathways connecting the states; and differences in the metacognitive integration of sense of self. Dissociative amnesias are conceptualized as profound forms of state-dependent learning and memory retrieval. Dissociative disturbances of identity result from differential accessibility of autobiographical memory and the development of highly state-dependent senses of self, which become progressively elaborated in the absence of normal metacognitive integrative functions. The chapter concludes with a tantalizing tie-in between the DBS model and the emerging field of nonlinear dynamics. The DBS model of pathological dissociation is elaborated in the chapters to follow.

Chapter Nine

The Developmental Basis of Dissociation

This chapter covers what is known about the development of normal and pathological dissociation. Although there are many theories and speculations about the developmental basis of dissociation, relatively little is known about it beyond the role of childhood trauma (see Chapter Four). Therefore, in addition to presenting the existing research data on the role of such factors as age, gender, genetics, culture, education/intelligence, and family environment, I discuss the DBS model's implications and predictions concerning these factors. I then move on to a discussion of research on the relation of normal developmental processes, such as attachment and fantasy/imagination, to the development of dissociation.

FACTORS INFLUENCING DISSOCIATIVE CAPACITY: RESEARCH FINDINGS

Age

Sweeping statements are commonly made to the effect that children are more dissociative than adults; the implication is that the greater dissociative capacity of normal childhood increases the vulnerability of children to developing dissociative disorders. What is the evidence?

Initially such statements were based on extrapolations of studies showing higher hypnotic capacity in children than in adults. Back when it was assumed that dissociativity and hypnotizability were synonymous processes, greater hypnotizability in children was considered evidence of greater dissociative capacity. Indeed, the experimental hypnotizability literature supports the observation that hypnotizability is higher in children than in adults (Plotnick, Payne, and O'Grady, 1991). On average, scores on standard hypnosis scales show a curvilinear relationship with age. They rise during middle childhood, peak at about 9–11 years of age, and decline during adolescence. (E.g., see the developmental curves for hypnotizability in Cooper and London, 1971; see also Putnam et al., 1994.) During adulthood hypnotizability is relatively stable, showing only a modest decline in later decades.

Measurement problems with young children make it difficult to quantitate hypnotizability below the ages 5–6 years, but studies suggest that preschoolers have significant capacities in some areas, which may exceed those of older children (Gardner and Olness, 1981). When specific hypnotic capacities or dimensions are examined, the developmental picture is actually a bit more complex. Different hypnotic phenomena (e.g., posthypnotic amnesia, hypnotic hallucinations, arm rigidity, etc.) show different developmental curves. For example, young children have little difficulty with standard posthypnotic amnesia or auditory hallucinations—test items that are difficult for older children, especially teenagers. However, they have problems with test items such as suggested dream or age regression, on which teenagers score much higher. However, as discussed in connection with the autohypnotic model of MPD in Chapter Seven, hypnosis does not appear to be the same process as pathological dissociation.

Nonetheless, data do support the belief that children are more dissociative than adults and that dissociation declines with age. Research with the Child Dissociative Checklist (CDC), which is presented in Appendix Two and discussed further in Chapter Twelve, found modest declines in dissociation with age in normal and maltreated children (Putnam et al., 1993; Putnam, 1996a). The rate of decline in CDC scores with age varied across groups. For the normal children the overall decline with age was small, in part because this group had very low scores to begin with. Incestuously abused girls showed a much steeper decline in CDC scores with age. (Putnam et al., 1993). Children diagnosed with DDNOS also showed a significant decline in CDC scores with age, but children with MPD did not. In part this was because the MPD children were more symptomatic and were significantly older than those with DDNOS (Hornstein and Putnam, 1992; Putnam et al., 1993; Coons, 1996). To summarize, research with the CDC indicates that dissociation is higher on average in younger children (ages 5–6 years), and that it declines with age for many (but not all) traumatized and nontraumatized children.

A meta-analysis of 14 DES studies has demonstrated a modest, but statistically significant, decline in scores with age (van IJzendoorn and Schuengel, 1996). The gradual decline in DES scores continues until the seventh decade of life, beyond which the data are too sparse (Ross et al.,

1989e). Similar decreases in age have been noted with other dissociation scales.

Thus we have evidence that dissociation scale scores decline with age for different age groups. It is difficult to establish definitively that children are more dissociative than adults, because different scales are required to cover the vast span of ages/developmental stages. To date, the DES is the only dissociation scale that has been used with both adults and juveniles as young as 11 or 12 years. If taken at face value, these data show significantly higher scores for younger ages (Ross, Ryan, Voigt, and Eide, 1989g). However, the DES is an adult measure, and there are reservations about its validity for children and early adolescents (Carlson and Putnam, 1993). At present, there are no data from a common measure across all age groups, which would be necessary to demonstrate convincingly that dissociation scores decline with age. However, within each group for which validated measures are available, there is a reliable (although often not statistically significant) decline in dissociation scores with increasing age.

A comparison of child and adult symptoms and behaviors that are considered dissociative provides another gauge of the changes in dissociative behavior with age. Although child dissociation scales assess the same general domains of amnesia, dissociative behaviors, and identity alterations as adult instruments, they also inquire about phenomena that would be considered absolutely pathognomonic of psychopathology in adults such as imaginary companions (ICs). In adults—Harvey, the 6-foot invisible rabbit, notwithstanding—the presence of ICs is considered pathological and even psychotic. In contrast, Ics are present in 30–60% of normal children, and are sometimes taken as signs of intelligence and creativity. (See the discussion later in this chapter.)

Gender

A meta-analysis of 19 DES studies ($n = 4,074$) found no gender differences in DES scores (van IJzendoorn and Schuengel, 1996). However, there are large gender effects for the diagnosis of dissociative disorders. That is, there are typically six to nine times more females than males in adult samples (e.g., Putnam et al., 1986; Coons et al., 1988; Ross et al., 1991). Analysis of a large juvenile sample ($n = 177$) divided into four age groups (preschoolers, school age, early adolescence, and late adolescence) found a steady increase in the percentage of female dissociative disorder cases with age (Putnam, Hornstein, & Peterson, 1996). (See further discussion in Chapter Twelve.)

The reasons for this gender effect in diagnosed cases are not well understood. Various hypotheses have been offered (Loewenstein and Putnam, 1990). These include (1) speculation that male MPD cases are not seen in the mental health system because their antisocial behaviors lead them into the criminal justice system; (2) arguments that there are quantitative and qualitative differences in the maltreatment experiences of males and females (e.g., girls have longer average durations of sexual abuse, and the primary perpetrators are more often immediate family members); and (3) the possibility that male dissociative presentations are more subtle, and that clinicians have a lower index of suspicion for males.

Genetic Factors

Genetic factors are given weight in some versions of the autohypnotic model (e.g., Kluft, 1986). However, research to date suggests that they probably do not contribute much to the development of pathological dissociation, but this remains to be determined. Twin research studies under way should help to clarify this issue. In California, Niels Waller is using the A-DES (see Appendix Three) to examine genetic and familial factors in teenage twins. The famous "twins reared apart" project at the University of Minnesota has also included the DES in its test battery.

Cultural Factors

Cultural factors undoubtedly play an important role in the expression of pathological dissociation. This is illustrated by the plethora of culture-specific dissociative reactions included under the DSM category of DDNOS (American Psychiatric Association, 1994). However, core components of pathological dissociation—as measured by the DES in translation—appear to be remarkably similar across different cultures (e.g., see Ensink and van Otterloo, 1989; Carlson and Rosser-Hogan, 1991; Boon and Draijer, 1993; Draijer and Boon, 1993; Berger, Onon, Nakajima, and Suematsu, 1994; Park et al., 1995).

When ethnic or racial differences are found, they often appear to reflect demographic and life experience differences (Carlson and Putnam, 1993; van IJzendoorn and Schuengel, 1996). For example, initial differences in DES scores among African-American, Hispanic-American, and European-American combat veterans disappeared when level of combat exposure was controlled for (Zatzick, Marmar, Weiss, and Metzler, 1994).

Education and Intelligence

Despite the widespread belief that MPD is a "creative defense" available only to highly intelligent, imaginative people, several studies find no significant deviations from normal IQ ranges in dissociative patients (e.g., Coons et al., 1988; Hornstein and Putnam, 1992; Rossini, Schwartz, and Braun, 1996). Nor, with one exception, have DES scores been found to have significant correlations with education or IQ (van IJzendoorn and Schuengel, 1996). Dunn, Paolo, Ryan, and Fleet (1993) did find a small negative correlation with education level. It has been noted that some items on the DES require a high school reading level (Paolo, Ryan, Dunn, and Fleet, 1993). Further research is required, but IQ and education (within limits) probably do not affect intrinsic dissociative capacity—although they may confound attempts to quantitate it.

Family Environment

There are few systematic data on how family environmental factors influence children's dissociative capacity. Much of what we "know" is generalized from clinical impressions and therefore limited. Opportunities for research on this topic have been opened by the validation of dissociation measures for different age groups.

Scattered through the clinical literature are impressions that dissociative patients' families of origin are pathological in a number of ways. Inconsistent parenting, typically defined as erratic reinforcement and punishment of the same behavior, has been noted (e.g., Kluft, 1984a; Braun and Sachs, 1985; Mann and Sanders, 1994; see also Chapter Fifteen). Mann and Sanders (1994) reported modest correlations between a measure of inconsistent discipline and parental dissociation scores. Nash et al. (1993) found that when a measure of family environment was used as a covariate, it explained much of the differences in dissociation scores between abused and comparison women. Alexander and Schaeffer (1994) clustered adult child abuse victims on variables of abuse characteristics and family environment. They found that individuals with pathological dissociation all belonged to the same cluster, characterized by severe abuse, conflicted and controlling families, and extremely violent parents.

In addition to finding inconsistent parenting and discipline, clinicians have characterized dissociative families as authoritarian, patriarchal, and religiously fundamental (e.g., Kluft, 1984a; Braun and Sachs, 1985; Spiegel, 1986; Mann and Sanders, 1994). To a large extent, these characterizations overlap with features attributed to maltreating families in general. Although there is truth to these generalizations, the magnitude of the contribution by parental characteristics and family environment to dissociation, both pathological and normal, remains to be systematically determined.

The role of pathological dissociation in the transgenerational transmission of child maltreatment has been a subject of speculation among clinicians for some time (e.g., Brown, 1983). In a unique study, Egland and Susman-Stillman (1996) investigated the contribution of parental dissociation to maltreatment. Egeland and colleagues are conducting a prospective longitudinal study of families at risk for child maltreatment. Mothers with histories of childhood maltreatment who maltreated their children were compared with mothers with similar maltreatment histories who were not maltreating and were providing adequate care. The maltreating mothers had DES scores more than twice as high as those of the nonmaltreating mothers. They also manifested more dissociation during interviews, as scored by raters who were unaware of the maltreating status of the mothers. Interestingly, those mothers who were maltreated themselves, but did not maltreat their children, were much more likely to have had treatment and to be able to discuss their own childhoods.

FACTORS INFLUENCING DISSOCIATIVE CAPACITY: MODEL-BASED PREDICTIONS

Age

According to the DBS model (see Chapter Eight), behavioral and cognitive maturation (i.e., growing up) are reflected in the addition of new discrete behavioral states; in refinement or replacement of developmentally earlier states; in the creation of new connections and behavioral pathways; and in increases in metacognitive inputs to self-modulation of states. New states add to the growing child's behavioral repertoire and facilitate encoding of new responses to an ever-enlarging world of experiences. Refinement and replacement of older states (e.g., feeding-related states) reflect maturing behavioral patterns evoked in response to basic needs and recurrent contexts. New connections increase behavioral flexibility, permitting more environmentally responsive shifts in behavior. Expansion of metacognitive functions increases volitional self-control.

The growing child's behavior becomes smoother and better modulated. The child acquires increasing control over emotions, attention, and behavior. There is corresponding increase in a sense of autonomy and differentiation of self. At older ages, self-observation and introspection further enhance these processes. The child is more resistant to and better able to recover from disruptions of behavioral state. Indeed, these state-related capacities are the essence of cognitive maturation. Their absence or loss (e.g., in cases of mental retardation, head injury, or senility) is viewed as "childlike." Growing cognitive capacities facilitate the creation of highly refined behavioral states, such as those associated with artistic performance.

Gender

Gender influences behavioral states through cultural and biological effects. In many cultures there are gender-specific experiences that produce unique behavioral states (e.g, coming-of-age rituals). Gender-specific biological effects (e.g., premenstrual tension) and experiences (e.g., pregnancy) also produce discrete states of consciousness not readily available to the opposite sex. The DBS model predicts that gender would interact directly (biological effects) and indirectly (cultural effects) to produce discrete behavioral states that would be largely restricted to one or the other gender. For example, psychophysiological states associated with bulimia are largely confined to females in our culture. An exception sometimes occurs for males involved in activities such as wrestling, where great emphasis is placed on meeting a specific body weight limitation prior to a match.

Genetic Factors

An individual's genetic predisposition undoubtedly influences the range and types of behavioral states that can potentially be experienced. Biologically heightened responses to certain substances may increase susceptibility to addictive behaviors (see the discussion of addiction in Chapter Ten). Extraordinary physical or artistic abilities may facilitate entry into performance-related mental states not available to most. In the DBS model, genetic predisposition defines the boundaries of behavioral state space available to an individual.

Cultural Factors

Culturally shared and sanctioned behavioral states are integral components of culture itself. From a Japanese tea ceremony to a Spanish bullfight, shared group experiences produce common states of consciousness that give each culture its special flavor. Basic affective states are universal, but each culture adds an overlay in the form of specific mental states and their nuances of expression. The DBS model predicts that there should be culturally unique affective, anxiety, and dissociative psychopathological states. Indeed, we find culture-specific "dissociative states" such as *ataque de nervios* in Hispanic cultures and *amok* in Southeast Asia.

Education and Intelligence

Together with heredity, education and intelligence open up possibilities or set limits on potential behavioral states. For example, absorptive states of imaginative involvement associated with reading poetry or rousing fiction are not accessible to the illiterate. The DBS model predicts that individuals differing greatly in intelligence and/or education probably differ in their use of detailed fantasy states as an escape from an overwhelming situation.

Family Environment

The DBS model suggests that children from families in which one or both parents undergo recurrent dramatic shifts in states of consciousness will exhibit deviations in their own modulation of behavioral states. Such a situation may arise in the context of a parental substance abuse problem, rapid-cycling bipolar illness, or dissociative disorder. Children in such situations must learn to cope with rapidly shifting and fundamentally different parental behavioral states. These extreme parental states are characterized by marked differences in parents' sense of self, relationship to their children, responsiveness to a given stimulus, and access to autobiographical memory (e.g., family history, myths, and coping styles).

Extreme, state-dependent parental behaviors can be expected to affect children in several ways. First, the powerful identification/introjection/imitation processes through which children incorporate aspects of parental behavior into their own behavioral repertoires are confounded by contradictory and contextually different versions of their parents. Using parental mood state as a salient cue, some children make remarkable sense out of their parents' radically different behavior. Other children, particularly younger ones, assign dramatic parental state-dependent differences to different, unintegrated percepts of their parents. Clinical experience suggests that these different parental variants are highly compartmentalized, particularly with respect to emotional issues. In addition, the discontinuous, unintegrated, and often self-contradictory behavioral style of such a parent may become a major working model for a child's own response to the world.

Second, a parent's radically different parental personae—be they intoxicated, depressed, manic, or dissociative—may stimulate the creation of complementary behavioral states in a child. Although this has not been systematically documented, experienced clinicians have encountered mutually complementary alter personalities/behavioral states in MPD parents and their children. That is, when an MPD parent and child are seen together in family sessions, the child will behave in highly specific ways in the presence of certain parental alter personality states. In cases in which both parent and child have MPD, specific parental alter personalities evoke the emergence of complementary child alters. For example, Kluft (1984a) describes observing a child switch personality states in response to a personality switch in the mother. I have witnessed similar examples and have frequently heard MPD patients relate seeing this happen with their children. It is likely that a similar phenomenon occurs in children of substance-abusing parents, who come to adopt different behavioral styles depending on whether the parents are intoxicated or sober.

Third, rapid and dramatic shifts in parental behavioral states produce inconsistent parenting and erratic reward and disciplinary behavior. For example, strong state dependency in accessibility of autobiographical memory may seriously impede the rule-making, precedent-generating, limit-setting, and privilege-negotiating processes that continually occur between parents and children. Dissociative parents have difficulty recalling the history of interactions centering around a particular parent–child issue. Consequently, their responses may be highly situation-dependent over time; this produces inconsistent and contradictory behavior. (See the discussion of family therapy in Chapter Fifteen.)

Inconsistent parenting also implies that parents are unable to integrate and contextualize children's experiences. Parents are supposed to share their larger perspective on life with their developing children, and to impart this perspective to the children in an appropriate fashion. One important aspect of this is to place specific experiences in context for the children. There are many kinds of contexts that can be brought to bear on a given experience, and parents must suggest and integrate among these as necessary.

Time is an example of what I mean by "context." Young children have limited capacities to conceptualize the flow of time; they also have difficulty chronologically organizing earlier memories. Parents help children to connect past experiences with present and future events and their consequences. They also help to contextualize fragmentary memories reported by the children within the larger family history ("Oh, that happened when you were 3 years old and we were living on Elm Street").

Adults with dissociative disorders have significant difficulties with such chronological tasks (Putnam, 1989a). It is predicted that these deficits will carry over to their parenting behaviors. We know little about the consequences of parental deficiencies in "contextualizing" experience and memory for children. However, I would suggest that extensive deficits in this area contribute to dissociative behaviors in children—in part through failure to help the children integrate their own autobiographical versions of self, and in part through failure to nurture the children's integrative capacities.

Stereotypic repetition is another important process for young children. For example, they demand that a story be read over and over again in *exactly* the same way ("No, Daddy, make the little pig say it in a squeaky voice"). Young children prefer familiar books, videos, and games to novel ones. Repetition serves many purposes, one of which is to help children integrate an important experience (such as a favorite story) across time, contexts, and behavioral states. The constancy of the repeated experience bridges the discontinuities of life for younger children. Dissociative parents are likely to have serious difficulties in providing the constancy of experience that young children seek. If a parent's state (e.g., alter personality, substance-induced state, mood state) impedes access to previous "performances" of the book or game, or simply is incompatible with the demands of the situation, a child is denied an important source of stability.

RESEARCH ON THE RELATION OF NORMAL DEVELOPMENTAL PROCESSES TO DISSOCIATION

Attachment

The earliest expressions of inconsistent parenting occur in a parent's different responses to the primary behavioral states and basic needs of an infant. This will disrupt attachment behaviors. As mentioned in Chapter Two, Bowlby's (1982) theory regards attachment behaviors as an evolutionary mechanism to increase the proximity of the infant to the primary caretaker, and thereby to increase the chances of the infant's survival. Attachment theory has proven to be of enormous value in understanding the sequelae and intergenerational manifestations of maltreatment (Cicchetti, 1989). Attachment theory has been applied to dissociative disorders by several investigators. Barach (1991) conceptualizes some clinical features of MPD as attachment responses. He equates dissociation with Bowlby's (1973) observations of "profound detachment" in children who lose their primary caretaker. Barach speculates that the loss or unresponsiveness of the primary caretaker may create a detached/dissociative state in maltreated children. Irwin (1994) has shown that, independent of maltreatment history, familial loss in childhood is associated with increased DES scores in adults.

Liotti (1992) extends Barach's theory by suggesting that a specific type of attachment behavior/disorder, Type D, increases vulnerability to developing a dissociative disorder. Type D behaviors, first described by

Main and Solomon (1986), are characterized by disorganized and conflicting movement patterns, contradictions in intention, lack of orientation to the environment, and periods of sudden immobility associated with a dazed expression or trance-like state. Up to 80% of maltreated infants and toddlers show type D attachment behavior (Cicchetti and Nurcombe, 1994). Liotti (1992) outlines three theoretical pathways through which type D attachment behaviors could contribute to the development of MPD. Main and Hesse (1996) have presented and published data indicating that a high DES score in the mother predicts type D attachment behaviors in her infant. Other researchers are beginning to focus on attachment in children and adults. The interest of attachment researchers in dissociative phenomena is stimulating a new and exciting area of developmental research.

Fantasy and Imagination

Fantasy play is increasingly being appreciated as a developmental arena of extraordinary complexity and subtlety. A comprehensive review is beyond the scope of this book. However, research on the development, nature, and functions of fantasy play is pertinent to informed clinical judgments about the presence or absence of dissociative psychopathology.

Fantasy play is a constantly changing process, delicately flitting back and forth between reality and nonreality. Bretherton (1989) observes that the creation of "subjunctive" or "would-be" realities through fantasy play blossoms during the preschool years, reflecting an increasing acquisition of symbolic functioning. Make-believe play requires (1) the ability to manage multiple roles or perspectives on self and situation; (2) the capacity to alter reality playfully through counterfactual thinking; and (3) the ability to play with the play frame itself (Bretherton, 1989). These are evolving metacognitive capacities, thought to follow a roughly predictable sequence in normal children.

Piaget's theory that the occurrence of pretend play follows an inverted-U-shaped function, peaking at about age 6 years, has received little scientific support (Fein, 1981). Instead, it is clear that there are important individual differences associated with such factors as innate fantasy predisposition, support of fantasy play by a significant adult, gender, social class, and family environmental factors. Studies suggest that children who watch a great deal of television have impoverished fantasy play (Fein, 1981).

Researchers often focus on a child's management of reality and nonreality as a crucial task for successful make-believe play (e.g., Fein, 1981; DiLalla and Watson, 1988; Bretherton, 1989; Harris et al., 1991). Fantasy–reality boundary management is hypothesized to develop in a stepwise fashion from "no boundary" to a "fuzzy boundary," which means that the child recognizes some differences but has poor control over the boundary. The next step is the development of a "rigid boundary," which means that the child acquires volitional control over shifts back and forth between fantasy and reality. The final step is the development of an "integrated boundary," meaning that the child can easily differentiate, control, and integrate fantasy and reality realms (DiLalla and Watson, 1988). This probably reflects the development of specific metacognitive capacities. As in many cognitive areas, girls appear to acquire these capacities earlier than boys.

Researchers are discovering the incredible complexity of children's fantasy. Make-believe is no simple thing. One pertinent aspect is the child's management of multiple roles of self and others. Adopting the language of the theater, developmental psychologists identify roles such as actor, playwright, director, and narrator (e.g., Bretherton, 1989; Wolf, 1990). The management of these roles, particularly in the context of shared pretend play, is both extraordinarily subtle and very sophisticated. Children usually signal role shifts to playmates by changes in voice. Although children playing together almost never miss a cue, researchers have failed to grasp the nature of these role switches until recently (Bretherton, 1989). Roles often reflect status among children.

The functions of pretend play are many and deeply interwoven. Increased predisposition to use fantasy is associated with cooperation, social competence, and peer acceptance (Bretherton, 1989). Fantasy play is an important arena for the mastery of emotion and the transformation of self-perspectives. The child's success in slaying make-believe dragons contributes toward mastery of anxiety provoked by real-life tasks. Fantasy also provides an important domain in which unpleasant aspects of reality can be "fixed" and painful affects can be safely and privately discharged.

Imaginary Companions

In my earlier book, I note that the relationship between ICs and MPD is tantalizing but ambiguous (Putnam, 1989a, p. 52). Many have speculated that the alter personality states of MPD patients evolve from ICs defensively elaborated by traumatized children (e.g., Bliss, 1983; Lovinger, 1983; Putnam, 1985b; McElroy, 1992; Sanders, 1992).

IC-like phenomena are frequently reported in child and adolescent dissociative disorders. For example, Peterson's (1991) review found ICs mentioned in 42% of case reports on children and adolescents with dissociative disorders. Our questionnaire study (Peterson and Putnam, 1994) found ICs in 56% of a sample of patients with dissociative disorders, including 71% of MPD cases. When systematic questions about ICs were included in the diagnostic evaluation, we (Hornstein and Putnam, 1992) found the 84% of child and adolescent dissociative cases had histories of vivid ICs.

In the most direct study to date, Trujillo, Lewis, Yeager, and Gidlow (1996) compared IC phenomena in 23 normal boys (aged 10–11 years) and 23 emotionally disturbed boys in a residential treatment center. In the latter group, 22 boys had been removed from their homes because of maltreatment, and 7 were diagnosed with MPD by semistructured interview. There were 7 boys with IC's (30%) in the normal sample, and 13 (57%) in the treatment group.

The prevalence rates of ICs reported in samples of children with dissociative disorders are at the upper ranges reported for normal children. Although plausible, the relatively high rates of ICs in DD patients do not constitute proof of an etiological relationship between ICs and MPD alter personalities. A substantial percentage (33–66%) of normal children between the ages of 3 and 10 years have ICs, with higher rates reported for girls than for boys (Svendson, 1934; Manosevitz, Fling, and Prentice, 1977). If ICs were integral to the development of alter personality states in MPD, we would expect to see them in close to 100% of juvenile MPD cases.

Studies indicate that virtually all normal children can distinguish the nonreality of their ICs (Taylor, Cartwright, and Carlson, 1991). Experimenter suggestion studies indicate that children with ICs tend to have greater fantasy capacities than those without ICs. In the laboratory, children with ICs are more willing or able to participate in pretend games and to use an imaginary tool instead of a real object to perform a pretend task, such as brushing their teeth (Taylor et al., 1991). Speculations that the presence of an IC is associated with higher intelligence, greater creativity, or increased ability to wait have not been substantiated by developmental researchers (Manosevitz et al., 1977).

We do have data suggesting that the ICs of MPD patients differ in certain ways from normal ICs. Sanders (1992) studied the frequency and characteristics of ICs retrospectively reported by adult MPD patients, and compared them with data from college students. Sixty-four percent of the MPD subjects reported having one or more ICs between the ages of 2 and 13 years. The most striking difference lay in the vividness of the IC experiences: Virtually all of the MPD patients reported seeing and hearing their ICs and frequently believing that the ICs were real entities. Significantly fewer (25%) of college students with ICs reported a similar degree of vividness.

Although partially retrospective, the Trujillo et al. (1996) study provides our best comparative look at the differences between ICs in normal and dissociative children. More traumatized children had ICs, but this difference was not statistically significant. The normal boys with ICs averaged 2.5 entities each, while the MPD boys with ICs averaged 6.4 entities each ($p = .01$). More important clinically were the qualitative differences between the ICs of the two groups. The ICs of the normal boys were benign and benevolent, and could be called forth volitionally. They had cute names such as "Thumper" and "Boom-Boom." Normal boys reported that their ICs helped them with difficult feelings (e.g., loneliness) and served as playmates. ICs first appeared between the ages of 2 and 4 years, and had all disappeared by age 8.

Most of the ICs reported by the MPD boys were similar to—if not identical with—alter personalities (Trujillo et al., 1996). With names like "Strong Jamie," "Superman," "Rattlesnake," "Guardian Angel," "God," and "Devil," these ICs served somewhat different functions for the MPD boys. They acted as (1) helpers/comforters/playmates, (2) powerful protectors, and (3) family members. A substantial percentage served as protectors that were activated when the boys were frightened or threatened. In a number of cases, protector ICs were behaviorally associated with fighting and aggression. One surprising findings was that six out of the seven MPD boys had an IC that was based on a family member. Family member ICs played a range of roles, from protectors to abusers.

In contrast to the normal boys, the MPD boys were not able to date the first emergence of their ICs. The ICs of the MPD boys were still present at the time of the study (mean age = 10.6 years). Definitively determining whether ICs form the basis for the alter personality states of MPD is not an easy problem, but the results reported by Trujillo et al. (1996) support this possibility.

Evaluation of the existence and nature of ICs should be an integral part of the evaluation of a child or adolescent for dissociative disorders. The degree of Ics' vividness and believability, particularly for older children, constitutes an important clinical feature for distinguishing normal IC phenomena from pathological dissociation. The degree to which a child feels controlled by ICs is another. Trujillo et al. (1996) make a crucial point when they note that children who report conversations with "God" or the "Devil" should not be dismissed as merely expressing religious beliefs. Such statements should alert a clinician to explore for possible hallucinatory and possessiform phenomena associated with pathological dissociation. If ICs in traumatized children represent embryonic alter personalities, therapeutic interventions directed toward their internalization and integration are called for.

Elaborated Play Identities

Closely related to ICs are what I call "elaborated play identities." A normal child sometimes develops an elaborated play identity that may persist for several years. This alter identity—often with magical powers or special abilities—is primarily adopted in specific play situations. When the child assumes the identity, he or she often takes on a specific way of speaking, behaving, and interacting. In normal identity states, the child may refer to the elaborated play identity as another person.

FRED AND "MAGIC CAT"

Between the ages of 3 and 7, Fred, a normal, highly imaginative child, would often assume the elaborated play identity of "Magic Cat"—a sort of supercat with magical powers who chased "bad guys" and righted wrongs. As "Magic Cat," Fred was hyperactive; spoke (as well as meowed, purred, and growled) in a rapid, high-pitched voice; could be silly and regressed; and ran around chasing imaginary bad guys in a semiorganized frenzy. In nursery school and kindergarten, Fred sometimes enticed his schoolmates into playing "Magic Cat" games, which he scripted and directed. At home, he played "Magic Cat" by himself or with his younger brother.

Fred also identified a specific Lego figure who was "Magic Cat." He built Lego houses, boats, airplanes, and other things for this figure, and played out cops-and-robbers themes in which "Magic Cat" prevailed. At times, Fred spoke of "Magic Cat" as if he/it were an actual individual. Occasionally, when stressed, Fred would assume his "Magic Cat" identity in a nonplay situation—much to the annoyance of his parents. Fred would also assume "Magic Cat" at times when he wanted to be physically affectionate with his parents or peers. He would rub himself against the other person in a cat-like manner, "purring" and pawing. As Fred grew older, he assumed the "Magic Cat" identity and played "Magic Cat" Lego games less and less.

Fred was always comfortable and largely in control of "Magic Cat," although his parents would have to intervene to disrupt the state when he was being obnoxious. "Magic Cat" was his imaginary friend/alter identity. Fred never reported that "Magic Cat" controlled him, or blamed "Magic Cat" for his misbehavior. "Magic Cat" was a fluid identity that he could either assume directly or displace into the Lego figure. In general, "Magic Cat" was a moral figure who protected the weak and vanquished the bad. Magical powers made "Magic Cat" invulnerable to danger; this seemed important to Fred, who was at heart a cautious child.

An elaborated play identity can look and sound similar to an MPD alter personality state, in that it is a relatively enduring identity that a child repeatedly assumes in specific contexts. Such identities may well overlap in some domains with childhood MPD alter personality states. However, elaborated play identities and ICs are normal phenomena and must be differentiated from pathological alter personality states. The critical difference seems to lie in (1) the playful nature of an IC or elaborated identity, and (2) the fact that it never comes to control a child's behavior, to intimidate or frighten the child, or to endanger the child by "forcing" him or her into risky behavior. (Compare "Magic Cat" with "Marcie, the boy dog" in Chapter Eleven.)

Elaborated Daydreams

Leslie (1988) makes the interesting metaobservation that descriptions of pretense are best understood in terms of reports of a mental state. Fantasy productions occur in and can come to define unique mental states for an individual. This is particularly true in the case of what I call "elaborated daydreams." Elaborated daydreams are fantasy productions that are repeatedly invoked and embellished by an individual over time. Such a daydream has a more or less continuous story line, enriched by a history of prior fantasy episodes. The individual volitionally summons up the daydream, often in specific contexts (e.g., boredom, masturbation), and continues to elaborate the story or revisits prior episodes. Elaborated fantasies may run for years and can come to represent a significant portion of an individual's mental life. Although this is a fascinating area of inquiry, I am unaware of a body of research on long-running fantasy.

Like ICs, elaborated daydreams are normal phenomena present in a substantial percentage of the population. Defining when this daydreaming process becomes pathologically dissociative is difficult. My own and others' clinical experience suggests that evaluation of several dimensions is helpful in determining whether an individual's elaborated fantasy life exceeds normal parameters. These dimensions include vividness, maintenance of reality–nonreality boundaries, degree of volition or intrusiveness, control over the direction of the fantasy, and the intensity of the wish/drive to act out the fantasy. Other relevant elements include abnormal content (although this can be difficult to judge) and the pairing of deviant fantasies with powerful reinforcers (e.g., orgasm or drug states).

Context is also a critical issue. All-consuming, elaborated daydreams are frequent in captives and represent an adaptation to continuous physical confinement and threats to life. Poignant examples of carefully nurtured daydreams can be found in accounts by hostages and Vietnam POWs. For example, among the U.S. and British hostages held in Lebanon in the late 1980s and early 1990s, Reed constructed buildings in Islesboro, Maine. Cicippio designed his dream home brick by brick. Polhill taught himself to play 37 instruments and conducted mental band concerts. Anderson, held captive the longest, took elaborate step-by-step walking tours of Tokyo in his mind (Boustany and Priest,

1992). In such situations, incredible obsession with detail seems to be an important factor—perhaps because it recruits more cognitive resources and contributes to the vividness of the fantasized experience. The content of the fantasy is, however, reality-oriented (e.g., building a house, playing an instrument).

Dissociative children often have secret places in their minds where they go when overwhelmed. These magical places often have evocative names (e.g., "the jewel garden," "toyland," "my island"). Typically they are zones of vivid, experiential fantasy without strong reality constraints. When a dissociative child enters into one of these fantasy states, observers note that the child has behaviorally "shut down" and assumed a vacant, trance-like stare. The child may curl up in a fetal position or rhythmically self-soothe by rocking, stroking, or bumping. These kinds of behaviors, which are sometimes misinterpreted as psychotic or autistic, can often be associated with specific triggers or events in the child's life.

Does Fantasy Influence Behavior?

Does the nature and degree of an individual's fantasies influence his or her behavior? I suspect that it does, although few empirical studies have examined this question. Prentky et al. (1989) compared the fantasy content of serial sexual murderers (three or more victims) with single-victim sexual murderers. They found that violent fantasy was present in 86% of the serial murderers, compared with 23% of the single-victim murderers. Serial sexual murderers also had more intrusive fantasies, with a higher prevalence of paraphilia. An analysis of the degree of disorganization of the crime scene indicated that serial murderers were significantly better organized than single-victim murderers. The authors speculated that this organization might reflect better planning—perhaps through fantasy rehearsal.

Briere, Smiljanich, and Henschel (1994) examined the impact of sexual molestation on the sexual fantasies of college students. In addition to gender effects noted in previous research (males had more fantasies of forcing intercourse, participating in orgies, and having sex with strangers), they found that women with histories of sexual abuse had significantly more fantasies of being sexually forced than did either nonabused women or men with or without an abuse history. Earlier onset of abuse was correlated with fantasies of being forced into sex. Duration of abuse was correlated with fantasies of participating in sexual orgies. Clinically, a number of therapists have commented on the prevalence of rape and bondage fantasies in sexual abuse victims. Determining whether such fantasies directly influence sexual behavior is complicated, especially since some people fantasize about what they have already done, rather than doing what they have first fantasized about.

Fantasy Proneness and Pathological Dissociation

A final line of evidence connecting extreme forms of fantasy with pathological dissociation is the research on "fantasy proneness." First described by Wilson and Barber (1983), fantasy proneness characterizes individuals who "live much of the time in a world of their own making—in a world of imagery, imagination and fantasy" (p. 133). Several studies link fantasy proneness with pathological dissociation (Lynn, Rhue, and Green, 1988). Measures of fantasy proneness are moderately to strongly correlated with measures of dissociation (Putnam and Carlson, in press). Fantasy proneness is also significantly associated with histories of maltreatment (Lynn et al., 1988). Further research is necessary to firmly establish the degree of correspondence between fantasy proneness and pathological dissociation, but this appears to be a fruitful linkage.

SUMMARY

Beyond the role of trauma in the etiology of pathological dissociation, little is known about the influence of other factors. Increasing age—which probably serves as a proxy for maturational cognitive changes—is associated with a decline in dissociation scores with time. Age-related declines in dissociation scores have been found in studies using child, adolescent, and adult scales. None of these scales, however, validly measures dissociation over the entire life span. Thus the developmental course and overall magnitude of this decline have not been precisely established.

Studies within a given population (e.g., patients with BPD or MPD) do not find evidence of gender differences in dissociation scores. However, there are usually many more females than males in dissociative disorder samples (typically six to nine female patients for every male). Preliminary data suggest that genetic contributions to pathological dissociation are minimal. Ethnic and cultural differences undoubtedly influence clinical presentations and confound measurement; nonetheless, core dissociative features are found in common across widely divergent cultures.

Current research indicates that family environmental factors make important contributions above and beyond maltreatment experiences. Preliminary studies suggest significant correlations between dissociation in parents and in children, although many relevant factors have not been controlled for as yet (e.g., sibship and birth order). Exciting work by Egeland and colleagues has identified a role for pathological dissociation in the transgenerational (vertical) transmission of maltreating behaviors—a possibility long suspected by clinicians.

The DBS model predicts that parent—child interactions have powerful effects on the development of pathological dissociation, both together with and independent of maltreatment. Pathological dissociation in parents confronts children with radically different percepts of the parents to introject and to interact with. Clinical experience suggests that children create complementary behavioral states that embody attributes and behaviors reciprocally adaptive to the parental behavioral states. Erratic dissociative or affective state changes significantly impair parental inputs, such as providing consistency over time and contextualizing children's experience. These parenting dysfunctions are hypothesized to have an impact on the child's metacognitive integrative functioning, impairing the developmental consolidation of self and behavior.

Research has begun to relate aspects of several normal developmental processes, such as attachment and fantasy/imagination, to dissociative developmental trajectories. In toddlers, a specific type of attachment disturbance, type D, is associated with increased dissociation in their mothers. The presence of ICs, a normal phenomenon in preschoolers, has features in common with the presence of MPD alter personality states in children. It is widely hypothesized that ICs provide a developmental kernel upon which pathological dissociative states are elaborated in traumatic contexts. Child alter personalities in MPD cases can be qualitatively differentiated from normal ICs on dimensions of vividness, volition, and benignness. Elaborated play identities and daydreams are also normal phenomena, becoming pathological in certain contexts when they interfere with functioning and distort reality testing.

Chapter Ten

Dissociative and Altered States in Everyday Life

If discrete states of consciousness form a basic building block of mental life and personality, then examples from everyday life should be readily available. This chapter examines several common domains of mental life from the perspective of the DBS model. The intention is to provide examples that the reader can compare with his or her own experiences. The examples chosen include religion, a powerful force in the lives of many people; drug-altered states of consciousness, many of which constitute major social, medical, and criminal problems; television watching, the most common activity (besides sleeping) for youths; and sex and athletics, two major mental preoccupations (at least for males).

ARE ALL ALTERED STATES OF CONSCIOUSNESS DISSOCIATIVE?

Before I plunge on into religion, drugs, sex, and so on, it is worth considering whether or not all altered states of consciousness are "dissociative." Altered (or "alternative," after the fashion of Zinberg, 1977) states of consciousness are often loosely equated with dissociative states of consciousness. However, if we define dissociative states more narrowly as those altered states of consciousness that are widely separated from more normal states on dimensions of autobiographical memory retrieval and fundamental aspects of identity integration, then it is clear that many altered states of consciousness are not dissociative per se. For example, an individual may be deeply changed by a religious conversion, but he or she retains a basic sense of continuity of identity through the experience.

Dissociative states of consciousness share many state-related properties with each other and with strong affective states. Similarly, dissociative states may overlap on some dimensions with hypnotic states, but this should not be construed as their being one and the *same* states. On other dimensions, there may be very little overlap—as shown, for example, by the physiological differences between MPD patients and hypnotized controls in our EDA study (Putnam et al., 1990). Mapping these differences is one of the tasks of the scientific study of discrete states of consciousness (Tart, 1972).

RELIGION

I make no claims to expertise in the study of religion. Nonetheless, I believe that religion is a fertile ground for the expression of altered and dissociative states of consciousness in everyday life. My way out of this dilemma is to hold tightly onto the coattails of a great scholar, William James.

One of the most famous psychologists of all time, James delivered a series of lectures at Edinburgh University in Scotland during the 1901–1902 term. These lectures, published in book form as *The Varieties of Religious Experience: A Study in Human Nature*, have become a classic text for psychology, philosophy, and religious studies (James, 1902/1958). Approaching religion from the twin perspectives of philosophy and experimental psychology, James addressed the variety and meaning of a range of religious experiences. He did so in the conceptual language of states of mind. One of the fathers of the DBS model, James stressed the dissociative nature of many religious experiences.

Religious Genius

In his first lecture, James (1902/1958) quickly drew a distinction between "second-hand" religion, practiced by the masses, and religious "genius," which serves as the fount for faith and inspiration. He dismissed second-hand religion as uninteresting because the practitioner is following a faith "made for him by others, communicated to him by tradition, determined to fixed forms by imitation and retained by habit" (p. 24). James was interested in religious genius as exhibited by the saints and the mystics, whose revelationary experiences have sparked new religions and transformed old ones.

From agony to ecstasy, religious genius is manifested in altered states of consciousness. In an understated foreshadowing of his subsequent lectures, James ventured: "There is no doubt that a religious life, exclusively pursued, tends to make the person exceptional and eccentric" (1902/1958, p. 24). However, James abhored reductionism, which he called "medical materialism," and actively refuted the argument that religious experience is merely physiology or psychopathology run amok. He believed that the meaning of religious experience is separable from the biological processes underlying it.

The Divided Mind

James focused his attention on the characteristics of the mental states that collectively constitute religious genius. Central to the religious character is the "divided mind," manifested by "a certain discordancy or heterogeneity in the native temperament of the subject, an incompletely unified moral and intellectual constitution" (1902/1958, p. 141). Acknowledging that a certain amount of dividedness is normal, James observed that "a stronger degree of heterogeneity may make havoc of the subject's life. There are persons whose existence is little more than a series of zigzags, as now one tendency and now another gets the upper hand" (p. 142). The manifestations of a divided mind include a number of phenomena universally recognized as dissociative; among these are automatisms (see Chapter Four). James bluntly stated:

> You will in point of fact hardly find a religious leader of any kind in whose life there is no record of automatisms. I speak not merely of savage priests and prophets, . . . [but] of leaders of thought and subjects of intellectualized experience. . . . The whole array of Christian saints . . . had their visions, voices, rapt conditions, guiding impressions and "openings." (p. 362)

Related to automatisms are experiences of "a sense of presence," in which the individual vividly feels as if he or she is in the company of a spiritual being. The highest form of such an experience is the visualization of God; however, the presence is not always beatific and may take the form of unspeakable evil that attempts to take possession of the individual. In either case, the effect is irrefutably to convince the individual of the reality of an unseen spiritual world. James noted that automatisms, hallucinations, and related dissociative experiences serve to strengthen belief:

> The inchoate sense of presence is infinitely stronger than conception, but strong as it may be, it is seldom equal to the evidence of hallucination. Saints who actually see or hear their Savior reach the acme of

assurance. Motor automatisms, though rarer, are, if possible even more convincing than sensations. The subjects here actually feel themselves played upon by powers beyond their will. (p. 262)

Religious Conversion

Religious conversion—the transformation from a lack of faith to a strong belief—was the centerpiece of James's lecture series. He saw conversion as the unification of a divided, conflicted, and unhappy state of self into a happy and consciously superior union. The psychology of the religious convert lies in the extreme dividedness of the subject's personality, according to James. He believed that most individuals have some degree of heterogeneity of personality, which is expressed by changes in their behavior across different contexts.

James quaintly illustrated this point with the image of the U.S. president at that time, Theodore Roosevelt, on a wilderness fishing trip far away from the issues and anxieties of the White House. James believed that contextualized versions of self are normal phenomena, becoming pathological only when the degree of inconsistency between different context-determined expressions of self is too extreme. In fact, the absence of the natural ebb and flow of the divided self is what calls attention to the unification of the converted individual.

James's Dichotomy of Mental Processes

James postulated two overriding types of mental processes: a conscious and voluntary type, and an unconscious and involuntary type. (In many respects, his formulations anticipated the "effortful–automatic" distinctions made by modern psychologists.) Thus James postulated two forms of conversion, the "volitional" and the "self-surrender." Volitional conversion proceeds gradually as the individual acquires the values and habits that lead to a religious life. Predictably, James was uninterested in the former, preferring the more passionate conversion of self-surrender. Drawing on a series of vivid first-person accounts, James devoted several lectures to the altered states of consciousness and dissociative experiences associated with religious conversion. In particular, he specifically linked these experiences to hysteria and dissociative disorders:

> In the wonderful explorations by Binet, Janet, Breuer, Freud, Mason, Prince and others, of the subliminal consciousness of patients with hysteria, we have revealed to us whole systems of underground life, in the shape of memories of a painful sort which lead a parasitic existence, buried outside of the primary fields of consciousness, and making irruptions thereinto with hallucinations, pains, convulsions, paral-

yses of feeling and of motion, and the whole procession of symptoms of hysteric disease of body and of mind. (p. 189)

Mystical States of Consciousness

Toward the end of the series (lectures 16 and 17), James turned his attention to mystical states, which he called the "root and centre" of personal religious experience (p. 292). Attentive to definition, James characterized mystical states as having four fundamental properties: "ineffability," "noetic quality," "transiency," and "passivity." By "ineffability," he meant that mystical states defy expression; there is no adequate way of communicating the experience in mere words. Mystical states are "noetic" in that they are special "states of insight into depths of truth unplumbed by the discursive intellect. They are illuminations, revelations, full of significance and importance" (p. 293). Mystical states are also "transient" in that they cannot be sustained. James noted that except in rare instances, they last at most an hour or two. When they have faded, however, their memory can still conjure up their spiritual quality, and when they recur, they are recognized instantly. As they recur, they grow in depth and meaning for the individual in "what is felt as inner richness and importance" (p. 293).

Finally, although they may be initiated by preparations or rituals, mystical states are largely "passive" experiences in which the individual acknowledges and surrenders to a will greater than his or her own. For James, their passivity links mystical states with "certain definite phenomena of secondary or alternative personality, such as prophetic speech, automatic writing, or the mediumistic trance" (p. 293); in modern terms, these would be described as the passive influence phenomena of MPD. However, he went on to qualify this, observing that mystical states differ from MPD and the like in that memories for the events of mystical experience are retained and modify the inner life of the individual. In dissociative states, by contrast there is often amnesia or denial of the experiences.

DRUG-ALTERED STATES OF CONSCIOUSNESS

A few readers may take exception to the juxtaposition of religious and drug-induced altered states of consciousness. I think that there are some "state" features that are shared in common by mystical and psychedelic experiences. However, most drug-induced altered states are not mystical and simply represent attempts to feel "good" in some fashion.

People use and abuse mind-altering drugs for many reasons, and a fuller discussion is beyond the scope of this book. However, in passing, I would like to say that both policy and research on substance abuse suffer from a failure to appreciate the contribution of discrete behavioral states to substance-abusing behavior. Here, I confine myself to certain cultural aspects of mind-altering drug use that are related to the pursuit of altered states of consciousness in Western society.

As I use the term here, "mind-altering drugs" are any pharmacological devices that change an individual's mental state. They are used for many reasons—including the induction of religious experiences—in virtually all cultures. Cultures that completely outlaw all forms of mind-altering drugs do so for religious reasons. In Western society, mind-altering drugs are generally taken to feel "good" or to feel "nothing." Most individuals regularly use one or more of the legal mind-altering drugs (e.g., alcohol, caffeine, nicotine). A considerable number augment these with illicit substances.

Experimentation with mind-altering experiences is a common feature of adolescence. Drug experimentation should be understood as a facet of a larger adolescent process of experimentation with altered states of mind and alternative versions of self. Within limits, this is a maturational process that must be lived through. But it holds risks and dangers. Adolescence typically provides unsupervised access to dangerous state-changing, mind-altering experiences. Alcohol, other drugs, sex, reckless driving, and thrill seeking are easily available and often rashly combined (Windle, 1994). It's a wonder that any of us survive to adulthood.

With maturation, most individuals manage to acquire an acceptable degree of temperance and volitional control with regard to mind-altering activities. Unfortunately, a sizeable minority do not or cannot acquire this form of self-control. Increasingly, we label the compulsion to engage in a state-altering behavior (e.g., drug use, sex, violence, gambling) as an "addiction." This formulation is something of a cliché, but I think it is worthwhile to conceptualize addiction from the perspective of the DBS model.

Drug and Other Addictions

"Drug addiction" may be defined as the "repeated and increased use of a drug or chemical substance, the deprivation of which gives rise to symptoms of distress and an irresistible urge to use the agent again" (Kaplan and Sadock, 1991, p. 4). In the DBS model, drug addiction reflects the creation of a set of discrete states induced by the substance (and/or by behavioral acts associated with use of the substance)—a set that becomes a dominant locus in the larger state space of the individual.

A simplified model of how drug or other addictions develop postulates that the individual creates an initially rewarding altered state of consciousness through the behavior in question (e.g., smoking crack, playing blackjack, or skydiving). With repeated induction, a set of discrete states with different versions of self, state-dependent memories, behaviors, and regulatory physiology is created. This set of states increasingly comes to dominate the individual's life. In the case of drug use, drug-related states of consciousness act in a competitive, dynamic fashion to displace more conventional states. Often they come to constitute an alternative, often secret life for the individual. We speak of a person as being "addicted" to a drug when this drug-related set of behavioral states comes to dominate a significant portion of the individual's behavior.

In some individuals, the addiction process itself forms the nidus for the dividing, alternative focus of behavior. In others, the mind-altering behavior is layered upon an already divided and conflicted self. In either case, an individual behaves as if he or she had two or more discrete ways of being. Working with families of substance abusers, one finds that they frequently draw sharp distinctions between the patients when sober and the patients when intoxicated (e.g., "drunk Daddy" and "real Daddy"). Talking with substance abusers, one hears them speak about an internal split: "Doc, there is one part of me listening to you, and another part planning how to get hold of a bottle when I leave." The question of whether polysubstance abuse creates "pharmacological MPD" is one I must leave for another day.

Treatment Implications

As discussed in Chapter Two, there is increasing evidence of an important linkage between childhood trauma and substance abuse. The DBS model predicts that traumatized individuals who have developmental deficits in metacognitive integrative functions will be especially vulnerable to developing addictive behaviors. This model also predicts that addictions characterized by the existence of a set of highly discrete behavioral states will be very difficult to treat.

Currently, most substance abuse treatment focuses on blocking the individual's entry into intoxicated states, rather than working directly with drug-state-related behavior. Treatment is conducted in the sober state, and patients must be thoroughly detoxified before therapy is initiated. However, from the perspective of the DBS model, this approach primarily addresses an individual in those behavioral states that are not directly involved in the addictive behavior. As research has demonstrated, drug-induced states often have powerful state-dependent aspects (Weingartner, 1978; Weingartner et al., 1995).

One consequence of state dependency is the partitioning of the individual's values and beliefs into separate, usually conflicting, moral systems that operate differentially when the person is sober or intoxicated. Because of this state dependency, psychotherapy aimed at changing the drug-related behaviors and beliefs is not likely to succeed in and of itself when delivered to the individual in the sober state. A few substance abuse counselors have speculated privately that, early in treatment, perhaps some psychotherapy should be conducted with the individual in intoxicated states.

Psychedelic Drugs

Psychedelic drug states are sometimes equated with mystical experiences. Certainly Aldous Huxley's (1954) famous description of a mescaline-altered state of consciousness is a classic example:

> I continued to look at the flowers, and in their living light I seemed to detect the qualitative equivalent of breathing—but a breathing without returns to a starting point, with no recurrent ebbs but only a repeated flow from beauty to heightened beauty, from deeper to ever deeper meaning. Words like "grace" and "transfiguration" came to my mind, and this, of course, was what, among other things, they stood for. (p. 18)

But, as William James learned from his own experimentation with nitrous oxide, "the truth fades out, however, or escapes, at the moment of coming to: and if any words remain over in which it seemed to clothe itself, they prove to be the veriest nonsense" (1902/1958, p. 298). Like mystical experiences drug-induced states of consciousness are transient, and the experiences contained therein do not readily translate back to normal states of consciousness. Unlike mystical experiences, however, they result in no *lasting* sense of truth or of "inner richness and importance"—as James discovered. The insularity of a drug-induced state requires the individual to use the drug recurrently to reevoke the state, which may prove increasingly difficult to recapture as physiological tolerance develops.

As discussed in Chapter Seven, dissociation-like states can be produced by drugs such as phencyclidine. They produce alterations in sense of self and environment, as well as features of a thought disorder. Distortions in body perception, depersonalization, and loss of control over thought processes are common phencyclidine-induced experiences. In my clinical experience, abusers report using phencyclidine to induce profound alterations in sense of identity. As one kid told me at the end of a long night in the emergency room, "You want to be a rock star? On dust [phencyclidine], you *are* a rock star!"

Over-the-Counter Medications as Represented on Television

My last point concerns the way in which over-the-counter medications are represented on television. The universal selling message is that they "make you feel better fast." How is this conveyed? Usually by portraying a state shift or switch.

In the first scene, the individual is suffering miserably from some ailment, be it headache or indigestion. In the second scene, we cut away to a spiel about the miraculous medication in question, perhaps including an animation of its magical action on the stomach lining or headache nerve endings. A few seconds later we cut back to our now transformed former sufferer. We see an astonishing change. The person looks and sounds 10 years younger; he or she has energy, humor, relatedness, sex appeal, and whatever else was lacking in the first scene. Now the person copes magnificently with whatever comes along and loves being with grandchildren, spouse, or coworkers. Over and over again, the basic message is that drugs "make you feel better fast."

TELEVISION WATCHING

Children's Television

It is estimated that by age 18 a child will have spent more time watching television than in any other single activity except sleep (Liebert and Sprafkin, 1988). Television has profoundly changed family life and continues to do so. Television has also had massive social and community effects. Even metropolitan water supply systems have had to be redesigned to compensate for the rapid pressure drop resulting from heavy bathroom use during commercial breaks for events such as the Super Bowl. Studies of remote regions prior to and after the arrival of television demonstrate dramatic decreases in community involvement and shared activities such as team sports, particularly as the number of channels increases (Williams, 1986; Liebert and Sprafkin, 1988). Thirty-plus years of research have amply documented that exposure to television profoundly changes people's behavior and the patterns of daily life.

Television has an especially strong impact on children. A review of these studies is very disturbing. Far too little is being done to protect children from the currently pervasive negative influences and to accentuate the powerful prosocial effects that television can exert. Not all children's programming is negative by any means; some wonderful, positive programs can be found on public television and certain cable channels. Unfortunately, much commercial children's programming is predicated on a few basic assumptions about child viewers. Children are considered to have short attention spans, and to require quick movement and loud noises to capture and hold their attention. (Some regard this assumption as a tragically self-fulfilling prophecy.)

Children's shows are aimed at very broad age ranges (typically 2- to 11-year-olds), to increase audience size. They feature common-denominator themes of crime and aggression, comedy, adventure, and romance. Animation is favored because of its lower cost and greater flexibility, especially for "superhero"-type shows.

In contrast to adult series, which may be rerun once during the off-season summer months, children's programming is planned to be rerun as often as four times a year. Child audiences are believed to have low recognition for old material, although young viewers themselves make it plain that this is not true. Producers argue that heavy rerunning is justified because profit margins are lower on children's television. That may be true initially, but repeated airing of episodes over many years, coupled with the integrated marketing of theme toys and accessories, yields considerable long-term profits.

State-Altering Effects of Television

Leaving many concerns unspoken, I focus on the "state" effects of television on children. Observers of children who are watching television frequently comment on the children's "hypnotic" or "trance-like" states. Even children with ADHD "zone out" passively in front of a television. While watching television, children are usually inert and inactive, except during moments of tension, when they may hide (e.g., watching from a doorway, behind furniture, or under covers). Even when a show is frightening, children remained transfixedly glued to the set. It can be difficult to break this state in a child. Indeed, attempts to interrupt television viewing are often responded to with disproportionate irritation and anger. Children have great difficulty volitionally initiating an exit from television-related states and frequently require repeated parental interactions to move on to other activities. Most parents are well aware of television's trance-like effects; indeed, many use it as a babysitter.

To my knowledge, there is no research on the properties of television-induced behavioral states in children. What I offer here is speculation. According to the DBS model, television-related states should manifest significant state dependency for some types of implicit memory. Recall that implicit memory describes a set of memories that can be shown to influence behavior without the individual's direct awareness (see Chapter Six).

Reality Testing and Television-Based Belief Systems

While in the passive, highly focused states of consciousness induced by television, children are being exposed to a large number of suppositions about what the world is like and how things work. They suspend reality testing and buy into artificial microcosms ranging from television "families" to intergalactic confederations. These pseudorealities, each with its own script-driven system of beliefs, values, cause–effect assumptions, and "logic," define the children's world view—at least for the length of the show. These experiences (and viewing a television program or a movie can be an intense emotional experience) may be difficult to discuss with parents or others. Often there is a "you have to have seen it to understand" effect, which compounds the usual difficulties children and adolescents have in discussing disturbing material.

I contend that television-based assumptive belief and value systems are powerful influences on children's thinking about the nature of the world. Elsewhere (Putnam, 1993a), I give examples of the reality-testing contradictions that I found inner-city children mired in with regard to television depictions of violence versus their own life experiences. Television strongly influences children's sense of "reality." The powerful "seeing is believing" effect—to which we are all susceptible—is especially influential because children have a much smaller set of experiences against which to compare what they see on television. Television spans the extremes of the reality–nonreality spectrum. It carries a complex mixture of reality and fantasy—from live, on-the-scene, real events to superhero cartoons.

Even more problematic is the fact that much of television programming freely mixes real and unreal elements. For instance, a live, on-the-spot news report is periodically interrupted by commercials in which animated, three-dimensional "productoids" run around performing their magic. With the advent of morphing and other computer-generated special effects, all sorts of magical transformations between "real" images and cartoon variants occur in the blink of an eye. (Watching television, I wonder whether there isn't a conspiracy among U.S. advertisers to undermine the entire country's reality testing.)

Children's programming is especially insidious in using a variety of techniques to blur reality–nonreality distinctions. For example, toy advertisements rely on a heavy blending of live actors with animated action. I recommend that readers who have not seen nationally syndicated children's programming for a while tune in next Saturday morning; they may be shocked. Many of the cartoons, in particular, eat away at the boundaries of reality. Gone are the simple, clearly fantasy-based cartoon animals and people. They have been replaced by far more lifelike characters who exist in worlds that seem to overlap with our own. The rendering of face and form is often very realistic. In querying preschoolers and young school-age children, I find that many have a difficult time determining whether or not certain characters well known to this age group exist outside of television. This is, of course, what the advertisers want. A natural outgrowth is that cartoon characters endorse a variety of products—as a stroll down the cereal aisle in any supermarket will make all too clear.

A Postscript on Virtual Reality

Included with this set of concerns are my apprehensions about the large-scale coming of "virtual reality" (VR) to the personal entertainment industry. Like television, VR technologies have enormous potential for education. And even more than television, VR can be a mind-altering—even addictive—negative influence. Already the first generation of VR games and gadgets is upon us. (A "generation" is about 12–18 months.) The large potential market will drive rapid advances in technology and decreases in price. In a few years, personal VR devices will be as common as Walkman-type music devices are today.

Virtual worlds are going to be increasingly realistic and so naturally interactive that one can connect *directly* with all manner of beings and environments. One of VR's attractions for adolescents is the ability to assume virtual identities with superpowers. In the near future, large numbers of youths will be wearing video helmets or goggles, stereo earphones, and sensor gloves or other gear that will allow them to experience all manner of fantasy worlds directly and intimately. Whether they are using their computerized magical powers in battles with supernatural demons, dogfights with alien spaceships, or dinosaur hunts, they will see, hear, and feel the entire "experience."

Even the simple equipment of today is capable of producing profound changes in mental state. Tart (1990) cites the disorientation produced in pilots when they step out of today's flight simulators as an example of the potential ability of a VR environment to alter mental states. Consider the mental state (not to mention the time–distance–velocity judgment) of a teenage boy who has just spent 3 hours blasting aliens in his virtual rocket fighter and then gets behind the wheel of the family car.

VR experiences are far more private than television, which at least is shared in some fashion by a larger audience and therefore can be reexamined with the input of others. VR is designed to create imaginary worlds experienced only by one individual, or at most a partner or two. There is thus a dangerous potential for generating emotionally intense, almost autistic altered states. Many VR games and simulators incorporate features that allow the user to self-generate individualized scenarios and to assume multiple different interactive identities with powers such as flying and superstrength.

In the words of one VR developer, "If you can dream it, you can do it." More enticing than plain old reality, these realistic, highly personalized worlds appeal strongly to adolescents. I predict that in 10 years we will be faced with a group of socially withdrawn teenagers who are "addicted" to living in their virtual worlds. The window of opportunity to anticipate this problem and to implement research, regulation, and prevention efforts is rapidly closing.

SEX AND SPORTS

In discussing altered states of consciousness in everyday life, I feel compelled to say a few words about two universal state-altering activities: sex and athletics. Sex and athletics are common activities for most people. Obviously they take a number of forms, even for the same individual, and change over the life span. Although both can be strenuous, they are often followed by a sense of relaxation. Both are influenced by a sense of internal tension, which may be triggered or heightened by specific stimuli. Often the sense of tension builds over time until discharged by the activity or suppressed by will or circumstances.

Sex and athletics both create and expand a set of alternative states of consciousness. These states are highly context-specific and rarely occur outside of the appropriate setting, be it bedroom or tennis court. In these states, marked physiological changes occur and typically serve to reinforce the experience of pleasure for the individual. Attention is highly focused on the moment and the activity at hand. Sense of time may be altered. Many metacognitive capacities are suspended or largely unavailable. (Judgment, in particular, seems to be a frequent casualty.)

Sex and athletics typically involve a sequence of short-lived states moving along a set of well-worn pathways. When things are going well, the individual passes from one to another of these states with increasing speed and intensity. When things are not going well, the individual can get "stuck" in a state—generally a frustrating experience. In the case of sex, orgasm brings an abrupt state transition manifested by the termination of one behavioral sequence and the initiation of another. In sports, "victory" often leads to hypomanic states of exaggerated self-esteem.

Peak experiences may occur in either sex or sports. The pursuit of ecstasy, real and imagined, drives a lot of experimentation. Finally, fantasy plays a major role in both activities, and among the central features of such fantasies are alterations in sense of self.

SUMMARY

Altered and alternative states of consciousness are part of human mental life. Most are not dissociative in nature, in that they do not involve profound alterations in identity and discontinuities of autobiographical memory. This chapter has examined several examples to highlight the larger role of discrete behavioral states in basic human behavior.

Borrowing heavily from William James, I consider profound religious experiences. Drug use and abuse provide more contemporary examples of the innate human drive to alter mental states. Television also provides powerful state-altering devices, which may prove "addictive" to some; this may be even more true of the rapidly emerging VR technologies. Finally, sex and sports, two important tension-discharging activities, are briefly examined within the DBS model. I have refrained from including gambling and rock-and-roll in this chapter, although there is compelling evidence of dissociation-like discrete behavioral states with both.

Chapter Eleven

Dissociative Presentations: Clinical Vignettes

Children and adolescents with pathological dissociation come to clinical attention in a variety of ways. Some critics protest that these varied presentations prove that dissociative disorders are not coherent psychiatric syndromes. Their mistaken assumption is that psychiatric disorders are legitimate only if they present in an invariant fashion. Few psychiatric (or medical) conditions have only a single clinical presentation, however. Indeed, regardless of the nature of their psychiatric problems, emotionally disturbed children and adolescents typically present for evaluation with mixed or ambiguous symptoms. Children in particular can be difficult to diagnose definitively, and often must be followed and reevaluated several times before it becomes clear what the problem is. The existence of multiple and atypical presentations for child and adolescent dissociative disorders is just a messy, real-life aspect of clinical work; it is not fundamentally different from the range of presentations associated with many child and adolescent psychiatric disorders.

Dissociative children and adolescents may present with severe behavioral problems, with psychotic-like symptoms, with affective symptoms, with compulsive self-injurious or violent antisocial behavior, or with florid dissociative symptoms. The differential diagnosis of children and adolescents presenting with significant behavioral problems should include pathological dissociation. Traditionally, child mental health professionals have a low index of suspicion for dissociative disorders (Kluft, 1984a); this is changing, however. Dissociative disorders are increasingly being recognized for what they are—a category of posttraumatic disorders. The development and validation of checklists, structured interviews, and psychological testing profiles for child and adolescent dissociative disorders are improving our ability to detect and document pathological dissociation (see Chapter Twelve). Informed clinical evaluation, however, remains central to diagnosis. This chapter contains a series of clinical vignettes to illustrate a range of clinical presentations of child and adolescent dissociative disorders.

A FUGUE

CARRIE

Carrie, a 15-year-old, said that she "woke up" squatting behind a trash dumpster. She was confused and frightened, and felt as if "years had passed." Her only possession was a backpack filled with dirty clothes, which she recognized as hers. Wandering around, she asked several people where she was, but they did not speak English. She concluded that she was in a foreign country until she found a pay phone with a San Diego directory. She attempted to call her mother; when there was no answer, she was frightened. She reached a friend and learned that she had been missing for several days. Arrangements were made for her to stay with local family friends until her mother arrived. When they met, her mother noted that Carrie seemed unusually relaxed and calm, compared with the period prior to her disappearance.

Carrie reported that she had no memory for the events of her cross-country travel. She had disappeared while at a shopping mall with friends. There was some evidence of premeditated planning: She had dyed her blond hair dark and had packed clothes prior to leaving for the mall. Pieces of a postcard addressed to her father, with a brief message saying that she was alive and well, were found in her backpack. Carrie denied memory for a number of salient events leading up to her disappearance, including attending a dinner party with her mother, at which they had had a nasty public fight. She denied other episodes of time loss or amnesias. She reported no fluctuations in skills or abilities, and no problems with concentration or memory at school, at home, or with friends. She described a few transient experiences of depersonalization, such as having her hands suddenly look strange to her. She denied passive influence/interference experiences, such as feeling made to do something that she did not want to do. She denied waking auditory and visual hallucinations or a sense that there were other parts to herself. She did report frequent hypnogogic experiences, such as hearing her name called as she was falling asleep.

Carrie's mother described her as a "dreamy" child and provided numerous examples of microdissociation-like behavior, where she became transiently confused about what she was doing or why she was doing it. She was continually forgetting to do her homework or to turn in what she had done, typically denying that she had been given a school assignment. She daydreamed a lot, often turning on the radio and going into a reverie. When she was in this state, it was difficult to get her attention unless she was touched.

Her parents had separated when Carries was 8 and divorced when she was 10. She took this very hard and had been especially hateful toward her mother, who had custody. She seldom saw her father, who moved out of state and traveled extensively. She had an unusually close relationship with her mother's boyfriend, often staying up late at night talking with him after her mother went to bed. He provided sleeping pills for the insomnia and nighttime restlessness that became problems prior to her disappearance.

An EEG and a thorough neurological workup were negative. On interview, Carrie was a well-groomed, petite girl appearing a few years younger than her age. She looked out from behind her hair, which was combed so that it fell over her eyes. She was alert and watchful, but cooperative and interested in understanding what had happened. She seemed to be of average intelligence, was well spoken, and gave coherent and logical answers. There was no evidence of a thought disorder or delusions. Abstractive capacity was age-appropriate. Judgment appeared intact on standard questions.

She volunteered the following explanation of the events: She had noticed that when she got "really, really mad" with her mother, she often felt "spaced out." Being "spaced out" meant feeling very detached—"as if I was standing very far away and seeing myself"—and emotionally numb. She recalled being angry with her mother and thinking over and over, "If she goes away, so will I." She did not remember any specific event that had triggered her leaving, but recalled a sense of building inner pressure that increased with each negative interaction that they had. She expressed concern that this kind of thing could happen again, but said that the prior sense of internal tension had not returned and that she was feeling safer with each passing day.

Carrie's case illustrates a form of adolescent dissociative presentation that I have seen on occasion. The presenting problem is usually dramatic—for Carrie, it was a cross-country fugue episode—but typically the child has a long history of being unusually "spacey" or daydreamy, with difficulties in memory and concentration at home and school. Other examples I have seen included a 12-year-old boy with outbursts of violence toward his mother and destructive behavior for which he claimed amnesia, and a 16-year-old girl who stole specimens from her school's science lab and later "discovered" them at home. Dramatic dissociative acting out appears to serve functions of expressing unacceptable anger and of drawing outside attention to a problem. The adolescent describes being largely amnesic, with the exception of some fragmentary or "blurry" mental images associated with the events.

Dissociative acting out can be dangerous. Shaw (1992) describes a case in which a teenager firebombed his home in a dissociative state, which was apparently precipitated by rage at his adoptive parents. I have participated in the psychological autopsies of two teenagers, each of whom was accidentally killed while in an apparent dissociative state triggered by a threatening stimulus. Both died while inappropriately fleeing after misunderstanding an apparently innocuous interaction with an authority figure (e.g., being asked for identification by a guard). Both had long histories of intense preoccupation with elaborate fantasy worlds, to the detriment of their school and social activities. One was believed to have had an extended homosexual sexual relationship with a coach, although the liaison supposedly started a year or more after she began to exhibit excessive daydreaming.

A PATHOLOGICAL ELABORATED IDENTITY

NANCY AND "MARCIE, THE BOY DOG"

Nancy was a 6-year old-white female referred for evaluation of a possible dissociative disorder, because at times she insisted that she was "Marcie, the boy dog." Now in the care of her paternal grandmother (PGM), Nancy had a sketchy early history. She was born out of wedlock; her parents married when she was 2. Shortly thereafter, she disappeared with her mother for 6–9 months. Finally located in an out-of-state foster home, she had been removed from her mother's care after being found unattended on several occasions. She bounced among a succession of foster placements, her mother, her father, and her maternal grandmother for about 2 years until her PGM was given custody of her when she was 4½. The PGM alleged that Nancy's mother was heavily involved in drugs and prostitution, and described the father as a "paranoid schizophrenic" who lived on the West Coast. Except for an occasional phone call, he showed little interest in Nancy.

The degree of maltreatment that Nancy had experienced was unclear. There was a suspicion of sexual abuse by some of the mother's boyfriends (e.g., Nancy said that one made her "bounce" on him while she was naked). At times she exhibited sexualized behaviors (e.g., spreading her legs and talking about her genitals). She did not compulsively masturbate or exhibit public eroticization. The PGM had been told by one of the mother's friends that the mother used to beat Nancy with a belt.

"Marcie, the boy dog" first appeared after one of the father's rare phone calls, which had ended badly, leaving Nancy disappointed and hurt. Shortly after the call, she appeared crawling on the floor, with a tail made from a sock tucked in the waistband of her pants. She refused to talk and only barked and growled. With time, this behavior became increasingly prominent; it frequently occurred following stress or disappointment, and lasted for 2 or 3 days at a time. While in the "Marcie, the boy dog" mode, Nancy crawled on the floor, panted and growled, would not speak, and would not respond when spoken to. She would only eat off the floor and lapped water from a bowl. The PGM reported that Nancy crawled so much she wore out the toes on her shoes, and that she had to wear mittens to protect her hands, which were skinned and bruised. The PGM never witnessed the transition into "Marcie, the boy dog," reporting instead that Nancy would emerge from her room in this state. Sometimes Nancy would fall asleep curled up dog-like on the floor would and awaken as Nancy. In the "Marcie, the boy dog" state, Nancy lost much of her toilet training.

The PGM reported occasional dissociation-like behaviors—frequent trance-like, "spacey" periods, as well as some perplexing forgetfulness, manifested in loss of skills or mistakes about well-known facts. The PGM believed that this was more willful oppositional behavior than genuine amnesia. In addition to "Marcie, the boy dog," Nancy sometimes exhibited rapid regression into a baby-like state, sucking her thumb, seeking to be held, and crying like a baby. There was a history of some PTSD-type symptoms, particularly nightmares and hyperstartle responses.

My first interview with Nancy was not particularly informative. I was primarily struck by how adept she was at controlling adults and indirectly avoiding questions. I did not see any evidence of "Marcie, the boy dog," and when asked, Nancy said that she only pretended to be "Marcie."

I discussed examples of dissociative behavior in children with the PGM, and we went over the CDC (see Appendix Two). I asked her to keep a written log of the appearances of "Marcie, the boy dog" and the circumstances surrounding them. Weekly administrations of the CDC revealed somewhat more dissociative behavior than described in our first interview. However, over several months there was a steady decrease in the appearance of "Marcie, the boy dog." This period of marked improvement was coincident with Nancy's legal adoption by the PGM and her entrance into kindergarten. The baby-like state decreased correspondingly with the disappearance of "Marcie, the boy dog." Over a 6-month period, Nancy gradually stopped appearing as "Marcie." She made progress in school, but remained significantly behind her younger classmates in many areas. Although not aggressive in general, she could become vindictively vengeful if insulted. She was described as hyperactive in the classroom. Her pediatrician tried a course of methylphenidate, which had little effect.

I have seen several "Marcie, the boy dog" types of presentations in traumatized or highly insecure 4- to 7-year-olds. To some extent, this presentation resembles the animal identities/ICs seen in some normal, well-adjusted children—for example, Fred's "Magic Cat," described in Chapter Nine. The clinical judgment that "Marcie, the boy dog" but not "Magic Cat" was a pathological dissociative behavior depended on the degree of impairment or harmful dysfunction each identity caused the child and his or her caretakers.

"Marcie, the boy dog" differed from "Magic Cat" in several important respects. Although both children activated their animal alter egos in response to stress, this happened much less frequently with "Magic Cat." Fred had other, age-appropriate ways of coping with stress and anxiety. "Magic Cat" was also obviously more under Fred's volitional control, primarily appeared in play contexts, and was sometimes externalized into a specific Lego figure. "Magic Cat" was interactive and socialized as well; Fred often involved his nursery school and kindergarten classmates in the "Magic Cat" game, in which they ran around interspersing "meows" with meaningful communication. By first grade, Fred found his classmates more resistant to joining in the "Magic Cat" game, and it became more of a solitary activity. By second grade, Fred rarely activated "Magic Cat" in any context, although he maintained a strong affection for cats and collected cat toys, pictures, and knick-knacks.

In contrast, "Marcie, the boy dog" appeared to be Nancy's only coping response to stress or disappointment. "Marcie, the boy dog" was persistently and inappropriately active for extended periods, and his/her/its appearances were usually terminated by a period of exhausted sleep. "Marcie" was also highly regressed (e.g., eating off the floor, communicating only nonverbally, losing toilet training, etc.) and unsocialized. In contrast to Fred's manic delight in being "Magic Cat," Nancy never played or appeared to be having fun as "Marcie, the boy dog."

It is difficult to be certain about dissociative experiences of amnesia, depersonalization, and passive influence in children aged 4–6 years, but behavioral examples volunteered by caretakers are generally congruent with dissociative disturbances of memory and identity. The decline in the appearance of "Marcie, the boy dog" appeared related to increased stability and security for Nancy and increased socialization with her peers. As noted in Chapter Nine, entities such as "Marcie, the boy dog" do not always disappear, and some seem to become the nucleus of one or more alter personalities in MPD (Trujillo et al., 1996).

PERSISTENT CHILDHOOD MULTIPLE
PERSONALITY DISORDER

PENNI

I first saw Penni when she was 6 years old. She was referred for consultation because she complained that a series of named "people" lived inside her. They spoke to her in lengthy conversations and controlled or influenced her behavior. In addition, she had an array of serious behavioral disturbances, including frequent masturbation, sexual acting out in school, marked oppositional behavior, temper tantrums, and hyperactivity.

It was alleged that Penni had been sexually molested frequently, perhaps daily, by her father. It was also alleged that she had sometimes been locked in a closet. It was established that her mother had violently attacked her on a number of occasions, once going after her with a kitchen knife. (This incident appeared to be the source of a recurrent nightmare that plagued Penni for years.) Both parents had a history of confirmed sexual abuse in their own families, stretching back several generations on her father's side. Her mother was addicted to multiple drugs, carried diagnoses of BPD and bipolar disorder, and had been hospitalized over 20 times since Penni's birth.

At age 4½ years, Penni was saved by a neighboring couple, Mr. and Mrs. R., who started watching her after they noted abnormal behavior and apparent neglect. Their attention was drawn by her foul language (e.g., talking about her "pussy") and poor hygiene. Mrs. R. described Penni at that time as being "clingy, dirty, licking herself, and in perpetual motion." She noted that Penni did not know the names of colors, letters, numbers, or other age-appropriate information. In one instance, Mrs. R. accompanied Penni to the bathroom after the child complained, "My pussy stinks." She found blood-like stains on Penni's underwear. Mr. and Mrs. R. enlisted their church to help Penni by providing day care. Subsequent interactions between the pastor and Penni's parents led to a child protective services investigation, which documented severe neglect and physical findings consistent with sexual abuse.

The R. family's home initially served as an emergency foster placement. Mr. and Mrs. R. were eventually able to adopt Penni when she was 9 years old. The experienced mother of two grown children, Mrs. R. had a clear idea of what was not normal behavior for a young girl. She sought further psychiatric evaluation after noting that Penni frequently yelled and screamed at an invisible person, especially around bathtime. Penni had been receiving methylphenidate for "hyperactivity," and was being seen at the county mental health clinic for her chronic masturbation, sexual acting out, oppositional behavior, and chronic nightmares. While in a therapy group for sexually abused children, Penni began to describe a number of imaginary "friends" and to talk about the "other Penni" and "bad Penni."

Increasingly Penni began to talk to and about her imaginary "friends." She produced a list of names and at times claimed to be one or another of these "friends," refusing to answer to the name Penni. Mrs. R. described abrupt changes in Penni's behavior, which were frequently associated with her refusal to acknowledge her name. She reported that Penni's affect, activity level, and behavior would suddenly shift for no apparent reason. Abrupt behavioral changes were often associated with rapid blinking and upward rolling of the eyes. There were also numerous examples of perplexing forgetfulness. For example, Mrs. R. reported that when claiming to be "Melissa," Penni seemed to forget where to put her dirty clothes—a long-standing household routine. Mr. and Mrs. R. spent long periods trying to teach her basic information (e.g., the alphabet, names of colors, and types of money). They noted that her ability to remember and use this information was associated with stereotypic ways of behaving. She also frequently "tranced out."

My first consultation consisted of two sessions, 2 weeks apart. Penni was a well-groomed, normal-appearing child, who alternated rapidly between bright, cheerful affect and sullen, oppositional behavior. She frequently tugged and scratched at her crotch area, and sat in ways that immodestly revealed her underwear. At one point she wrote her name with her left hand. Because she had previously favored her right hand, I remarked on this. Penni, evincing surprise and confusion, appeared to "trance out" for a moment. She was then unable to write further with her left hand, and subsequently wrote and drew with her right hand. Her therapist (who was present during this evaluation) and Mrs. R. reported that they had never seen her write left-handed. Comparison of the left- and right-handed examples showed the left to be distinctly more legible.

On the first visit Penni refused to talk about her imaginary "friends," retreating into angry silence when I raised the topic. On the second visit, however, she spontaneously began to describe them to me. She called them "friends and cousins" and said that they lived inside of her. They had names, including "Princess Elena," "Michelle," "Melissa," "Glanny," "Chainy," "Zany," and "Amy." She said that she hated them and had put them all in a plastic bag. I noted that this would suffocate them. She said that she wanted them all dead.

I did not see any distinct alter personalities, although Penni's behavior during the handwriting episode was consistent with a covert personality switch. I provided Mrs. R. with a stack of copies of the 16 item CDC's (Version 2.2), to be completed monthly. I also asked her to keep a record of Penni's dissociation-like behaviors.

My primary recommendation was "to observe her and document evidence of dissociation and possible alter personalities, but not to aggressively seek out alters." In my initial note, I optimistically discussed how dissociative behavior may decline or disappear in many maltreated children when they are placed in a truly safe and stable living situation. Mrs. R. agreed to fill out the CDC on a monthly basis. (See "Dissociation Screening Measures," below.)

Six months later I saw Penni for a third time. She was in weekly psychotherapy through the county mental health clinic, and was showing some improvement in aggression and sexual behaviors at school and home. However, she talked more than ever about her "inside friends." In particular, she said that they were telling her not to do well in school. "Amy" was particularly active, writing letters and lists of names of the others. Penni continued to talk and argue with her "inside friends" on a nightly basis. She was also having frequent nightmares about kidnappers' coming after her or her biological parents dying. She was regularly observed to stare into space for prolonged periods, a "dark, pensive look on her face." Abrupt behavioral shifts were associated with striking facial changes. Mrs. R. said that she could tell which of the "inside friends" was active by the way Penni looked and moved.

During the interview, I saw an alter personality state appear while Penni was examining a doll. She compulsively stripped it of clothes, and upon pulling down the underpants, she froze with a blank stare. Bolting out of her frozen state about 30 seconds later, she looked at the doll in her hand and then threw it hard against the wall. She began crawling around on the floor, giggling and acting silly. "I'm 'Zany,'" she said. Observing the interview, her therapist commented that she had seen "Zany" before. "Zany" was manifested in silly and regressed behavior that had an oppositional quality, in that Penni could or would not cooperate to do what needed to be done at the moment. I have subsequently seen "Zany" several times, as well as several of Penni's other alter personality states. Although their relative overtness has waxed and waned over the years, these discrete behavioral states have exhibited strong consistency over time in terms of affect, behavior, age/developmental stage, skills, and abilities. Mrs. R. has recorded many interactions with these alter personality states. Penni's various therapists over the years have also observed and documented the same set of alter personality states.

Subsequent to this consultation, Penni continued in individual and group therapy, and received methylphenidate (15 mg twice a day) and diphenhydramine (25 mg as needed to control her nighttime agitation). Review of her individual therapist's progress notes for the period January 1990 through March 1991 revealed fluctuating problems with dissociative behavior, but some decrease in observed personality switches and arguments with her "inside friends."

However, Penni began to sleepwalk frequently. Her school performance waxed and waned, but was consistently below grade and IQ level. Periodically, her sexual behavior toward other children was out of control. Penni's behavior problems appeared to be connected with delays in the termination of her biological parents' rights and the initiation of adoption proceedings by Mr. and Mrs. R. On several occasions, the announcement of another postponement of legal proceedings was followed by headaches, stomachaches, irritability, impulsivity, and oppositional defiant behavior.

I saw Penni again in July 1990, following an incident at summer camp provoked by being teased by other children. At that time, "Glanny," a male alter personality state, emerged and caused problems. Mrs. R. provided numerous examples of Penni's amnesias and perplexing shifts in availability of knowledge (e.g., wildly erratic ability to play the same song on the piano). She also brought in Penni's diary which exhibited marked shifts in handwriting and the spelling of the same word (e.g., "end," "eand," and "ennd"). She also provided examples of drawings that showed clear differences in skill and style. During this interview I observed Penni switch into "Zany" and "Amy"; the latter gave her age as 9 years (more than a year older than Penni), and provided a different birth date. Diary entries signed "Amy" were characterized by better writing and drawing skills than entries signed with other names.

I did not see Penni again for 2 years. Her therapy records for this period indicate that she was seen monthly, primarily to review and renew her methylphenidate prescription. Her school problems were the focus of attention, although comments attributed to Penni in the notes were primarily related to the ongoing court proceedings. In March 1992, at age 9 years, Penni was legally adopted by the R. family. In July 1992, she was reevaluated by the clinic psychiatrist after her behavior markedly worsened. The psychiatrist noted "spacey-like behaviors in which she seems out of touch with reality and has a number of motor automatisms." These included rocking in a fetal position and pelvic gyrations against objects. There were also long pauses during which she stared off into space.

Mrs. R. contacted me in October 1992 for a consultation because of Penni's continued behavior problems. Penni was now receiving 15 mg of methylphenidate three times a day, but was having serious problems with hyperactivity, attention, agitation, aggression, anger, and nightmares. She was talking about running away or killing herself. She also remained highly sexualized, with frequent masturbation and genital-stimulating activities. Mrs. R reported a number of sexualized interactions with a younger adopted sibling now living with the R. family, including once licking the younger child's crotch area. At times Penni assumed a personality state characterized by an "angry, red-faced, evil look"; in this state, she threw objects, bit people, and talked to adults as if they were children. This could occur "out of the blue" or could be precipitated by trivial things, and generally lasted from 5 minutes to an hour.

Switch-like behaviors were associated with amnesias, different voices, and different behavior. Penni also described passive influence/interference phenomena: She complained that she was being forced to masturbate by the "people inside," and that it was painful. She also said that she did not want to make many of the hurtful comments, but that she was told to by the people in her head. In the interview, I again met "Zany," "Amy," and "Glanny." For the first time, Penni complained about feelings of depersonalization and derealization, saying, "I feel like this is not real. I don't feel like I am here." I also noted marked hyperstartle responses to background noises.

In June 1993, Penni was hospitalized for 2 weeks on a child psychiatric unit. The reason for admission was given as "out-of-control behavior"—that is, aggression and inappropriate sexual touching at school and home. Her psychotherapist (a psychologist) and the psychiatrist who provided her medication felt that there were subtle signs of a thought disorder emerging. Despite an inauspicious start, Penni did well in the hospital, adjusting to the milieu and becoming popular with the other children. Both the attending psychiatrist and a consultant confirmed the diagnosis of MPD. They also felt that her affect was blunted and her thinking "disjointed." She was placed on haloperidol (2 mg twice a day), clonazepam (5 mg per day—2 mg twice a day and 1 mg at bedtime), methylphenidate, and benztropine. At discharge, some improvement was reported in her thinking, and her aggression and hypersexuality had disappeared in the hospital. As is often the case, these improvements were short-lived at home. She was subsequently tapered off the haloperidol without noticeable change in her behavior or the quality of her thinking.

I next saw Penni, now aged 12 years, in December 1994. Again the request for consultation was prompted by an exacerbation in her behavior; this time it involved sexual acting out at school. Now in a level 5 school placement, she had to ride the bus almost 2 hours each way. For a while, Penni was barred from the bus because of her aggression and sexuality (the only other riders were two boys, also significantly disturbed), but was being permitted back on a trial basis. She was in twice-weekly therapy with an MPD-oriented psychologist, who was working directly with her alter personality states. This was the first time that she had received a treatment focused on her dissociative disorder. Several "integrations" had been attempted, but none had lasted more than a few days. Mrs. R. reported continuing to observe switching behaviors, although she thought that these had become more subtle. Penni was still taking methylphenidate and clonazepam, and had been started on sertraline.

Now a maturely developed young woman (she had started puberty at age 9), Penni was animated and friendly. She remembered the last visit 2 years earlier, and asked whether she could play with a certain toy that she had enjoyed then. In the interview, she talked about developing her coconsciousness (i.e., the sense that several of her alter personalities were simultaneously present). Still, there were many angry inner voices, and at times she could not think "'cause of the noise inside." She talked about her boyfriends and claimed that she was the "most popular girl in school" (there were only a half dozen girls in this special educational placement). At one point, when I refused to let her play with my computer, she switched into "Glanny." "His" distinctive pouting profile and deeper "male" voice were similar to his characteristics at prior meetings.

Dissociation Screening Measures. Figure 11.1 presents the scores on the CDC as completed by Mrs. R. at three time points spanning the period from July 1989 to December 1994. Penni's average 16-item CDC score was 23.44 ± 2.8 (well within the MPD range for her age). Her average 20-item score was 31.25 ± 3.5 (the 20-item CDC presented in Appendix Two, Version 3.0, was introduced in February 1990). In December 1994, Penni completed an A-DES with a mean score of 7.83 (a significant elevation). Although she was below our recommended age range, I asked her to complete a DES during the December 1994 interview as part of talking about

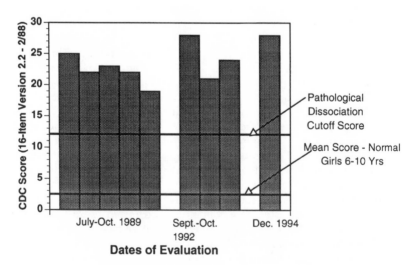

Figure 11.1. Penni's CDC scores over time.

her experiences. She scored a 73.2 (in the far upper pathological range). The item profiles of each measure were indicative of pathological dissociation.

Over a 5½-year period, there was good consistency in Penni's 16-item CDC scores and in the individual item scores. Strongly endorsed CDC items (i.e., average score of 1.5 or greater) included 2 (trance-like states), 3 (rapid changes in personality), 4 (unusual forgetfulness of information child should know), 6 (marked variations in skills, knowledge, and preferences), 8 (difficulty learning from experience), 9 (lying or denial of obvious behavior), 12 (unusual sexual precociousness), and 15 (vivid imaginary companionship). On the 20-item CDC, items 18 (unusual nighttime experiences), 19 (frequent conversations with self, perhaps using different voice or arguing with self), and 20 (two or more distinct and separate personalities that take control over behavior) were maximally endorsed at every time point.

Penni's self-reports of dissociative experiences on the A-DES and DES were also consistent with pathological dissociation. Penni strongly endorsed items related to periods of amnesia (recent and long-term autobiographical memory), depersonalization, passive influence experiences, and difficulty distinguishing actual events from thought and imagination.

Psychological and School Testing. Over the years, Penni received numerous psychological and academic evaluations for her behavioral and school problems. At age 6, her Wechsler Preschool and Primary Scale of Intelligence (WPPSI) indicated a Full Scale IQ of 105, with "significant scatter" (subscale scores ranging from low average to very superior). At age 9, she obtained a Full Scale IQ of 107 on the Wechsler Intelligence Scale for Children—Revised (WISC-R), again with "considerable scatter" reported on the subscale scores (e.g., 80 on Object Assembly and 125 on Vocabulary Picture Completion). At age 11, she had a WISC-R Full Scale IQ of 94, with "considerable variance between subtest scores." Her Wide Range Achievement Test—Revised (WRAT-R) indicated that she was 2 or more academic years behind in most areas. Penni also received yearly occupational therapy evaluations by the school system; these likewise evidenced considerable variation. Figure 11.2 is an example of the variations in Penni's ability to copy standard figures over four evaluations.

Penni's case was an example of persistent childhood MPD documented by different clinicians—as well as her adoptive parents and teachers—across many settings, over an extended length of time. Despite initial attempts to ignore and not reinforce her alter personality

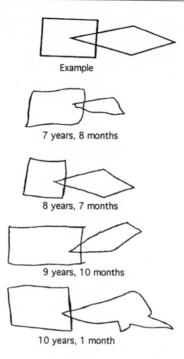

Example

7 years, 8 months

8 years, 7 months

9 years, 10 months

10 years, 1 month

Figure 11.2. Variations in Penni's copied figures over time.

states, these and other pathological dissociative symptoms persisted and came to play a major role in her psychological and behavioral problems. The case of Penni illustrates the consistency and chronicity of established alter personality states in some children.

CRYSTALLIZED ADOLESCENT MULTIPLE PERSONALITY DISORDER

TINA AND "GO-GO IN THE MIX"

Tina, a 15-year-old European-American 10th-grader, was hospitalized for sexual promiscuity, running away, mood swings, episodes of explosive anger, suicidal ideation, and the "delusional" conviction that she was an African-American. Her early history was marked by extreme poverty, family violence, and a history of alleged sexual abuse by her paternal grandfather. Most of her life had been spent in a house without running water. Her father was chronically unemployed, and the annual family income was estimated at $3,000. Tina and her sister were left in the care of her paternal grandparents while the mother worked. Her father was physically abusive toward the children and violently battered their mother. On several occasions, Tina witnessed potentially lethal assaults on her mother with knives and other weapons. When she was 7, her mother began treatment for depression at a community clinic, divorcing her husband shortly thereafter. Tina now lived with her mother and stepfather, who ran a "graphic arts" business. (I suspected, from the mother's extensive dermatological decorations, that this meant a tattoo parlor.)

Tina's sexual molestation was reported to have occurred between the ages of 4 and 10, while she stayed with the paternal grandparents; it allegedly included fondling and oral sex. Tina denied intercourse, but said that she had trouble remembering many details about the abuse. She said that she "blanked out" when she was near her grandfather. During the period of the alleged abuse, the mother remembered Tina as being obsessed with getting herself clean—difficult in a home without indoor plumbing.

Tina was a stocky adolescent with short hair; at the interview, she was dressed in jeans, a T-shirt, and a denim jacket. She appeared relaxed and willing to talk with me. She said that she was in the hospital to "get some things out." When I asked, "What sort of things?", she said that her grandfather had abused her. Then she volunteered that she could not remember much about it. I took a time loss history, asking for a couple of examples whenever Tina responded positively to a question. She described losing periods of time, often several times a day, particularly during school. She found herself in strange places with no memory of having gone there. The most dramatic example was finding herself talking with friends 2 days after she remembered having an argument with her stepfather. She said that she had some hazy memories, but that most of the time was unaccounted for. A recent example involved talking with her stepsister the day before, blanking out for a few moments, and finding the stepsister leaving angrily because of something Tina had said. She attributed this to "Taz" (which I learned was short for "Tasmanian Devil"), an alter personality state that said hurtful things.

We discussed the other "parts" of her. Tina said that she blanked out when they appeared, and that she only knew what people told her about them. "Go-Go in the Mix" was an African-American girl who was "not afraid of anything." Tina said that she was frightened whenever she found herself with "Go-Go"'s friends. "Go-Go" usually came out only around these friends, but occasionally got into fights with her parents, who were against her friendships with black people. "Go-Go" had many enemies, and Tina was fearful that they would find her instead of "Go-Go." "Taz" apparently only emerged for brief periods to do or say something hostile that would complicate Tina's life.

I asked whether it would be possible for me to meet with "Go-Go." Tina said that this was unlikely, because "Go-Go" would not come out in the hospital. Then she dropped her head, momentarily obscuring her face, and said in a different voice, "Why? So you can get rid of me?" Her voice and accent were not exactly African-American, but had some of those qualities. "Go-Go" described herself as half black and half white, with "sort of reddish skin." During this part of the interview, Tina developed a marked, blotchy, reddish rash that first appeared on her throat and spread to her face and arms. Following the reappearance of Tina, the rash began to fade. After we finished the interview, I showed the rash to her mother, who remarked that Tina always got that way when she was "upset."

"Go-Go" said that she was 15 and had first appeared when Tina was 13. She described herself as an "associate" of Tina's and was not angry with Tina, but also not very interested in her. "Go-Go" liked to "mess around" and especially enjoyed having sex with other girls' boyfriends, which she regarded as a personal challenge. She was concerned that the purpose of treatment was to get rid of her. "Go-Go" denied awareness of other parts of her mind; like Tina, she too lost time and found herself in strange places with no idea of what had happened. I asked for Tina to return, which prompted a discernible switch. Tina complained of dizziness and denied awareness of the conversation with "Go-Go."

Tina's case was one of crystallized adolescent MPD. The admitting psychiatrist said that he had never seen such a case before, but that he had no difficulty in making the diagnosis. In Tina's case there was ample preexisting evidence and independent corroboration of her shifts in identity states, complete with dermatological stigmata, language and accent changes, and dramatic alterations in self-image. Tina was lost to long-term follow-up when her family moved out of state.

NARCOLEPSY MISDIAGNOSED AS
MULTIPLE PERSONALITY DISORDER

Yvonne

Yvonne, an 11-year-old-girl, was diagnosed with MPD. She was referred for consultation because her therapist could find no evidence of abuse or trauma. Yvonne's problems began at approximately 8 years of age, when she complained of frightening nightmares that would not go away after she woke up. She was observed to have "falling-out" spells, during which she became limp and unresponsive for periods of seconds up to a few minutes. The spells could occur spontaneously, but were more often associated with sudden emotion (e.g., laughter or surprise). After a spell, there was a noticeable difference in Yvonne's personality: She would change from an even-tempered and compliant child to an argumentative and oppositional one, with anger, impulsivity, and poor frustration tolerance. She was also noted to be clumsier with decreased dexterity and sloppier handwriting. Although her IQ was found to be in the bright normal range, she was having serious academic difficulties at school. Prior to her being labeled as having MPD, Yvonne had received diagnoses of ADHD, dysthymia, and oppositional defiant disorder. At various points she had been treated with methylphenidate and amitriptyline, with some apparent improvement. All medication was discontinued when she was diagnosed as having MPD. Her therapist based the diagnosis of MPD on the presence of hallucinations, blanking out spells, and changes in personality associated with differences in motor skills.

Hearing the history, I arranged for Yvonne to have a neurological examination with a sleep-deprived EEG prior to seeing me. Her EEG was normal. During the examination she had an unresponsive spell, which the neurologist concluded was not a seizure because he could arouse her. He diagnosed a conversion disorder.

Yvonne was obese. She related well and talked easily about her symptoms. When asked about nightmares, she described seeing staring faces of dead people floating in the air. She also said that sometimes she could feel them touch her. The hallucinations primarily occurred at night while she was lying in the dark. Sometimes she had brief "nightmares" in school. These hallucinatory experiences were preceded by a "dizzy" feeling, which sounded more like a generalized weakness than like vertigo or syncope. She denied auditory hallucinations, amnesias, depersonalization, derealization, and passive influence experiences. She did not feel as if there were other parts to her that influenced or controlled her behavior.

Her parents, obviously aware of the child maltreatment implications of MPD, responded to my questions in a defensive manner. They denied any evidence of amnesias or memory problems, although Yvonne did have problems concentrating on her schoolwork. She was noted to fall asleep easily when riding in the car, watching television, or engaging in quiet activities at school. The personality changes typically followed a period of limp unresponsiveness, which was interpreted as willful and oppositional withdrawal. Each personality change was the same, and her mother likened it to the way Yvonne acted if she had been awakened with too little sleep. The behavioral shifts lasted 10–15 minutes, with the irritability and oppositionality gradually abating. No one had met a separate and discrete alter personality state. Yvonne always responded to her name and never insisted that she was someone else.

I felt that Yvonne did not have MPD, and that her symptoms

reflected either a complex partial seizure disorder or possibly narcolepsy, which I mistakenly believed to be rare in children. A second neurological evaluation was also negative, but she was referred to a sleep laboratory, where polysomnographic studies were consistent with narcolepsy. Yvonne's symptoms decreased markedly on protriptyline.

Yvonne's presenting "MPD" symptoms actually reflected hypnagogic hallucinations and cataplexy—two of the classic tetrad of narcolepsy symptoms. (The other two symptoms are excessive sleepiness and sleep paralysis [Aldrich, 1992]). Hypnagogic hallucinations occasionally occur during the "twilight state" between sleeping and waking in about 10% of people. They are considered normal and usually consist of visual images or simple auditory hallucinations, such as hearing one's name called. They are much more common in narcolepsy and can occur in the waking state during the day (e.g., Yvonne's "nightmares" at school). They are believed to be caused by dyscontrol of the REM dreaming mechanism. Cataplexy is a sudden temporary loss of muscle tone often precipitated by strong emotion. It is frequently followed by a brief period of sleep. Yvonne's personality changes and associated changes in coordination and motor skills following attacks of cataplexy probably reflected postsleep irritability and residual decreased muscle tone.

Yvonne's case reinforces that not everything that smacks of MPD is MPD. Child and adolescent narcolepsy is not nearly as rare as I once believed (Kavey, 1992; Dahl, Holttum, and Trubnick, 1994). Lifetime prevalence may be as common as 1 per 1,000, and roughly half of afflicted individuals report an onset of their condition during childhood or adolescence, although diagnosis is often not made until adulthood. The therapist who diagnosed Yvonne as having MPD made an all-too-common mistake of not exploring the symptoms and behaviors in depth. Atypical migraine headaches may also produce confused, dreamy states, disturbances in reality testing, and amnesias (Pelletier, Legendre-Roberge, Boileau, Geoffroy, and Leveille, 1995). On the other hand, children with MPD have been misdiagnosed as having narcolepsy (Lewis, 1996), and migraine headaches are extremely common in dissociative patients. Every child deserves a careful evaluation.

SUMMARY

Clinical presentations of pathological dissociation in children and adolescents resemble those of adults in taking on a variety of forms. Severe behavior problems, violence and aggression, self-injurious and suicidal behavior, depression and anxiety, and psychotic-like behavior are all encountered, separately and together. Cases may also present with classic dissociative symptoms, such as fugues (Carrie), pathological elaborated identities (Nancy/"the boy dog"), and crystallized alter personality states (Penni and Tina/"Go-Go in the Mix"). Several disorders, however, may be mistaken for pathological dissociation. These include narcolepsy (Yvonne), complex partial seizures, parasomnias, rapid-cycling bipolar disorder, atypical psychoses, and atypical migraines.

Chapter Twelve

Clinical Phenomenology and Diagnosis

A PHENOMENOLOGICAL APPROACH TO PEDIATRIC DISSOCIATIVE DISORDERS

Clinical phenomenology—the study of symptoms and behaviors in their own right, rather than from a theoretical point of view—has repeatedly proven itself as a useful starting place for the investigation of medical and psychiatric disorders. Clinical phenomenology, in the form of definitive syndromic descriptions, is also a core element of psychiatric diagnostic validity (Robins and Barrett, 1989). A well-replicated clinical phenomenology has been established for adult MPD. Smaller (but largely convergent) data bases exist for dissociative amnesia, dissociative fugue, and depersonalization disorder. Following the lead of adult investigations, child clinicians began the modern era of pediatric dissociative disorders with phenomenological studies.

Symptoms and Behaviors

More than a dozen clinical series and reviews have tabulated and discussed the range of clinical presentations of pathological dissociation in children and adolescents (e.g., see Vincent and Pickering, 1988; Dell and Eisenhower, 1990; Peterson, 1990, 1991; Hornstein and Putnam, 1992; Hornstein, 1993; Putnam, 1993c, 1994; Fleischer and Anderson, 1995; Pinegar, 1995; Lewis, 1996; Steinberg, 1996). Many contain lists or tables of symptoms and behaviors. Comparisons across studies find a high degree of overlap in profiles for what I have described in Chapter Five as primary dissociative, associated posttraumatic, secondary, and tertiary symptoms and behaviors (e.g., Vincent and Pickering, 1988; Peterson, 1991; Hornstein, 1993). Table 12.1 is a distillation of the literature and recent research data; the table is similar in structure to Table 5.1, but the emphasis here is on the symptoms and behaviors seen specifically in the *juvenile* population.

We (Hornstein and Putnam, 1992) examined 64 children and adolescents diagnosed by NIMH research criteria as having MPD or DDNOS. The average child had received 2.7 ± 1.3 psychiatric diagnoses prior to the dissociative disorder diagnosis. Affective and anxiety symptoms were prominent, including depression, affective lability, withdrawal/hopelessness, self-blame, and low self-esteem. Serious suicidal ideation was found in over half of the children. Almost half of the children diagnosed as having MPD had made a suicide attempt. Self-mutilation was also common in children diagnosed with MPD.

Conduct problems were present in over two-thirds of the cases, particularly aggression, explosive temper, disruptive and oppositional behaviors, hyperactivity, and truancy. Sexual behavior problems were present in about half of the cases. Teachers, parents, and foster parents described an array of academic difficulties, including reading problems, learning problems, distractibility, and difficulty concentrating. Posttraumatic symptoms—particularly intrusive symptoms, such as flashbacks, traumatic nightmares, and intrusive thoughts—were present in about three-quarters of cases. Hyperstartle and hypervigilance were also frequent clinical features.

Amnesias and dissociative memory problems were common, particularly for traumatic experiences. Trance-like states and rapid behavioral regression were present in virtually 100% of cases; rapid changes in demeanor were also common. Auditory hallucinations were reported in over three-quarters of the cases. Visual hallucinations were described in about half. Delusional or paranoid thinking was present in almost 20% of cases and could often be traced to intrusive and disturbing dissociative experiences (e.g., Hornstein and Putnam, 1992; Putnam, 1993c).

The numbers and types of dissociative symptoms differed somewhat by diagnosis. In general, MPD patients were far more symptomatic than patients diagnosed with DDNOS. Similar differences in the severity of dissociative symptoms were found in several studies (e.g., Hornstein and Putnam, 1992; Peterson and Putnam, 1994; Coons, 1996). MPD children were more likely to manifest amnesia for behaviors not related to traumatic or stressful situations. Passive influence/interference symptoms (e.g., "made" thoughts and feelings, automatisms) were seen in 60% of MPD cases, but were rare in DDNOS. There was a trend for MPD children to exhibit more of a dissociative "thought disorder" (see Chapter Five for a discussion).

By definition (i.e., NIMH dissociative disorder research criteria),

TABLE 12.1. Symptoms and Behaviors in Youths with Pathological Dissociation

Primary dissociative symptoms

Amnesias and memory symptoms

Amnesias, blackouts, time loss for complex behavior (e.g., emotional outbursts, fights, social activities)

Perplexing forgetfulness for basic information (e.g., names of best friends, ownership of possessions, asking permission to do something that they just did)

Inconsistent and fluctuating skills and abilities (e.g., academic, athletic, artistic, musical, social)

Inconsistent and dramatically alternating habits and preferences (e.g., different favorite colors, foods, or clothes)

Fugue episodes (generally involving travel for short distances)

Flashbacks and intrusive memories (may include abrupt disabling somatic symptoms)

Amnesias for the source of information (e.g., surprised by knowledge displayed on a test, musical, or language abilities)

Autobiographical information (inability to recall salient personal information or relevant prior personal history)

Dissociative process symptoms

Trance-like absence states (blanking out, vacant staring spells, excessive daydreaming)

Auditory hallucinations (distinct voices with gender, age, and affect attributes—usually, but not always, internalized)

Rapid behavioral regression (baby-like behavioral states)

Passive influence/interference experiences (inability to control behavior despite sincere efforts, physical struggles with self, compulsive masturbation, or self-mutilation, despite efforts to stop)

Distinct alter personality states; pathological elaborated indentities; persistent, vivid imaginary companionship with passive influence/interference effects)

Associated posttraumatic symptoms

Reexperiencing symptoms (may overlap with dissociative flashbacks and intrusive memories, reenactments, traumatic play, dreams without recognizable content, night terrors)

Avoidant symptoms (constriction of play, social withdrawal, decreased range of affect, behavioral regression, or loss of developmental skills and milestones)

Hyperarousal (ADHD-like behaviors, new fears, anxieties, or aggression)

Secondary symptoms

Depression

Anxiety

Affective lability (irritability, rapidly fluctuating mood states)

Low self-esteem

Somatization (rapidly fluctuating physical complaints—e.g., headaches, stomachaches, unusual pains without clear organic etiology)

TABLE 12.1. *(Continued)*

Tertiary symptoms

Suicidal ideation or attempts
Self-mutilation
Conduct problems (aggression, oppositional or disruptive behaviors)
Sexual behavior problems
Academic problems (learning problems, problems with concentration and distractibility, difficulties with problem solving that utilizes previously acquired information)

MPD cases had distinct alter personality states seen on three or more occasions. One or more alter personality state switches were witnessed by the examiner. Switch-like rapid behavioral shifts, such as changes in demeanor or marked behavioral regression, were common to both groups, but did not take the form of an identifiable personality state in the DDNOS children. The alter personalities of the MPD children included a range of protectors, helpers, and companions. Although not tabulated, nonhuman alter personalities (e.g., animals, robots, superheroes) were common.

Age and Gender Differences

To explore possible age and gender differences in dissociative and related symptoms, we combined cases from two separate studies that used the same symptom checklist (Putnam, Hornstein, and Peterson, 1996b). This yielded a sample of 177 children and adolescents (mean age = 10.7 ± 4.2 years). Cases were grouped into four age groups: preschoolers (2.5–5.9 years), school age (6–11.9 years), early adolescence (12–15.9 years), and late adolescence (16–20 years). These analyses were cross-sectional; therefore, developmental trajectories are only inferred, not demonstrated. Longitudinal studies, not available to date, are required for a true sorting out of developmental pathways.

A comparison of the female-to-male ratios across age groups found a steady increase in the percentage of females with age. By late adolescence, 83% of cases were female—a finding congruent with the high (6:1–9:1) female-to-male ratios reported in adult samples (e.g., Putnam et al., 1986; Coons et al., 1988; Ross et al., 1991). As discussed in Chapter Nine, the reasons for the preponderance of females in adolescent and adult samples are not well understood.

Analysis of gender differences found females to have more anxiety symptoms, posttraumatic symptoms, sleep problems, sexual behavior problems, and somatic complaints than males had. There was a trend for females to have more eating problems, whereas males showed a trend toward more conduct problems. There were no gender differences in dissociative symptoms.

Other age-related symptomatic differences were not striking or surprising. In general, older subjects were more symptomatic than younger children. For example, late adolescents had more eating disorder symptoms, amnesias, passive influence/interference symptoms, and somatization than preschoolers and school-age children. Dissociative and posttraumatic symptoms showed a tendency to increase steadily with age—albeit not significantly in many instances (Putnam et al., 1996b). The percentages of many symptoms appeared to peak in early adolescence and then to decline somewhat by late adolescence. This may reflect a social desirability effect, as older adolescents often deny having "crazy" symptoms such as hallucinations and self-mutilation.

Differential Diagnosis

Virtually all studies of the clinical phenomenology of dissociative disorder patients report significant psychiatric comorbidity, prolonged treatment histories, and multiple past psychiatric, neurological, and medical diagnoses (e.g., Putnam et al., 1986; Coons et al., 1988; Ross et al., 1989d, 1990; Schultz et al., 1989; Loewenstein and Putnam, 1990). Retrospectively sorting out legitimate comorbid diagnoses from misdiagnoses of pathological dissociation is impossible. What can be concluded from this well-replicated finding is that all age groups with pathological dissociation acquire a relatively large number of diagnoses. A history of polydiagnosis should be regarded as a clinical sign and should increase the index of suspicion for pathological dissociation.

Table 12.2 lists differential diagnoses to be considered together with pathological dissociation. Dissociative symptoms and behaviors that may resemble the primary condition are given in parentheses. Children with pathological dissociation may have acquired one or more of these diagnoses. In some instances, this reflects genuine comorbidity of two or more disorders; in other instances, it is likely that dissociative symptoms are being mistakenly attributed to another process (e.g., rapid-cycling bipolar illness). Pathological dissociation should be considered in the differential diagnosis of each of these conditions; and each of these conditions should be considered in the differential diagnosis of pathological dissociation. In a few instances, the DSM will flag dissociative disorders in the differential diagnosis; for example, dissociative disorders are listed in the rule-out criterion for ADHD (American Psychiatric Association, 1994). In most instances, however, clinicians are on their own.

TABLE 12.2. Differential Diagnosis of Pathological Dissociation in Youths

Attention-deficit/hyperactivity disorder (ADHD)

Restlessness; difficulty concentrating; fluctuating academic abilities; memory impairments; distractions produced by dissociative hallucinations and passive influence/interference experiences

Conduct disorder

Denial of misbehaviors secondary to amnesias (apparent lying); explosive anger; apparent lack of remorse for misbehavior and aggression

Rapid-cycling bipolar disorder

Alter personality switches misinterpreted as "mood swings"; irritability and anger; suicidal behaviors; hypersexuality; grandiosity; depression

Schizophrenia and other psychotic disorders

Auditory hallucinations; passive influence/interference experiences; dissociative "thought disorder"; thought insertion–withdrawal

Seizure disorder

Amnesia for complex behavior; depersonalization; automatisms

Borderline personality disorder (BPD)

Disturbances in identity and integrity of self; mood swings; suicidal and self-mutilating behavior; transient psychotic-like symptoms

---

Unusual cases should also raise a suspicion of dissociative disorders. For example, Jacobsen (1995) describes a 15-year-old with selective mutism in school. This was a response to threats made to him after he witnessed the murder of a sibling. Treatment for dissociation led to resolution of the mutism and improved academic performance.

DIAGNOSTIC APPROACHES

General Principles and Aims

The diagnosis of pathological dissociation in children and adolescents rests on four general principles. First, there must be a thorough evaluation according to the standards of psychiatric practice to rule out other conditions (American Academy of Child and Adolescent Psychiatry, 1995). Second, there must be good evidence of persistent pathological dissociation documented through multiple informants. Third, pathological dissociative symptoms must cross at least two major domains of a child's or adolescent's life (e.g., home, school, peer relationships). Finally, pathological dissociation must provide a parsimonious explanation for the troubling symptoms and behavior.

I would emphasize the first two principles in particular. That is, a dissociative disorder diagnosis should never be made without a careful evaluation and documentation of persistent pathological dissociation. A thorough workup is especially necessary in children and adolescents. In too many instances, dissociative disorder diagnoses—particularly MPD—are bestowed cavalierly. Just as all hallucinations do not signify schizophrenia, all dissociation does not equal MPD. Significant dissociation occurs in about half of PTSD patients and may be present to a lesser extent in other psychiatric disorders (Putnam et al., 1996a). Transient dissociation occurs in some acute stress responses.

The diagnostic approach differs to some extent, depending on whether a clinician is serving as an outside consultant for a time-limited evaluation or is seeing a child or adolescent as a potential patient/client for treatment. Although some maintain that there can be no distinction between evaluation and treatment, in reality there often must be. By and large, therapy for pathological dissociation is a long-term proposition. Consultants should not attempt treatment or major therapeutic interventions. Appropriate clarification and explanation during the course of an evaluation are helpful for a child and family, but attempts to work with alter personality states or to initiate major treatment regimens should be left to the designated clinicians. Too many therapists spoil the therapy.

The aims of diagnostic assessment include (1) determination of the reasons and causes for the referral; (2) determination of the nature and severity of the symptoms, behavioral problems, and impairments, and the level of the child's distress; and (3) identification of those factors (individual, family, and environmental) that may contribute to or mitigate the situation (American Academy of Child and Adolescent Psychiatry, 1995).

Gathering Information Prior to the First Interview

Outside information (e.g., school records, medical records, psychological testing, agency and juvenile system reports, etc.) should always be requested—and pursued when it is not immediately provided. Whenever possible, these records should be obtained and reviewed prior to the first meeting. I organize the information chronically and read forward in time, cross-checking among the different sources at given time points (e.g., school records against hospital discharge summaries for the child at the same age). This provides a rudimentary life course scaffold, alerts me to salient issues, and flags discrepancies. Often various working hypotheses emerge that give me a head start.

Interviewing Parents

Children do not bring themselves in for psychiatric evaluation; they are brought in by those responsible for them. With young children, it is best to interview the parents or relevant caretakers first. The reasons and circumstances leading up to an evaluation are usually best obtained from a child's primary caretaker. Some clinical models stress seeing the whole family as the unit of evaluation; however, I prefer to interview the parents or primary caretaker first. Later, if I feel that it is indicated, I will include siblings, grandparents, or other relevant individuals. Usually more than one interview is required for an adequate understanding of the situation.

What to Look For

The clinician needs to obtain a clear and explicit description of the problems that have led to the evaluation, followed by a history of the development of the problems, and a description of their impact on individual family members and on the family as a whole. The child's development must be understood in the context of the family. The clinician is generating a working picture of the child, parents, and family, including their level of functioning, their medical and psychiatric problems, and their community and cultural setting.

Questions should be asked with tact and sensitivity, particularly with respect to cultural and ethnic differences in child-rearing practices. Pertinent historical information (e.g., age, birth history, developmental milestones, and prior treatment) is best obtained by asking specific questions. Information about symptoms and behaviors should at first be elicited with general, open-ended questions. As much as possible, parents should be allowed to talk freely, but time constraints often require a more narrowly focused interview after a while. The clinician must always remember that in addition to gathering information, he or she is seeking rapport and a working relationship with the most important people in the child's life.

The clinician should listen carefully to the content and to the affect of the parents' answers. In addition, the parents' general health and grooming, intelligence and education, self-esteem, competency, and attitudes toward the child should be observed throughout the interview. The clinician is looking in particular for parenting difficulties, such as punitive parenting, major parental psychopathology, or serious deficits in the ability to care for the child. It is also important to be alert for less serious problems, such as intermittent parental depressions or serious marital conflicts that disrupt continuity of adequate care.

Checking Parents' Reports against Other Information

Unfortunately, parents may be poor historians. Yarrow, Campbell, and Burton (1970) prospectively showed that normal parents misrecalled many salient facts about their children's behavior and abilities over periods as short as 36 months. The clinician should always be alert to the possibility (in some families, the likelihood) that important information is being omitted, either deliberately or "unconsciously." Discrepancies in parental reports about symptoms and problems are common. These are usually attributable to differences in the parents' exposure to their child's behaviors, access to the child's subjective feelings, differences in how they perceive and interpret events, and differences in their abilities to conceptualize and articulate information.

In practice, information is frequently obtained from prior records, as noted above. Whenever possible, clinicians should make independent inquiries to gather information and to confirm the accuracy of records. Too exclusive a reliance on "records" is a serious mistake, however; all too often, they contain misinformation and/or are missing the really important information.

Checking with multiple informants is always a good practice in child evaluations. It is critical for the diagnosis of pathological dissociation. Teachers are often good sources of information. Grades may show remarkable fluctuations (e.g., A's to D's from one marking period to the next). Teachers' comments, however, are usually the most revealing (Lewis, 1996). They will remark on a child's perplexing forgetfulnesses, trance-like or daydreaming states, behavioral regressions, identity alterations, and variations in skills and knowledge. Teachers can be given the CDC to complete, although several questions pertain to behaviors that are not likely to be encountered in the classroom (e.g., sleepwalking or vivid ICs). Dissociative children are frequently very different in the classroom than they are at home, so there may be significant discrepancies between parent and teacher reports for some behaviors. It is important to weigh and resolve such discrepancies before making a definitive diagnosis.

Developmental History

Developmental history covers a large number of topics. The American Academy of Child and Adolescent Psychiatry (1995) details these in its assessment guidelines. The basic list includes (1) cognitive functioning; (2) school history; (3) peer relations; (4) family relationships; (5) physical development and medical history; (6) temperament and emotional development; (7) values, morals, and conscience; and (8) interests, talents, and hobbies. The clinician needs to get some idea of the child's general social skills, as well as the quality of his or her play alone and with others. A history of significant events is mandatory, including witnessed and experienced trauma, separations, losses, accidents, moves, school changes, and so on.

Family and Community History

A history of the family is important—that is, marriages, divorces, deaths, and siblings' lives. In addition, what is the family's educational, occupational, and financial situation? What social and community resources are available? Family pathology (e.g., alcoholism, mental and physical illness, legal problems, etc.) must also be inquired about. Genograms, supplemented with pertinent notations, are a useful way of summarizing this information.

Interviewing Children

A preschooler or young child should be present during the first interview with the parents or primary caretaker. This provides an excellent opportunity to observe caretaking/state-modulating behavior toward the child under stressful circumstances that divide the parents' attention. The clinician is looking at the quality of the parent–child interactions, the "goodness of fit" or lack thereof, and the ability of the parents/caretaker to recognize and respond to the child's needs and behavior. Children, including preschoolers, are keen listeners; a child will be registering the content of the interview and reacting to the parents' affect and attitudes, even when the child appears oblivious to the adult conversation. The clinician should discreetly observe the changes in the child's behavior and play as the parents talk about different issues and problems. It may also be necessary to see the parents alone, to talk about specific issues with them and to allow them to say things about the child in private.

After the parents are interviewed, it is important to see the child alone. Techniques for interviewing children and adolescents are well reviewed elsewhere (e.g., Lewis, 1991; American Academy of Child and Adolescent Psychiatry, 1995). Infants and toddlers require special techniques, especially direct observation of caretaker–child interactions. Overall goals include history taking, assessment of the child's developmental levels, and examination of his or her mental status.

Getting the Child's View of the Problem

A child should not be expected to provide a coherent statement about what the problem is or why he or she has been brought for evaluation. Rather, the clinician should look for a symbolic representation of the child's understanding of the problem in his or her play and/or interactions with the parents or clinician.

WILSON

Wilson, a 4-year-old boy with extensive congenital hand deformities, was referred for evaluation of violent, self-abusive, possibly dissociative temper tantrums. His parents were engaged in a protracted lawsuit against the obstetrician for prescribing an allegedly teratogenic medication. The mother did not accompany the father to the first interview. As he related the problem and history, the father's affect was wooden—until he broke into tears as he talked about not being able to play baseball or football with his only son. (Wilson had two normal sisters who were active in sports.)

Alone with me, Wilson spent his time separating and grouping various toy figures. The groupings did not make obvious sense; they included figures of different races, styles, and sizes. When I asked why certain figures were placed together, Wilson showed me their hands. This key determined who belonged in which "families." Play figures were grouped according to how completely their fingers were represented. By this criterion, Wilson did not belong in his family. He proved not to have a dissociative disorder.

Wilson's perception of his situation was readily discernible because of his physical representation of belonging. Unfortunately, children's "play" expressions of their world and their problems are not always as transparent as Wilson's. Children are always trying to tell adults something, but exactly what is often open to interpretation. A clinician has to take in what a child presents, but must refrain from jumping to conclusions. The possibilities of misunderstanding, overinterpretation, and downright projection of the therapist's concerns into the "meaning" of the child's play are always present.

The Evaluation Setting

When a clinician controls his or her clinical environment, it is possible to create a coherent and therapeutic clinical space in which to conduct evaluations and treatment. (See the discussion of "therapeutic space" in Chapter Thirteen.) Unfortunately, many of us share our clinical space with others, or it must double for other purposes. In some instances I see children in my office, which is cluttered with research in progress. Occasionally I can schedule the use of a playroom; however, this is shared with numerous others, and thus is continually changing in content and configuration. The best I can do is to create a consistent subspace within the larger space, as I describe in more detail in Chapter Thirteen. Only a few simple toys are necessary: paper and crayons, a doll, a few neutral Lego-type figures (i.e., no thematic action figures such as GI Joe), a toy house of some sort, a pair of friendly-looking puppets (one for the clinician and one for the child), and some blocks. Computers—now common in clinic settings—are a big distraction. I make sure to turn them off and clearly designate them as off limits.

In some cases, I must travel to a hospital or residential facility to evaluate a child who is restricted as a suicide or elopement risk. Here things are even less controlled. For example, Tina ("Go-Go in the Mix"; see Chapter Eleven) was interviewed in a medical examination room. I brought in two chairs and placed them so as to screen off the examination table and medical paraphernalia as much as possible. Confidentiality is especially important to adolescents, and this was the only truly private place on the ward. I began our interview by commenting on the nature of the interview room and wondering what she thought of it. She said that she preferred it to the other options offered us by the staff. For some children, such a setting with its medical implications may be frightening, and another arrangement will be necessary. The clinician should do whatever is possible to provide a safe, private, and conducive evaluation environment.

Asking Children about Pathological Dissociative Experiences

I remain skeptical that clinicians can reliably ask children younger than 7–8 years of age meaningful questions about dissociative experiences and be reasonably certain of what their answers mean. This does not mean that younger children cannot be assessed for pathological dissociation; it does mean that evaluation depends more on behavioral observations and interactions than on the answers to an interviewer's questions. A similar age limitation is encountered in structured interview research with children. Most child researchers do not trust structured diagnostic interview data on children younger than about 9 years of age.

Older children and adolescents can and should be asked about dissociative experiences during a psychiatric evaluation, but clinicians must carefully weigh positive answers against other clinical data. No set of questions encompasses the range of developmental, cultural, and intellectual differences routinely encountered by professionals working with traumatized children. The following examples are meant to illustrate types of questions that have proven fruitful in clinical situations. I do not make any proprietary claims, and freely acknowledge that I borrow a good clinical probe any time I hear one.

Amnesias and perplexing forgetfulness

"Do you get back tests or homework that you don't remember doing?" [If yes:] "Can you give me an example?" or "Can you tell me more about that?"

"Have you gone to do something and found that you have already done it?"

"Do you find yourself doing something or going somewhere and you don't know why?"

"Do you surprise yourself because you know something and you don't know where you learned it?"

"Do you have a problem deciding whether you have already done something or just thought about doing it?"

"Do you go to do something and find that you have forgotten what you were going to do?"

"Are you so good at acting or lying that you fool yourself?"

"Do you find that you can't remember things that you think that you should be able to remember?"

"Do people tell you about things that you think that you should remember, but you can't?"

Depersonalization/derealization

"Do you ever feel that you are in a fog, or that things around you seem unreal, as in a dream?"

"Do you ever not recognize yourself when you look in a mirror?"

"Do you feel like you are standing outside of your body, watching yourself as if you were watching another person?"

"Does your body, or parts of your body (like your hands), ever look or feel as if it or they do not belong to you?"

Passive influence/interference experiences

"Do you have strong feelings that do not feel as if they are your feelings?"

"Do you find that you can't make your body do what you want to do?"

"Do you find yourself doing something that you don't want to do, but you can't stop yourself?"

Identity alteration

"Do you ever not recognize your own name when someone calls you?"

"Do you act so differently at times that you feel like a different person?"

"Do you have a special or secret friend who goes with you everywhere and that other people can't see?"

Trance states and "spacing out"

"Does it sometimes seem that everyone else in school was told something that you weren't?"

"Do you find that the class has moved on to another subject and you didn't notice the change?"

"Do you notice that time has gone by and you don't remember what has happened?"

"Do you have a special place in your mind that you go to if things are not going well?"

Auditory hallucinations

"Do you argue with yourself out loud?"

"Do you hear voices in your head?"

"Sometimes children who are frightened or lonely can talk with someone in their minds. Has this ever happened to you?"

Whenever a child or adolescent gives a positive or seemingly positive answer, it is critical to follow up by asking for more information and examples. These examples are the real data. They must be carefully examined and, whenever possible, corroborated. The examples and elaborations will indicate whether the youngster has correctly understood the question and is having pathological dissociative experiences. The questions and examples should be recorded as close to verbatim as possible, as they provide important documentation.

Observing Dissociative Behaviors during an Interview

Dissociative symptoms during an interview are typically manifested in marked shifts and/or discontinuities in ongoing behavior. For example, a child may stop and stare blankly, be unresponsive to the interviewer, or engage in perseverative repetitive movements. If this happens, the interviewer should gently but persistently attempt to get the child's attention, and should note any circumstances that may be associated with the onset of the episode. (Videotapes of such behavior make it clear that sometimes the triggering stimulus is not directly related to the interviewer's behavior, but occurs in response to the child's own play sequence or to a background event.)

When the child becomes available again, the clinician should gently ask about what was happening, or what he or she was thinking about just a moment ago. Often the child cannot describe what has happened. Sometimes, however, dissociative children describe a passive influence/interference experience that impedes their volitional behavior. For example, one MPD boy described being made to wait for a mental traffic light to turn green before he could talk again.

Intrainterview amnesias may also be manifested in the child's repeatedly asking a question that has been previously answered, or by a sudden discontinuity in or preplexity about the current interview/play sequence. When asked what they remember about the immediately preceding events, dissociative children often can provide little or no information, or just say that they "forgot." Questions about similar experiences may help clarify the frequency of such time loss experiences.

Sometimes a child exhibits a marked change in demeanor—for instance, suddenly going from quiet and withdrawn to loud and boisterous, or from age-appropriate to markedly regressed. The child can be asked directly about such differences: "Just a minute ago, you were walking around yelling loudly. Now you are sitting and sucking your thumb. Did you feel different when you were yelling then you do now?" Apparent intrainterview examples of dissociative behavior provide an important opportunity to ask the child about what is happening and to inquire about similar experiences elsewhere. The intention is to clarify what is happening with the immediate example, and how it may relate to other experiences the child has at home or school.

Play and Projective Interview Techniques

Many child therapists use interactive play techniques to interview children. Typically these include imaginative play with puppets, dolls, or small figures. Interactive imaginative play can be an important means of assessing social interactions, as well as the range and regulation of affects and impulses. An experienced professional can often make significant inferences about the child's concerns and perceptions (American Academy of Child and Adolescent Psychiatry, 1995).

Formal and informal projective techniques are also helpful. A common technique is drawing a picture and talking about it; asking the child what kind of animal he or she would most like to be and least like to be is another simple projective approach. "What would you wish for if you could have three wishes?" and "Who and what would you take to a desert island?" are other traditional child interview questions. A child can also be asked to complete a story stem, such as what happens when a baby bird falls out of its nest. Having the child describe a dream, book, or television show may tap the child's interests, concerns, and preoccupations.

Projective and play techniques are often informative and may be rapport-building. However, the clinician must be careful not to overinterpret the content or to introduce distortions. In my opinion, some child therapists give too much weight to their interpretation of a few drawings or a therapeutic play sequence, and not enough to systematically documenting dissociative symptoms and behaviors across different contexts. I do not believe that pathological dissociation can be diagnosed from artwork or play sequences alone. Diagnosis must rest on the principles enumerated above.

Physical Examination

Psychiatrists and psychologists tend to neglect the physical examination as part of the diagnostic evaluation. This is unfortunate, since even a "normal" examination often contains useful information (e.g., surgical scars, presence or absence of cutting or bruising) that may be factored into the evaluation. For children and adolescents, the physical examination is important, because they are much less likely than adults to volunteer pertinent information or to make connections between physical problems and psychological symptoms. Lewis (1996) observes that for maltreated children, the physical examination is especially important for a number of reasons. These include assessing the physical basis for any somatic symptoms and complaints; providing assurance to the child that his or her body is intact and not irreparably damaged; and documenting any signs of physical or sexual abuse. A physical exam at the time of evaluation also establishes a baseline for monitoring medication side effects.

In many instances, it is likely that the therapist will refer the examination to a pediatrician or physician's assistant. It is important to brief this examiner ahead of time, and tactfully to reinforce a sensitivity to the child's concerns and responses. The examination should be explained to the child both beforehand and on a step-by-step basis as it is being conducted. Whenever possible, the child's assent should be obtained. The exam should be conducted in the presence of an adult not suspected to be associated with maltreatment. Restraint or force should be avoided.

The physical examination should include measurements of height and weight, which should be entered on standard growth charts to determine whether the child is growing normally. Head size is important to rule out microcephaly or hydrocephaly. The examiner should be alert to physical stigmata, particularly those associated with chromosomal abnormalities or prenatal toxicity. Secondary sex characteristics can be coded by Tanner stage, providing another index of development.

The skin should be inspected for scarring and bruising; hair and nails should be examined for pulling, picking, and biting. Nutritional state is important to detect anorexia or neglect. Gait, gross and fine motor coordination, balance, left–right discrimination, reflexes, muscle strength, and eye tracking should all be assessed. Neurological "soft signs" are of interest, because they suggest possible organicity or neurodevelopmental immaturity. It has been suggested that asymmetry of reflexes or motor tone may be associated with deprivational states (Lewis, 1991). Dental examinations may also provide critical evidence of abuse. An analysis of the sites of injury in abused children found that the largest percentage occurred to the face and mouth (Jessee, 1995).

The examiner should be prepared either to collect all necessary forensic evidence, or to stop the examination to avoid contaminating evidence until a properly equipped and trained examiner can complete the exam. Forensic evidence includes physical specimens (e.g., semen, hair, blood), photographic evidence (both color and black-and-white photos that include a scale to document size of injuries, etc.), and laboratory data (e.g., blood work, vaginal cultures). The examiner must be prepared to establish a "chain of custody" for all evidence. The American Medical Association (1993) has published detailed guidelines for conducting physical examinations of suspected child abuse.

SCREENING MEASURES AND INTERVIEWS FOR PATHOLOGICAL DISSOCIATION IN YOUTHS

An essential feature of the Robins and Guze (1970) model for the validity of a disorder is the existence of "laboratory tests" that serve as external validators for a given diagnosis (see the discussion of validity in Chapter Five). Unfortunately, no one has yet developed a reliable and valid laboratory test for any major psychiatric disorder. In the absence of laboratory standards, clinicians employ dimensional scales and questionnaires, as well as structured diagnostic interviews. Such measures improve the reliability of psychiatric classification and insure a greater consistency in the way in which psychiatric diagnosis is conducted. Nonetheless, psychiatric diagnosis still leaves much to be desired.

Validated dissociative screening measures and structured diagnostic interviews for adults have reshaped the field. (See the discussion of the measurement of dissociation in Chapter Four.) In the early to mid-1980s, a number of clinicians independently generated symptom profiles to aid in identifying dissociative children and adolescents (e.g., Elliot, 1982; Fagan and McMahon, 1984; Kluft, 1985a; Putnam, 1985b). Comparisons revealed many similarities in the features that their authors thought salient to pathological dissociation in children (see discussions in Putnam, 1986b; Peterson, 1990). Items from these early predictor lists constitute the core of current child and adolescent dissociation scales and interviews (Evers-Szostak and Sanders, 1992; Reagor et al., 1992; Tyson, 1992; Putnam et al., 1993). Here, I focus the bulk of my discussion on those measures with which I am most familiar—namely, those that I have authored or coauthored.

The Child Dissociative Checklist

The CDC is derived from a symptom profile that I circulated among child protection workers in 1981. Early versions were published as footnotes or tables by other authors (e.g., Elliot, 1982; Kluft, 1985a) prior to our validation article (Putnam et al., 1993). The most commonly encountered versions are labeled "2.2—2/88" and "3.0—2/90." The former is a 16-item checklist. The latter has 20 items, which include all of the Version 2.2 items in the same order, permitting easy comparison. I encourage readers to copy and use the CDC. It is a public domain document and may be reproduced and distributed without special permission. A reproducible copy is included in Appendix Two. (Readers who wish to tinker with it should change the name to reduce confusion for others.)

The CDC is an observer report measure and uses a 3-point scale response format (i.e., 2 = "very true," 1 = "somewhat or sometimes true," and 0 = "not true"). The time frame in the instructions covers the present and the prior 12 months. Clinicians are free to specify another time frame as appropriate (e.g., the preceding week) when the CDC is completed weekly as part of a longitudinal evaluation or treatment outcome measure.

The CDC score is the sum of all of the item scores and can range from 0 to 40 on Version 3.0. Table 12.3 gives scores for different groups of children by age. The table shows that healthy, nonmaltreated normal children generally score very low on the CDC, with younger children scoring slightly higher. As a group, maltreated children score significantly higher than normals; however, they score significantly below children with diagnosable dissociative disorders. MPD children score uniformly high at each age point, with DDNOS children falling close below on average. The large standard deviations in the pathological groups indicate

TABLE 12.3. CDC Scores for Different Groups by Age

Group	Age (years)	Mean	SD	n
Normal	5–8	3.2	2.9	54
	9–11	2.9	1.0	42
	12–16	1.9	1.9	96
Maltreated	5–8	10.3	8.7	39
	9–11	6.1	6.5	87
	12–16	4.2	1.9	129
MPD	5–8	24.1	8.5	9
	9–11	23.8	9.7	12
	12–16	22.3	9.1	26
DDNOS	5–8	21.4	9.1	19
	9–11	16.5	6.9	8
	12–16	20.0	8.0	19

that a wide range of scores can be expected with a subgroup of high scorers. As a general rule of thumb, a score of 12 or higher is considered an indication of pathological dissociation, and further evaluation is warranted.

Reliability and Validity

Several studies of the reliability and validity show the CDC to be a reliable instrument. For example, the mean Cronbach's alpha was .86 in three studies, and the mean test–retest reliability was .74 in two studies (Malinosky-Rummell and Hoier, 1991; Putnam et al., 1993; Putnam and Peterson, 1994; Wherry, Jolly, Feldman, Adam, and Manjanatha, 1994).

The validity of the CDC has been primarily assessed in terms of its ability to discriminate among groups. Studies to date have found that sexually abused children score significantly higher than nonabused comparison children (Malinosky-Rummell and Hoier, 1991; Putnam et al., 1993; Wherry et al., 1994). Three studies indicate that the CDC can discriminate children with dissociative disorders from abused and nonabused children without dissociative disorders. In three studies (Hornstein and Putnam, 1992; Putnam et al., 1993; Putnam and Peterson, 1994), children with MPD had median scores of 25, 24, and 25, respectively, whereas children with DDNOS had median scores of 16.8, 16.5, and 18.2, respectively. In one study (Putnam and Peterson, 1994), scores on the CDC as completed by parents and caretakers were significantly correlated with scores on item-equivalent dissociation scales completed by the children's primary therapists. Clinicians using the CDC typically report similar results. For example, the mean scores for diagnostically mixed groups of child and adolescent dissociative patients were 16.6 and 23, respectively, in two recent studies (Coons, 1996; Yeager and Lewis, 1996). In sum, the CDC has proven to be internally consistent, reliable over time, and generally able to discriminate children with pathological dissociation from those without.

Cautions

A number of cautions should be kept in mind. First, the CDC scores reported in Table 12.3 are means; they reflect the "average" child in a given group. Second, individual children (both traumatized and nontraumatized) can and do exhibit variation on the CDC, as well as on other measures. Thus a high score does not prove that a child has a dissociative disorder; nor does a low score guarantee that a child does not have a dissociative disorder. In addition, there is variability in the way in which adult report measures such as the CDC are completed by parents, foster parents, teachers, and other informants. This problem exists for all adult report child measures. Finally, the CDC is but an indicator of the presence or absence of pathological dissociation. High and low scores must be weighed within the larger clinical context. Therefore, the CDC is best used as a screening instrument for detection of possible pathological dissociation during evaluation, and as an index of a degree of dissociation for purposes of research and treatment evaluation.

Factors Influencing Scores

Developmental and individual variables (e.g., age, gender, ethnicity, parental education, etc.) must be factored into an interpretation of a CDC score. (See the discussion of age and gender effects in Chapter Nine.) In general, CDC scores decrease with age (Putnam, 1996a). Current data suggest that the rate of this decline varies across normal and clinical groups. Our findings indicate that nontraumatized children, even at young ages, have very low scores. Between the ages of 6 and 16, the decline in CDC scores is modest but significant, $r (134) = -.19$, $p = .02$. The age-related decline in scores for maltreated children is actually somewhat steeper, $r (121) = -.34$, $p = .0001$. Children with dissociative disorders (MPD and DDNOS), particularly those with MPD, show essentially no decline in CDC scores over the same age range. Thus, for most groups CDC scores do decline with age, but in the most extreme cases they do not.

We know less about the effects of gender and culture on CDC scores. I am certain that these factors influence reported scores in some cases, and probably more so for children than for adults. Certain social behaviors that the CDC inquires about (e.g., sexual and aggressive behaviors) also differ significantly by gender and probably often by culture, although little is known about these factors.

Research Uses

The CDC is designed to be both a clinical and a research tool. As new information is rapidly accruing, researchers should review the most current literature before embarking on a CDC study. In general, the CDC can be used to quantify dissociative behavior for dimensional approaches and to generate cutoff scores to categorize children into low- and high-dissociation groups.

Clinical Uses

The CDC is employed clinically in three basic ways. Its first use is as a routine screening instrument given in a clinical setting. For example, parents can be asked to fill out the CDC, together with other parent report measures such as the Child Behavior Checklist (CBCL), when they bring their child for evaluation/treatment. In selected cases, the CDC can be sent to teachers or others who know the child reasonably well. When filling out the scale, teachers should be told to ignore items 17 and 18, which inquire about nocturnal behavior. After a period of observation on inpatient units, designated staff members can complete the CDC for an assigned child. Again, allowances should be made for an observer's familiarity with the child, particularly across different staff shifts. As noted above, the source and reliability of all scores need to be considered in the clinical context.

Second, for finer-grained screening, the CDC can be serially completed by a designated observer. For children in whom there is reason to suspect pathological dissociative behaviors, parents, foster parents, or others can complete the CDC weekly or monthly for a period of time. In nondissociative children, there is often a small increase (1–3 points) over the first few completions, because the questions draw attention to minor dissociative behaviors that were previously ignored. Clinicians should be looking for evidence of sustained pathological dissociation—that is, for CDC scores that are consistently 12 or higher (e.g., see the case of Penni, Chapter Eleven and Figure 11.1).

When using the CDC in this fashion, I ask parents to keep a log of examples of the behaviors that they are endorsing on the CDC. I review this with them as a quality check on how they are completing the scale. As with any measure, questions on the CDC can be misunderstood. However, I find that parents use the scale pretty much as intended, and that they rarely endorse items inappropriately. The consistently low scores for normal subjects across different studies support this.

Lastly, the CDC can be used as a rough index of treatment progress. There is less experience with this mode, but preliminary results indicate that the CDC provides a reasonable indication of whether or not a child is improving with time or treatment. In several acute trauma cases elevated CDC scores declined to normal ranges over a 2- to 3-month period, supporting clinical observations that the children were improving. In other instances (e.g., the case of Penni), repeated administations of the CDC over several years suggested that little improvement occurred.

The Adolescent Dissociative Experiences Scale

As experience with the CDC accumulated, it became apparent that its utility during adolescence is limited. This is a result of parents' rapidly decreasing familiarity with the details of a teenager's life, compared with the life of a younger child. Adolescents are also (somewhat) better observers of their own behavior than children; thus, for teenagers, a self-report scale offers a reasonable approach to screening for pathological dissociation.

The A-DES was designed to fill this need. The A-DES is a collaborative effort among a number of individuals organized by Judith Armstrong, Eve Bernstein Carlson, and myself (see Armstrong, Putnam, and Carlson, in press). A reproducible, public domain copy of the A-DES is included in Appendix Three. The 30-item A-DES surveys dissociative amnesias; absorption and imaginative involvement (including confusion between reality and fantasy); depersonalization and derealization; passive influence/interference experiences; and dissociated identity experiences. Items are neutrally worded so as not to upset adolescents. The answer response format is a 0–10 scale, anchored at the ends with "never" (0) and "always" (10).

Items are generally worded in the present tense, and the temporal frame of reference is the present and recent past—in accordance with the "anything before yesterday is ancient history" adolescent frame of reference. The subject circles the number that best describes how often a given experience happens. On the face sheet, respondents are instructed not to count experiences that occur under the influence of alcohol or drugs. As with the CDC, readers are requested to rename any modifications of the A-DES, in order to distinguish them from the original.

Preliminary studies indicate that the A-DES is a reliable and valid measure of pathological dissociation in adolescents. Cronbach's alpha was .93 for the whole scale, with good subscale reliabilities (Armstrong et al., in press). Split-half reliability was .92, and 2-week test–retest reliability was .77 for normal junior and high school students. The A-DES differentiated abused and nonabused psychiatric patients. Dissociative adolescents (diagnosed independently of A-DES scores) scored significantly higher than other adolescent inpatients (Armstrong et al., in press). However, scores of older adolescents with psychotic disorders approached those of dissociative adolescents. Table 12.4 lists A-DES scores by diagnostic category.

The A-DES is scored by summing item scores and dividing by 30 (number of items). Thus the overall score ranges from 0 to 10. When the A-DES and DES are given to the same subjects, the scores are well correlated ($r = .77$ in a college sample; Armstrong et al., in press). As a rule of thumb, the A-DES score is approximately the DES score divided by 10. Until further data accrue, this provides a reasonable guide for interpreting results. A-DES scores of 4.0 or greater suggest pathological levels of dissociation. Scores of 4–7 are typically found in adolescents with MPD (Armstrong et al., in press). These are preliminary results, however, and more data are needed. Interested readers should consult recent journal articles or contact me for further information.

TABLE 12.4. A-DES Scores for Different Groups

Group[a]	Mean	SD	n
Dissociative disorders	4.9	1.1	13
Abused	3.5	1.8	54
Psychotic disorders	3.8	2.2	8
Nonabused	2.1	1.6	47
Substance use disorders	2.4	1.3	18
Affective disorders	2.2	1.4	24
Conduct disorder	2.0	1.9	16
Normal	2.4	1.4	60

Note. Data from Armstrong et al. (in press). Used by permission from the authors.
[a]Members of all groups excepts the "normal" group were psychiatric inpatients.

Diagnostic Interviews

Structured diagnostic interviews play an important role in research on dissociative disorders. Clinically, they can be useful in a number of ways. For clinicians inexperienced in the art of inquiring about dissociation, diagnostic interviews provide a systematic way to ask about dissociative symptoms. Some dissociative patients report that structured interviews are helpful in articulating experiences that they find difficult to put into words. A videotape of a properly administered structured diagnostic interview can be an important forensic document. In daily practice, however, structured diagnostic interviews are cumbersome for children and adolescents, and are usually reserved for exceptional circumstances.

As discussed in Chapter Four, two structured interviews are used for diagnosis of DSM dissociative disorders in adults: the DDIS (Ross et al., 1989b) and the SCID-D-R (Steinberg, 1994). Neither is specifically adapted for children or adolescents, but both have been used with some success with older adolescents.

The DDIS has 131 items, and covers dissociative disorders, major depression, somatization, and BPD. Many DDIS questions simply restate DSM criteria and use a yes–no answer format. An abuse and trauma interview—which some patients find emotionally difficult—is embedded within the interview. The DDIS generally takes 30–45 minutes to administer, and may be given by a clinician or a competent staff member.

The SCID-D-R is regarded as the more comprehensive of the two diagnostic interviews. However, it has more than 250 items and demands considerable time; it often requires 2–3 hours to complete. Officially supervised training is required, and the semistructured format, though allowing flexibility, requires greater clinical sophistication on the part of the interviewer. The SCID-D-R assesses five dissociative symptom areas: amnesia, depersonalization, derealization, identity confusion, and identity alteration. Symptom severity is graded on a 4-point scale, permitting better quantification for research. Concrete examples of positive symptoms are required, and the interviewer also scores dissociative behaviors observed during administration. The SCID-D-R has been used with adolescents as young as 14 years (A. Steinberg and Steinberg, 1994; M. Steinberg and Steinberg, 1995).

Dorothy O. Lewis and her colleagues have developed the Bellevue Diagnostic Interview for Dissociation in Children (BDID-C; Lewis, 1996). This is the first sophisticated dissociative interview specifically designed for children. It benefits from extensive experience with dissociative and behaviorally disturbed traumatized children. The BDID-C uses a television analogy to frame questions inquiring about dissociative experiences (e.g., channel changing as a metaphor for switching experiences). It is also flexibly organized, to allow the interviewer to tailor its administration to the child's ability (or inability) to stay on task and talk about difficult subjects. The BDID-C inquires about (1) states of awareness; (2) problems with memory; (3) imaginative experiences; (4) auditory and visual hallucinations; (5) temper and aggression; (6) disciplinary experiences; (7) sexual experiences; (8) alterations in skills and abilities; (9) identity disturbances and alterations; and (10) medical complaints. Pilot data indicate that the BDID-C has good interrater reliability with satisfactory agreement even when questions are administered in different sequences.

Psychological Testing

The Testing Process

Psychological testing for dissociative disorders emphasizes the testing process as well as test content. Psychological testing is stressful for many patients, and therefore more likely to elicit dissociative and posttraumatic behaviors. Testers typically spend several hours with patients, focusing on tasks that highlight attentional and cognitive difficulties and shifts in behavior and affect. Therefore, psychological testing is a prime arena for the detection and documentation of pathological dissociation. Judith Armstrong, in particular, has been instrumental in drawing attention to the value of systematically assessing dissociative behaviors during administration of standard measures in adults (Armstrong and Loewenstein, 1990; Armstrong, 1991, 1996). Joyanna Silberg (1996) has played a similar role for children.

Test-triggered dissociative behaviors take the form of amnesias and perplexing forgetfulness (e.g., patients' apparently forgetting testing instructions or their own responses immediately afterwards). "Spacing-out" and staring episodes; rapid behavioral and affective shifts; and perplexing changes in style, content, or developmental level of responses should be noted, particularly when they appear unrelated to or inappropriate for the situation. Sometimes test items elicit powerful dissociative reactions, such as partial or full flashbacks in which a subject's responses are discrepant to the item's content and may show disorientation to time, place, or situation. Over time, dissociative patients often show gross inconsistencies with repeated testing.

Based on extensive experience, Armstrong and colleagues developed the Dissociative Behaviors Checklist—II, a list of dissociative behaviors typically exhibited during psychological testing of adults (Armstrong et al., 1990; Armstrong and Loewenstein, 1990). This checklist covers a range of dissociative and dissociation-related behaviors, such as sudden shifts in affect, amnesias, eye rolls, auditory hallucinations, odd self-references, changes in skills/styles, unresponsive states, and changes in handwriting. When a tester observes unusual or apparent dissociative behavior, the simplest, least suggestive approach to clarification is to ask the subject in a neutral manner what is happening (Armstrong, 1996).

Silberg (1996) has developed and validated a comparable list for children. Comparing young general psychiatric subjects with child and adolescent dissociative patients, Silberg documented a set of dissociative behaviors frequently displayed during psychological testing. Dissociative children had more amnesias and forgetting responses for their own answers; exhibited more staring spells and trance-like states; had more odd movements (e.g., tics, grimaces, repetitive leg movements, and odd hand gestures); and showed more fluctuations in activity, relatedness, language level and usage, affect, and physical complaints. In addition they displayed more fearfulness and angry responses to test material, supporting the idea that test content may act as a traumatic trigger for some patients. The dissociative children also frequently generated multiple, conflicting responses to a test item (something my colleagues and I routinely encounter when dissociative patients complete self-report measures). These findings have been incorporated into a child–adolescent psychological test instrument, the Dissociative Features Profile (Silberg, 1996).

Test Content

Standard psychological tests, primarily the Minnesota Multiphasic Personality Inventory (MMPI; Coons and Fine, 1990) and the Millon Clinical Multiaxial Inventory—II (MCMI-II; Ellason, Ross, and Fuchs, 1995), have proven useful in probing for pathological dissociation. For the MMPI, the most characteristic features include (1) high F and Sc scales; (2) critical items 156 and 251, which involve dissociative symptoms; and (3) polysymptomatic profile similar to that seen in borderline personality disorder patients (Coons and Fine, 1990). No psychological test, personality inventory, or projective measure can as yet definitively diagnose a dissociative disorder. Research using various measures finds that patients with pathological dissociation often simultaneously fulfill criteria for several Axis I and Axis II disorders (Armstrong, 1996).

Projective testing, particularly the Rorschach, is being actively investigated in research on PTSD (van der Kolk and Ducey, 1989) and the dissociative disorders (Carlson and Armstrong, 1994; Armstrong,

1996). In a number of studies, dissociative and PTSD subjects show marked increases in "blood and aggression" responses, which are generally rare (Carlson and Armstrong, 1994). Armstrong and Loewenstein (1990) have developed a Traumatic Content Index to quantify these. Morbid responses, traditionally interpreted as evidence of psychosis or regression, are conceptualized as evidence of intrusive traumatic memories triggered by the inkblots.

Psychological testing is helpful in ruling out significant cognitive or organic problems. It may also provide important indications of pathological dissociation, in terms of both the testing process and the test content. When psychological testing is indicated, the referring clinician should alert the tester to the possibility of pathological dissociation and request the tester to be alert for dissociative behaviors during the testing session.

Longitudinal Observation

In general, I believe that diagnosis of psychiatric disorders in children and adolescents is a multistage process that may require weeks to months. Unfortunately, mental health professionals are increasingly forced to bestow a diagnosis after the first (or, at most, second) session. Third-party payers demand a DSM label or they withhold payment. This managed care practice has done a lot of damage, especially to the validity of psychiatric diagnoses contained in medical records. Whenever possible, it is important to withhold a dissociative diagnosis until other conditions are eliminated and sufficient evidence of persistent pathological dissociation across multiple contexts has been collected.

Longitudinal observation plays an important role in establishing the presence of pathological dissociation in children and adolescents. In many instances, dissociative children live in a setting where responsible adults can be enlisted as longitudinal observers. Parents, foster parents, group home personnel, residential placement staffers, concerned teachers, coaches, and counselors can all be tapped to provide helpful information.

The basic approach is to have each designated observer keep a log of dissociative behaviors that he or she observes in the child. Entries should include time, place, circumstances, and a description of the event/behavior. Examples of target behaviors include evidence of amnesia/perplexing forgetfulness, significant alterations of identity, auditory or visual hallucinations, self-injurious behaviors, trance-like behavior, conduct problems, and potential dissociative behaviors (e.g., lying). Observers should be instructed to record the questionable behavior and circumstances as objectively as possible.

Here are some examples from a log kept by the adoptive mother of a 16-year-old Cambodian-born girl with MPD.

JANICE

3/8/93. 4 p.m.: Found Janice curled up in closet. Crying like a baby. Doesn't seem to know who I am . . . [or] understand English. Minutes before, talking with Rachel on phone.

3/11/93. 2 p.m.: Call from school. Janice told her teacher that she felt like someone was trying to make her walk into traffic. Said someone inside was trying to kill her.

3/19/93.5:30 p.m.: In closet. For hours? Angry when I got her out. Saying, "What do you want?" Denied lying on floor.

Cooperative adolescents can keep a diary of unusual or distressing experiences. They can also complete the A-DES on a serial basis. In MPD, diaries often prove useful as supportive documentation because they contain entries in different handwriting (sometimes signed by the alter personality states), with different grammar and spelling, and opinions that a patient does not recognize or disavows. (See the examples of differences in writing and drawings in Lewis, 1996.)

Hypnotic and Drug-Facilitated Interviews

There is a limited role for hypnotic or drug-facilitated (e.g., amytal-enhanced) diagnostic interviews for adult dissociative disorders. However, the acrimonious debate regarding an interviewer's potential suggestive influence on a patient in a hypnotic or drug-induced altered mental state has cast doubt (mostly unreasonable) on the credibility of dissociative disorder diagnoses made under these conditions. Hence, I recommend keeping the diagnostic evaluation process as "pure" and rigorous as possible; this will enhance the credibility of a given child's dissociative disorder diagnosis for the many professionals who will probably work with that child in the years to come. I feel that hypnotic and drug-facilitated interviews should not be used in diagnostic evaluation for dissociative disorders in children and adolescents. If persistent pathological dissociation is present, it will be evident in everyday behaviors.

SUMMARY

Literature reviews and clinical case series have found common features in child and adolescent dissociative patients. Dissociative children and adolescents are usually highly symptomatic and have histories of prior contacts with mental health and social services. They have usually acquired two or three psychiatric diagnoses, commonly including ADHD, conduct disorder, bipolar disorder, schizophrenia or other psychotic disorders, epilepsy, and BPD (see Table 12.2). Affect and anxiety symptoms are prominent presenting features, as is serious suicide potential. Conduct problems occur in about two-thirds of cases. Sexual acting out is present in about half of cases. School performance and learning problems are common and provide an important alternative source of information that must be fully explored. Females appear to have more anxiety and posttraumatic symptoms, sleep problems, sexual behavior problems, and somatization than males. The percentage of female cases increases steadily with age; the female-to-male ratio is about 8:1 by middle to late adolescence. Older children and adolescents are usually more symptomatic than younger children.

The diagnosis of pathological dissociation requires a thorough evaluation to rule out other disorders. Persistent pathological dissociation must be documented across two or more major domains of the child's life (e.g., home, school, and peer activities). Diagnostic evaluation must include multiple informants. Parents and caretakers are often the principal sources of information. Much can be learned from observing parent–child interactions during evaluation. Children can provide information directly through questions and answers, and indirectly through behavioral interactions and play or projective sequences. A comprehensive physical examination is important for children suspected of having been maltreated. Pathological dissociation can be screened for with parent/adult report measures, such as the CDC (ages 5–12), or self-report scales, such as the A-DES (ages 11–20). Adult structured dissociative disorder diagnostic interviews, such as the SCID-D-R, are being adapted for adolescents. Promising child-oriented, semistructured interviews (e.g., the BDID-C) are becoming available.

Psychological testing provides both an important screening function and a way to document pathological dissociation systematically. Quantification of dissociative behaviors manifested during the testing process provides information in addition to the test results. Longitudinal observation by informed observers (e.g., caretakers, teachers, group home staffers) is an important source of information about the persistence of pathological dissociative behaviors. Behavioral logs or diaries are convenient ways to collect this information. Serial completion of the CDC or a similar measure offers a simple, standardized method of gathering data longitudinally.

Hypnosis, although useful in some treatments, is not advisable for diagnosis. Both hypnosis and drug facilitation are widely viewed (largely incorrectly) as contaminating the diagnostic evaluation. A clinician should always be aware that he or she is only one of many professionals who will be involved with a dissociative child over the years to come. Therefore, the diagnostic evaluation must be conducted in a manner that preserves the credibility of the diagnosis.

Chapter Thirteen

Philosophy and Principles of Treatment

When a person is identified as an "expert," there is pressure to behave as if he or she were somehow omniscient. This comes in the form of questions, pleas, and expectations to provide "*the* answer" to the many difficulties, dilemmas, and controversies confronting patients, families, and therapists. Yet a person who has acquired a modicum of expertise is all too aware how much he or she does *not* know or understand—especially concerning the complexities of any given case. The tension between the sometimes pressing expectations of others and the "expert's" awareness of the limits of his or her knowledge can be awkward.

This is especially true in the area of teaching. My experience in giving lectures and workshops has taught me that there is inevitably strong pressure (from both organizers and participants) to present a prescriptive, omnibus treatment model organized in a simple, stepwise fashion. Sounds great! However, most treatments rarely proceed in this manner. Although they garner high ratings on evaluation forms for continuing medical education, simplistic treatment models are of limited use in real life. They can be detrimental when they deceive us into believing that there is a easy, foolproof way to conduct therapies.

In particular, it must be understood that the treatment of traumatized individuals, whether children or adults, is complex, demanding, and not straightforward. Some general principles and broad rules apply, but each person is different and must be worked with individually in a manner that is cognizant of and sensitive to the circumstances of his or her life. Thus, this chapter and Chapter Fourteen serve as an introduction to the principles, problems, and issues raised by therapeutic work with traumatized and dissociative children and adolescents. The lack of simple, definitive prescriptions may prove disappointing to some. I too have wished that the "experts" I consult would be more authoritative and conclusive. However, to present my ideas this way would be misleading. Rather, it is my intention to lay out basic guidelines and to suggest broad strategies. Every therapist is responsible for formulating a patient's particular problems and for devising interventions that consider the patient's unique situation.

MEETING THE NEEDS OF CHILDREN

Children have basic needs that must be met if they are to develop properly. Some are material such as food, clothing, medical care, and shelter. Others are abstract, such as love, a sense of security, and a sense of self-possibility. The latter are more difficult to appreciate and to provide, but they are equally important to a child's healthy development.

Children need love and security. This need is met by reliable, caring relationships and a stable environment. Children also need a sense of future and possibility. They need to experience new things and to be allowed to grow. They need recognition and praise. Finally, they need to be permitted and encouraged to assume appropriate responsibility for and control of their own lives. Therapists must look for ways to facilitate the meeting of these needs in the lives of the children with whom they work.

SUPPORTING THE NATURAL RESILIENCY OF CHILDREN

To clinicians working with children across a range of settings, it is apparent that despite severe trauma and loss, many youngsters exhibit a remarkable natural capacity to restore order and function in their lives. Resiliency is often overlooked in the evaluation and treatment of traumatized children. Generally the therapeutic focus is on dealing with these children's problems and misbehaviors. One rarely hears much about supporting their strengths and their capacity to recover from disappointment, loss, injury, violation, and setback. Yet an understanding of the nature of resiliency, and of how a therapist can support and nurture this capacity, informs interventions that are important over the long run.

Our knowledge of resiliency owes much to Norman Garmezy and the generations of researchers whom he has mentored. Garmezy has continually emphasized that no matter how high the risks, morbidity never reaches 100%. There are always children who are "defying the voice of doom" (Chess, 1989, p. 179).

The study of resiliency is complex, and much has been written about it (Cicchetti and Cohen, 1995b). A key principle emerging from this research is that the child brings to the situation the basic capacities that interact with the environment to produce resiliency. But much can still be done to nurture and develop these intrinsic capacities, and to compensate for deficient or poorly developed abilities in some children. Resiliency is a multidimensional capacity that emerges from a developmental network of abilities and capacities operating independently and synthetically.

The first crucial ability is a child's capacity to take an active stance toward obstacles and problems. Resiliency—the capacity to bounce back, to change things for the better, to persevere despite difficulties—requires by definition the child's persistence in trying to improve the situation. The child must keep trying, endure, and be sustained by a vision or belief that things can and will improve. The child who gives up or gives in will not have a positive outcome.

But resiliency requires an aware and informed persistence, not mindless, robotic perseveration. The child's efforts must improve and grow with experience and in accord with changing circumstances. A therapist can support the child's initiatives by processing experiences and results, and by helping and encouraging the child to develop a larger repertoire of skills and strategies. The therapist should help to inform, nurture, and support the child's vision of what life can and should be. At times the therapist must become the continuing source of hope that things can and will get better.

The child's various intelligences are also critical to the process of resiliency. Smarter children have a better chance. But high intellect alone is not sufficient, for the child must have a broad range of interests, skills, and strategies (Demos, 1989). The broader and better developed the child's repertoire, the more options and the greater flexibility he or she will have.

Flexibility—the ability to know when to use what—is a key feature of resiliency (Demos, 1989). A therapist can support and encourage a child to explore and to add to or improve capacities and abilities. For many children, this first and foremost entails actively working to create and support the best school situation possible. In the case of deeply troubled children, this demands active, ongoing, long-term communication with teachers and administrators. School is the major source of new skills, experience, interests, and abilities for most children. Unfortunately, schools are sometimes willing to give up on maltreated children because of their disruptive behavior.

Resiliency requires further that a child be able to analyze problems and to discriminate selectively among options. Here a therapist and others can help the child to understand the circumstances and to think through responses. They must first have an empathetic understanding of the child's understanding of the situation before helping the child process the options. A therapist should help a traumatized child to develop problem-solving abilities that are useful in the here and now, and that are consonant with the child's capacities and developmental levels. To do this, the therapist must work to keep pace with the child's growth and development, so that the child's newly emerging capacities can be identified, nurtured, and integrated.

Finally, resiliency requires that the child receive reinforcement and gratification from his or her efforts and from the improvements—however small—that these efforts produce. The child's experiences of actively working to change the situation must be intrinsically motivating (Demos, 1989). Children can produce change in their lives only in small increments. Unrealistic expectations, which all too often generate feelings of failure and overwhelming disappointment, can kill initiative and stifle resiliency.

Unfortunately, children and adolescents often have grossly unrealistic expectations, frequently shaped by the distortions of reality commonplace in the mass media. (See the discussion of television watching in Chapter Ten.) A therapist must identify and reinforce a child's experience of success, however it is manifested, in a way that promotes a sense of satisfaction and enhances the child's self-esteem. And the therapist must come to understand the child's expectations and to ground these gently in hard reality. This is a tricky process, greatly complicated by the profound misunderstandings and distrust that can occur between children and adults. Children, and especially adolescents, don't care to hear how adults think that their world works; this is a big turnoff for them. The problem is particularly acute when there are differences in culture and ethnicity between a child and a therapist. Finding good ways to talk about these issues with hurt, suspicious, and angry minority kids is one of the hardest things I know.

The characteristics and circumstances of a child's family and environment are crucial to the expression of resiliency. The child's temperament, intellect, and innate endowment of abilities, capacities, and talents interact with the characteristics of his or her family and of others in the immediate environment, such as peers and teachers. Regardless of the child's abilities, the resiliency and flexibility of those individuals (and their institutions) also strongly influence the child's outcome. Frequently the most effective interventions involve working with the family, school, and others to achieve a better fit between the strengths and weaknesses of these crucial supports and those of the child.

One important intervention is simply helping others who work with the child understand the child's strengths, problems, pathology, and potential. If the child is viewed as too hopeless, too badly damaged, or somehow defective because of genetic and familial ties, there will be little recognition of or support for the child's compensatory initiatives. With dissociative children, it is important to spend a large percentage of time working with family, teachers, therapists, caseworkers, and others to help them to understand what dissociation is like and how it is triggered by the demands and stresses routinely imposed on children. Enhancing the understanding and flexibility of the people and institutions involved with such a child is a major part of therapy.

There are still other factors that affect the expression of resiliency. Racism and poverty are especially destructive social problems that crush generations of children, no matter how bright, adaptive, or persistent they are. Racism in particular is a terrible problem in Western society, severely limiting the opportunities available to minority children. Alcoholism and drug abuse—highly associated with social problems and family chaos—are also extremely destructive processes that bury resiliency and condemn families to generations of pain and poverty (Long and Vaillant, 1989).

SIZE, TIME, AND POWER: UNDERSTANDING CHILDREN'S PERSPECTIVE

One of the larger gaps in many adults' empathy for children is a failure to appreciate the scale of a young child's world. Time, size, and power are different for children. By and large, the human-made world is scaled for adults; all kinds of things are made optimal for adult size, strength, coordination, and cognition. Like Tom Thumb or Jack and the Beanstalk, children continually struggle with giant-sized objects and contend with devices (e.g., doorknobs and soda can poptops) that are designed for adults. The skills and knowledge necessary to operate in this world belong to adults, who rarely consider how physically difficult things can be for children. Indeed, children often know much more than they can do. For example, even young children demonstrate surprising abilities to use computers, VCRs, and electronic gadgets that daunt adults. They can display their abilities because the controls (i.e., button pushing or mouse clicks) do not require adult dexterity or strength.

In working with children, adults are frequently focused on *what* the children should do, whereas the children are frequently focused on the *how* of it. This can be an unrecognized sticking point, as many children withdraw or become oppositional when they are overwhelmed with the question of *how* to do something. It is important to be open to a child's concerns about how things are done and how he or she can do what needs to be done. Often this requires exploring problems in a very concrete, step-by-step way with the child. Frequently a therapist or another adult is surprised by the conceptual obstacles or concerns raised by the child. Yet these concerns are often very compelling when considered from the child's perspective.

Adults are especially ignorant about the ways in which children perceive and conceptualize time. Adults operate on a clock-based model, which assumes the steady, uniform, and linear forward progression of time. However, for younger children especially, time is not experienced as smooth and linear; it moves quickly at some points and slowly at others, and it jumps abruptly, with gaps in continuity. Children also do not chronologically sequence events in the same fashion as adults do. Eventually a more conventional sense of time emerges with metacognitive development and socialization, but even older adolescents' experiences of duration and continuity differ markedly from those of adults. Capacities such as the ability to delay gratification and the degree of future orientation reflect a child's experience of time.

In the novel *Gravity's Rainbow*, Thomas Pynchon (1973) introduced the notion of "temporal bandwidth"—the amount of time an individual spends thinking about the past, present, and future. Young children tend to have narrow temporal bandwidths that are centered on the present, with fringes of the very near future and recent past. Adults are generally much less focused on the immediate present and are more concerned about past or future events.

Mismatches in temporal bandwidth lead to misunderstandings and to adults' failure to appreciate why children seem so concerned with things that will obviously (to the adults) disappear or change in the near future. Children demand action in the immediate now, because the present dominates their experience of time. A narrow temporal bandwidth also acts to obscure cause-and-effect relationships, so that things that happened in the past are not connected with the overriding experience of the immediate present. For most children and many adolescents, if it happened yesterday, "it's history"—and therefore not of much interest.

Although it is empathetic, enlightening, and even fun to be able to enter into children's or adolescents' time frame, it is more helpful to try gently to broaden their temporal bandwidth. Making temporal and causal connections among the past, present, and future enlarges their world and provides a scaffolding within which events can be linked and anticipations of the future can be framed.

INSURING CHILDREN'S SAFETY

In her landmark book *Trauma and Recovery,* Judith Herman (1992) identifies insuring safety as the central task of beginning therapy. Safety is both a physical condition and a state of mind. All too often, the basic issues of safety are overlooked in the treatment of traumatized children. Because of their powerlessness in an adult world, younger children in particular face great obstacles in trying to insure their own safety. From first contact, a therapist must be actively involved with the issues and problems of a child's safety.

In cases where the trauma is understandable (e.g., earthquake, hurricane, or accident) and the source of distress is external to the family, it is generally not too difficult to create a safe environment and a sense of safety. However, in cases where the trauma is intrinsic to the home (e.g., neglect and abuse) it is much more difficult to establish physical and psychological safety. The first task is to ascertain whether a child is in danger of further trauma. This is frequently the case. If a clinician has concerns about the child's safety, the situation should be immediately reported to the appropriate child protective service agency. (See the discussion in Chapter Two.)

For many reasons, reporting suspected neglect or abuse does not always produce a definitive response. A case may have to be built over time before it becomes clear exactly what is happening and what action should be taken. However, a clinician should not rationalize a failure to report a suspected situation because it may not be investigated and responded to. Repeated reporting may be the most important step in building a child protective services case. Even when a child is safe from physical risk, it is likely that he or she will continue to feel profoundly unsafe; paradoxically, the child may even do things that place him or her in jeopardy. The therapist must be alert to the child's fears about safety. Excess investment in special hiding places—either actual external surroundings or internal fantasy worlds—indicates that the child remains fearful and only feels safe in limited contexts. Vivid fantasy and/or dissociation is often the only viable escape for children trapped in chronically traumatic situations.

Clinicians must be always be alert to self-endangering behaviors, especially in adolescents. Suicidality, self-mutilation, risk taking, and abusive peer relationships are frequent in maltreated adolescents. Since teenagers rarely volunteer this type of information, clinicians must repeatedly probe these areas. Surprisingly, however, adolescents will often honestly answer direct questions about such behavior. Therapists should be alert for and inquire about peer groups' risk-taking games, such as Russian roulette (Denny, 1995).

Some risky behaviors take on the guise of personality style. Ruth Mausert-Mooney's (1992) research on appeal and vulnerability behaviors in sexually abused adolescent girls provides an example. Mausert-Mooney found that in the presence of a strange man (i.e., a neutrally behaving male psychologist, who was unaware of whether a girl had been abused or not), sexually abused girls differed significantly from nonabused comparison girls in having more "flirtatious" and "vulnerable" behaviors, as determined by a standardized coding of videotapes. Certain body language gestures (e.g., touching the inner thigh and crotch area) were almost never exhibited by the nonabused comparison girls. Other behaviors—especially behaviors that signal passivity and submission, such as increased head bowing or gaze aversion—were significantly more frequently and inappropriately displayed by the sexually abused girls.

Many such behaviors are viewed as "seductive" in our culture and are considered part of the eroticization of sexually abused children. (See the discussion in Chapter Two). An alternative interpretation is that they are part of misguided attempts at social affiliation (Mausert-Mooney, 1992). In either case, behaviors that place a child at greater risk for revictimization must be addressed as part of a therapist's concerns about safety. Supportive feedback about such behavior can take creative forms, including joint viewing of videotapes of therapy sessions. (I think these behaviors could also be addressed by a focused, time-limited therapeutic intervention in early adolescence, perhaps involving a peer group and/or videotape modeling techniques.)

Younger children often express concerns about safety in play themes and artwork. Although wishes for omnipotence are common in normal young children, an excessive focus on superheroes, or an insatiable need to be all-powerful, invisible, or invulnerable, can be a sign of fears about safety. Risk taking may be symbolically expressed by placing play figures in dangerous situations or toys in places where they are likely to be broken. Sometimes risk taking is evident in board games such as chess or checkers, when the child sacrifices important pieces or makes obviously self-detrimental moves for no apparent reason and with little (or an incongruent) affect. (See the description of Reginald's chess games in Chapter Fourteen.) Concerns about safety can often be fruitfully explored and addressed in play therapy with younger children. One of the advantages of play therapy is its ability to allow a child to set up dangerous or troubling situations and then to explore and resolve them—perhaps by trying a variety of different endings to explore cause-and-effect sequences.

UNDERSTANDING CHILDREN'S LOGICAL BINDS
AND LANGUAGE PROBLEMS

Near the end of my child psychiatry fellowship, I read a draft of *Healing the Hurt Child* (Donovan and McIntyre, 1990). It was enlightening in many respects. For me, the most useful insight lay in the portrayal of young children as "obligatory slaves of logic"—in stark contrast to the traditional Freudian–Piagetian dogma of young children as "prelogical" beings. Through a series of compelling vignettes, Donovan and McIntyre demonstrate how young children operate within closed systems of "logical" interrelating propositions. The premises of a child's system may or may not be true, but the child is conceptually bound by the "logic" of these premises, regardless of their truth. I have confirmed this observation on many occasions, both clinically and parentally. Young children are in fact often driven to certain behaviors—adaptive or maladaptive—by their "logical" reasoning about a given situation. Effective therapeutic interventions sometimes involve understanding and correcting the "logical binds" that children find themselves in.

Logical binds originate in the intense need of children to understand and make sense of how things happen. (How are babies born? How do germs cause disease? How does Santa Claus get down the chimney?) By and large, children do not tolerate an explanatory void for the questions and concerns that are important to them. Instead, they invent a "logical" explanation that is consistent with their understanding of the world. Adults regard such explanations as cute examples of children's "fantasy."

Donovan and McIntyre (1990, p. 28) argue that such explanations are better understood as expressions of a "logical" belief system in operation. They regard such "fantasies" as operational hypotheses about the structure of reality. When one grasps this, certain previously incomprehensible symptoms or behaviors make perfect sense. The adult idea of "fantasy" as a charming, playful, and volitional manipulation of reality is frequently misapplied to children, who are struggling to understand the (sometimes terrible) reality of their lives.

Logical binds develop in numerous ways. Some originate in the vagueness of spoken language, in which so much of the meaning of what is said depends upon context, tone of voice, affect, and body language. Different words sound alike to a child. Consider "to," "two," and "too," or the various meanings of "jam." How is a young child, who hears them as the same word, to reconcile their various meanings? Substituting one meaning for another can produce significant differences in what is being said—and thus significant differences in what the child "logically" concludes about how something came to be.

Other logical binds arise as a child attempts to reconcile the various explanations, direct and indirect, that have been offered at various times by various people in various contexts. We forget how many influential sources of information and misinformation bombard even preschool children: relatives and family friends, peers, television, movies, stories, and (surprisingly often) strangers overheard by chance. Adults are often unaware that children are listening to, observing, and absorbing adult interactions all the time. They do this while seemingly obliviously involved with play or peers. Religious teachings, with their mystical and authoritarian imagery, also powerfully influence younger children's understandings of cause and effect.

Many of the explanations and models of the world that children receive are adult versions of fantasy as we imagine that it is experienced by children. Movies, television, theme toys, books, and stories are based on increasingly commercialized adult fantasy productions, which are cynically imposed on children. Although even young children can make some distinctions between "real" and "pretend" phenomena, very often they include entertainment-media-based models of the world in their thinking and problem solving. (See the discussion in Chapter Ten.)

Logical binds manifest themselves in many ways, and the reader is urged to seek out further examples in *Healing the Hurt Child* (Donovan and McIntyre, 1990). Therapists should be aware of the power of logical binds and misunderstandings of language to produce powerful behavioral responses in children. A child usually does not recognize that his or her symptoms or behaviors arise in response to some painful "logical" conclusion that he or she has reached. Nor do the therapist's interventions have to produce an awareness or verbalization of this process. In fact, attempting to make this process "conscious" often has negative consequences or undoes a successful nonverbal therapeutic intervention, as noted below. It is usually sufficient to address and correct the logical bind within the context of the child's responses in therapy, but in such a way as to undo the bind.

INTERVENING IN IMPLICIT VERSUS EXPLICIT WAYS

Adult models of psychotherapy are predicated on the principle of producing therapeutic change by making explicitly conscious previously "unconscious" ideation, behaviors, and motives. This approach is generally counterproductive with children, for two reasons. First, adult forms of psychotherapy require a reasonably well-developed self-monitoring capacity or "observing ego." Metacognitive self-monitoring and reflective capacities develop over time and do not become well integrated into behavior until adulthood (if then). And, as previously discussed in Chapters Three and Nine, metacognitive functions appear to be disrupted in dissociative individuals.

Second, one must be psychologically minded for such insights to "make sense," and therefore to become working mental models influencing one's understanding of one's own behavior. Children do not conceptualize themselves and their behavior in adult psychological terms. Attempts to have a child explicitly verbalize his or her psychological understanding of a therapeutic intervention usually undercut the efficacy of that intervention. With children and many adolescents, much therapeutic work takes place in nonverbal ways. Efficacious interventions often leave their mark implicitly. Therapists working with children must be comfortable operating in the implicit and "unconscious" domains.

At times, a therapist or another adult may resort to "magical" interventions to correct logical binds and implicit beliefs that are crippling for a preschooler. This can take the form of a ceremony in which the frightening or maladaptive issue is symbolically neutralized.

JAYSON

Jayson, a 3-year-old, presented with insect phobias and nighttime fears about being bitten by bugs. He had a history of being bitten by "red ants," and had once been stung by a wasp. It became apparent that Jayson believed that dangerous insects lived inside his father's computer. (It seems likely that this idea originated from hearing someone talk about computer "bugs.") All the dangerous bugs in his father's computer were "killed" in a ceremony in which his father squirted compressed air into the computer's orifices and then took the top off to show him that the bugs were all gone and could never come back. After this, Jayson's phobias markedly eased.

Unfortunately, most frightening things are all too real and cannot be banished with a therapeutic ritual.

CREATING THERAPEUTIC SPACE

I am also indebted to Donovan and McIntyre (1990) for their thoughtful articulation of the nature and rules of "therapeutic space." As a child fellow, working in an overburdened clinic setting in which many therapists shared a few offices, I frequently observed the impact on a child of returning to find that the therapy room was not the same as when he or she left it. Toys that had played important roles in the last session were nowhere to be found. When I raised concerns about the effects of never seeing a child in the same setting twice, some of my supervisors acted as if I were mentally deficient. Their position was that a good therapist should be able to work with a child at any time, in any place, with nothing. One pulled out a chewed-up toy soldier and said that this was the only toy that he had *ever* used in treating children. Like many trainees, I concluded that the problem lay with me. It was liberating to discover Donovan and McIntyre (1990) affirming the nature and importance of the "therapeutic space" in conducting treatment.

Space has a special role in the life of a child. Children are exquisitely sensitive to the space around them. They imaginatively restructure it to meet their needs. In play, they create whole worlds in a sandbox or under the kitchen table. (Children especially like to play at the edges of adult "turf.") In therapy, space should become a special place with strength, structure, and stability—a place that can be utilized and internalized as an alternative to the chaotic and unstable world many children inhabit.

"Therapeutic space" is operationally defined as the physical, temporal, and interpersonal environment created by the therapist (Donovan and McIntyre, 1990). In many respects, it is a contractual virtual space, created by careful and consistent adherence to a set of rules and principles. Donovan and McIntyre lay down a number of specific rules about the nature and structure of therapeutic space. I do not agree with all of their stipulations, but their thoughtful articulation of the structure and role of space in the conduct of therapy is informative for child clinicians.

In summary, they regard therapeutic space as being created through a consistent, principled adherence to rules and boundaries about how a child interacts with the objects and space in which the therapist works with the child. The goal is to create a safe, consistent, and dependable environment in which the child can address and work through concerns and problems. The space should be for the child and therapist alone. Specifically, Donovan and McIntyre do not permit parents in their play therapy room. What the child says and does in the play therapy room is confidential, except when genuine concerns or danger dictate sharing this information. The child cannot bring anything into the therapy room or take anything out. Everything in the room has its own place, and that place does not change. At the end of a session, everything is returned to its place; if the child chooses not to participate in this process, then he or she must remain and watch it. Toys should be generic (i.e., they should not be highly commercialized or theme toys). They should be as sturdy and unbreakable as possible. When toys are broken, they should be repaired in front of the child. No toy should suggest or invite aggression. No harm to self or others is permitted. No undressing, even taking off of shoes, is permitted.

Even if therapists accept these rules in principle, they may not have the control and freedom to create and protect the space in which they practice, as I have noted in Chapter Twelve. Those of us who work in public settings usually share space with others, whom we may never have even met. Even within institutional limitations, however, it is still possible to create a therapeutic space by consistent adherence to many of the principles advocated by Donovan and McIntyre (1990). I have never had the luxury of completely controlling my therapy space, but I have found that viable therapeutic space can be created by consistent enforcement of rules and boundaries, and by the communication of respect and regard for the setting as a special place where a child and I meet.

Although many of the rules described above (such as keeping adults out of the room and respecting confidentiality) can be maintained by a therapist, when the therapist arrives only minutes ahead of the child, the overall state of the room is impossible to control. My solution is to have a drawer or shelf defined as exclusively mine, which I consistently structure and maintain. When possible, I use a lockable drawer or cabinet to create a protected, stable space within the larger shared space. I explain that I share this room with other therapists who also see children here, but that this is a special space for our things only. I find that children quickly understand this boundary and relate to the stability of this small protected space in the midst of the ever-changing larger space. In many ways it is analogous to their lives, where only a very small part of the world is under their control.

I allow children to bring things into the therapy room, as long as they ask permission and give a reason why the objects should be included in a session. They must take the objects with them at the end of the session. The things that children bring to therapy are often expressions of their concerns. A therapist should be alert to attempts to smuggle objects into or out of the therapy room. This is common in abused children, who are testing the sanctity of the therapeutic space, the therapist's consistency in enforcing rules, and the therapist's ability to detect secret behavior.

Violations of the therapeutic space should not be permitted. The therapist's ability to protect and maintain the therapy setting assures the child of his or her own value and of his or her protection within that setting. For a traumatized child, the nature of the therapy setting is inseparable from the child's perception of the therapist and is inextricably bound to the child's understanding of what is supposed to occur between them.

SUMMARY

The principles and philosophy of psychotherapy with dissociative children are surveyed in this chapter. The goal here and in the next chapter is to provide a broad perspective that each therapist can shape as necessary. This chapter begins with an enumeration of children's basic needs, and goes on to note that children are often more resilient than we give them credit for. Resiliency emerges from children's intrinsic capacities; therapists and caretakers must help the children to identify these and to make the best use of them. Persistence in trying to improve the situation is central to resiliency. Intelligence, both in specific domains and more broadly, also makes a critical contribution. Adults must help children toward realistic expectations about what can be achieved with how much effort in what span of time. Equally important is helping children appreciate their success, however small, as improvement. Involved adults should also help others, who may view dissociative children very negatively, to see the children's promise and to understand the effects of pathological dissociation on behavior.

Children are smaller, weaker, less experienced, and less knowledgeable than adults. They see and experience the world differently. We cannot change that, nor should we try. We can appreciate that their concerns are not always apparent to us and do not necessarily overlap with ours. We must also strive to insure the safety of the children whom we work with; they must be protected both from further victimization and from their own risky and self-destructive impulses.

Children are sometimes the victims of their own "logic," which dictates certain interpretations and responses to situations that adults view very differently. Logical binds can be undone, but often this undoing must be handled implicitly to be therapeutic. Therapy must take place in a principled and private space that a therapist defines and protects—and that a child experiences as an extension of the therapist's personality.

Chapter Fourteen

Individual Therapy

I begin this chapter with an overview of treatment outcomes for maltreated and dissociative children and adolescents. This is intended to inform the reader up front that there is little to point to in the way of empirical data. Nonetheless, clinical experience indicates that treatment does make a difference for at least a subset of children. Drawing on this experience, I focus in the remainder of the chapter on basic sets of treatment issues and techniques.

The first set of issues involves the therapeutic alliance. Transference themes such as trust and control, and countertransference problems such as setting limits and feeling responsible for a child's behavior, are common threads that run through therapy. The next set consists of treatment process issues, which include working with problem behaviors; trauma; loss and mourning; guilt and self-blame; and low self-esteem. These are framed for maltreated children in general. Issues and interventions for pathological dissociation are framed in terms of the DBS model. I conclude with a discussion of play therapy, a therapeutic modality unique to child treatment.

TREATMENT OUTCOMES

Maltreated Children in General

In the United States, millions of children have been and are being maltreated—even by conservative estimates. We spend enormous sums on the delivery of services to these children. Yet we know little about the effectiveness of these services. In general, it appears that many maltreated children improve with treatment. Lanktree and Briere (1995) found that time in treatment was more predictive of symptomatic improvement than was passage of time between the end of abuse and the beginning of treatment. Finkelhor and Berliner's (1995) review of research on the treatment of sexually abused children concludes that on the whole, treatment is efficacious, particularly when it is abuse-specific. Although we have accumulated some clinical knowledge about the treatment of child abuse, there are few well-designed treatment outcome studies to validate current approaches. For example, Finkelhor and Berliner's (1995) review found only 29 studies of five or more children evaluated at two or more time points during treatment. Many used simple pre- to posttreatment designs, which make it difficult to distinguish between treatment responses and basic passage-of-time effects.

However, certain symptoms, especially externalizing behavioral problems, appear to be resistant to therapeutic interventions. Sexualized and aggressive behaviors are prime examples (Finkelhor and Berliner, 1995). Symptoms may also show exacerbations at various points prior to sustained improvement, especially early in treatment.

A great many factors, both independent of and interdependent with treatment, influence outcome. For example, family functioning variables such as cohesion and conflict management styles are reliable predictors of rate of improvement (Finkelhor and Berliner, 1995). Family distress (particularly parental symptoms) has a strong negative impact—as has been proven for other forms of trauma in children (e.g., Handford et al., 1986; Laor et al., 1996). Emerging data indicate that parents (both parents, when available) must be included in abuse-oriented treatments to maximize success rates (Finkelhor and Berliner, 1995; Cohen and Mannarino, 1996).

Children with Pathological Dissociation

Beyond a few descriptive case reports (e.g., Fagan and McMahon, 1984; Kluft, 1985a, 1985c, 1986; Weiss et al., 1985; Riley and Mead, 1988; LaPorta, 1992; Putnam, 1993a; Jacobsen, 1995), little is known about the outcomes of children treated for pathological dissociation. Somewhat more is known about adult dissociative disorder treatment outcomes (e.g., Kluft, 1984b, 1988; Coons, 1986; Putnam, 1986b; Choe and Kluft, 1995). Fortunately, studies in progress will begin to fill this void. However, until "definitive" studies can be conducted (i.e., random assignment of subjects to two or more different treatment conditions), claims of success must be regarded with appropriate skepticism by practitioners—and remain open to question by critics.

A few basic outcomes appear to be repeatedly observed in dissociative children and adolescents. In young children, a "meltaway" phenomenon has been reported in some instances (e.g., Fagan and McMahon, 1984; Kluft, 1985a; Peterson, in press). That is, prominent dissociative symptoms apparent during initial evaluations rapidly disappeared when the children were established in a safe and supportive environment.

JOHNNIE

Johnnie, a 4-year-old girl, was caught in a contentious custody battle, which included allegations that her father sexually abused her by fondling and digital penetration. Johnnie was referred because she talked about another girl living "inside of me." She was observed to have rapid, regressive behavioral shifts, and at times told her mother that she was the other girl. These symptoms were prominent for at least a month prior to evaluation. She was also observed to have "spacey," vacant staring states. During the first evaluation, several brief unresponsive spells were noted. She also referred to herself in the third person, but no distinct alter personalities were identifiable. When I asked her about what she heard her mother tell me in the mother–child evaluation session, she would say very little about the girl "inside of me."

Prior to the second session, the court required that Johnnie's father submit to supervised visitation. During the second clinic visit, she said that the other "girl inside of me" had gone away. She now identified this girl as a girl with superpowers from a favorite cartoon show, who had come to protect her (against what remained unclear). By the third visit about a month later, Johnnie's mother reported no further references to an inside girl, fewer behavioral problems, and fewer "spacey" spells. Follow-up at about 15 months revealed no significant problems. The father had also moved out of the area.

In several clinical cases, serial administrations of the CDC have supported the clinical observation that many dissociative behaviors decline with time and/or treatment. In our longitudinal study of sexually abused and nonabused comparison girls, CDC scores declined most sharply in the sexually abused group (see Chapter Twelve). However, in our prospective longitudinal study, about 6% of sexually abused girls continue to have pathological dissociative behaviors (i.e., CDC scores $\geq$ 12) at least 2 years after the cessation of abuse (Putnam and Trickett, 1997).

Adolescents with Persistent Pathological Dissociation

Adolescents appear to be more refractory to treatment, and also show fewer general passage-of-time improvement effects. A number of clinicians offer pessimistic appraisals of therapeutic efforts with adolescent

MPD cases (e.g., Dell and Eisenhower, 1990; Hornstein and Putnam, 1992; Kluft and Schultz, 1993; Putnam, 1993a). In addition, dissociative adolescents are more likely to have full-fledged MPD with crystallized alter personality states (Putnam et al., 1996b). Clinicians working with adolescent MPD cases often comment that teenagers are not motivated to engage in therapy. They have not yet come up hard against the problems produced by dissociative discontinuities in cognition and behavior. (After all, who really cares if they behave very differently in math class compared with English or with different groups of friends?) Adolescents also have a difficult time acknowledging that they are different from peers, especially with respect to emotional problems. The hot developmental issues of adolescent rebellion, generational distrust, and cynicism about adult values further color teenagers' cost–benefit appraisals of what they really need. Some clinicians appear to do well with dissociative adolescents, but I, for one, find them difficult to treat.

Factors Influencing Prognosis

Many factors influence prognosis and outcome. As yet, we have little idea of how much weight to give each one, particularly in a given case. Various child-specific factors are undoubtedly important. Many have been discussed in Chapter Thirteen as important for resiliency; they include the child's active efforts to improve things, intellectual capacities, and interpersonal skills. Temperament, physical health, and genetic factors also probably make meaningful contributions. Family environment makes a strong contribution, for better or for worse. Over time, supportive families with one or more involved caretakers can do much to correct trauma-related psychopathology. Conversely, poor parenting impedes development of metacognitive integrative functions and further increases dissociative behaviors. The nature and timing of the traumatic experiences is probably also critical (see the discussion of the diversity of maltreatment outcomes in Chapter Three). Finally, the presence (or absence) of other resources and opportunities (e.g., school activities, sports, and social groups such as Scouting or church groups) also shape function and health.

Some children known to have been exposed to significant traumas appear asymptomatic when evaluated. These children pose a dilemma (Finkelhor and Berliner, 1995). Is something being missed? Should some kind of preventive intervention be made? If so, what kind and how much, given that there are no target symptoms to monitor? Will the children deteriorate at a future point? Little is known about asymptomatic children, except that 10–20% of them will be markedly worse when evaluated a year or two later (Finkelhor and Berliner, 1995). So-called "sleeper effects" have been documented, in which children who appeared to be the least symptomatic on initial evaluation are the most symptomatic at a later point (e.g., Mannarino, Cohen, Smith, and Moore-Motily, 1991; Finkelhor and Berliner, 1995). Such effects limit the confidence that we can place in short-term treatment studies reporting improvement.

Treatment dropout is another factor that influences outcome. Little research has explored the utilization of treatment by maltreating families. What is known indicates that treatment dropout is influenced by child gender (boys are more likely to drop out), family minority status, family symptomatology, and whether or not a parent receives treatment (Finkelhor and Berliner, 1995; Horowitz, Putnam, Noll, and Trickett, 1997). The continuing presence of the offender in the home also decreases the utilization of services. If dropouts were fully represented in treatment outcome studies, it is likely that reported success rates would be significantly lower. Finding out why people do and do not utilize services is an important area of treatment outcome research that is just beginning to be addressed for maltreating families (Horowitz et al., 1997).

The State of the Art

One of the biggest mistakes made (in my opinion) during the early years of the modern MPD movement (circa 1978 to 1988) was the overselling of positive treatment outcome (Putnam, 1986b, 1989a, 1993b). The implicit (and often explicitly stated) notion that every MPD patient who entered into a dissociative-disorder-focused treatment would become a psychologically healthy, integrated individual was routinely communicated in training workshops and professional meetings. In fact, there was little evidence for this notion beyond the glowing accounts of a few clinicians reporting large numbers of successful integrations. By 1990 these optimistic reports were being questioned by others, who were achieving more modest improvements. Although I believe that there is much of value in reports of clinical experience, such reports do suffer from the natural tendency of their authors to emphasize successes, to minimize failures, and to overgeneralize outcomes from memorable cases.

We need systematic research to assess treatment outcomes scientifically. This is expensive and requires a supportive clinical–research infrastructure. Through no fault of their own, researchers in child maltreatment and dissociative disorders lack resources. The field of PTSD research has benefited greatly from the long-standing connection between the Department of Veterans Affairs and academia. Yet, even with these considerable resources at researchers' disposal, surprisingly few systematic treatment outcome data are available for PTSD (e.g., see review in Solomon et al., 1992). In comparison with PTSD, child maltreatment and dissociative disorders are largely orphans without a similar sophisticated research infrastructure. I hope that this will change for the better in the next century—although I would not rule out the possibility that things could get even worse.

THERAPEUTIC ALLIANCE ISSUES

Trust

Although trust is a basic component of human relationships, it is not well understood. Trust is multidimensional; it also waxes and wanes dynamically across contexts and over time. The capacity to trust can be grievously damaged by maltreatment experiences, but it may be reparable—at least for some individuals. When trust is damaged, other fundamental aspects of an individual's relationships and basic assumptions about the world are also altered. Restitution of the capacity to trust takes place in small increments, and usually with frequent testing.

An individual's capacity to trust others is believed to be strongly influenced by his or her primary attachment relationship. Maltreated children generally have significantly disturbed attachment relationships (see Chapters Two and Nine). It may be possible for a therapist to modify a child's attachment relationship, but it is slow work. What therapy does best is to offer the child an opportunity to explore attachment issues. This can be done in person (i.e., family therapy with the primary caretaker), or, more often, in an indirect fashion (e.g., doll or puppet play, or drawing and talking about pictures of families).

In the course of therapy, much early work centers around the development or "building" of trust between patient and therapist. It is implicitly assumed that it is the child who must "build" trust, because it has been "shattered" by life experiences. However, in the context of therapy (as in other relationships), development of trust is a mutual, interactive process. It grows out of the large and small exchanges that occur between two individuals, and between the individuals and their shared environment. Some view a patient's trust as a prize that can be won or an obstacle that can be overcome once and for all; then the therapy can move on to the "really important stuff." In fact, therapy with maltreated individuals is always concerned with trust and never moves very far from this basic issue.

The chemistry of trust is an unfathomable mixture of the individuals involved and the history and circumstances that they share. There is no sure way to teach anyone how to develop a positive, trusting therapeutic relationship with someone else. Caring and consistency are important components, but by themselves they do not insure success. With a traumatized child, trust is nurtured through honesty, consistency, and fairness. The child's experience of the safety and stability of therapeutic space, which is an extension of the therapist's personality, is also pivotal.

Trust can rapidly become a major countertransference problem. Anyone who has tried hard to be trustworthy resents feeling mistrusted. In particular, therapists seeking flattering reflections of themselves from patients may perceive mistrust as an insult. Attempts to resolve issues of trust rapidly are doomed to failure.

The Therapist's Assumption of Risk and Responsibility

One of the most anxiety-provoking aspects of clinically managing a behaviorally disturbed, traumatized child is the question of just how much control to allow the child in a given situation. As children grow older, adults must turn over control of more and more areas of their lives to them. For better or for worse, it is inevitable; it is also necessary to help children to grow into healthy adults. But how and when to do this are difficult decisions for those bearing responsibility to and for the children.

Some dissociative children and adolescents are dangerous (see the discussion in Chapter Fifteen). Some are suicidal. Most are impulsive, interpersonally hypersensitive, prone to misperceptions, and affectively labile. Many are frighteningly headstrong and just will not or cannot listen to adults. Each is a uniquely complex person, defying generalizations, and requiring on-the-spot decision making. Balancing such a child's needs against the larger risks to the child and others requires tolerating the anxieties that come with such responsibilities. Judgment tempered with experience is crucial. But often a therapist (or another caring adult) just has to accept some risks and see what happens. It can be therapeutic to pass control to a child or teenager on some issues. Occasionally, however, doing so ends badly—and people and the press are quick to blame the therapist (or the foster parent, caseworker, teacher, etc.). We need to understand, and to make it clear to society at large, that there are serious risks involved in working with maltreated children. We must find ways to support those individuals who are called upon to accept these risks and responsibilities, and must realize that they cannot be expected to control their charges completely.

Being a "Hardass"

There is a long-standing therapeutic tradition of taking a firm, limit-setting, boundary-managing stance toward dissociative adults (e.g., see discussions in Putnam, 1989a, and Kluft, 1994). This applies equally to dissociative youths. Any therapist working with disturbed, traumatized children is sometimes put in the uncomfortable position of having to be a "hardass." This can occur in many ways, but however it happens, the therapist must take a position that sets firm boundaries with strong and definitive consequences for transgression. The issue involved is often a choice between the child's interests and the welfare of others. Occasionally a tough stand appears to create a tragic, self-fulfilling prophecy. I don't know any rule for deciding when and how to be a "hardass," but sometimes it must be done—and it can be therapeutic.

Persistence and Patience

Traumatized, dissociative children wear down the patience of therapists and others with their erratic ability to learn from experience and their frequent inability to make use of previously established rules and plans. The sense of going over the same ground repeatedly, with no apparent improvement, is frustrating. Sometimes, just when therapists think they are getting somewhere, the children revert to the way they were before therapy began—without any apparent benefit from past efforts. This profound inability to incorporate learning into reliably accessible behavioral responses is a result of traumatized children's state dependency of learning and memory, as well as of their metacognitive integrative deficits.

More than anything else, patience and persistence are necessary to make progress—not thoughtless patience and persistence, but informed, creative, humorous, philosophical, and even religious patience and persistence. Caretakers, group home personnel, residential staff members, teachers, and others must be convinced of the necessity of going over and over the same material again and again. A dissociative child should be presented with the same basic explanations and expectations, regardless of the behavioral state he or she happens to be in at the moment. The manner of delivery can be varied somewhat to accommodate the child's shifts in affect and developmental level, but the basic message should always be the same. Consistency and constancy are important factors in bridging pathological dissociative state dependency.

Patience and persistence produce a cumulative impact on a dissociative child's behavior, although it may take some time before this is manifested. The constancy of the information, and the constancy of the adult imparting that information, do indeed register—although the child may show no sign of this at the time. I view this as a Zen-like task of chipping away at a mountain. But I admit that I too lose my patience and "blow my cool" from time to time.

TREATMENT PROCESS ISSUES

Control of Behavior

Behavioral problems—for example, aggression, suicide attempts, self-destructive and risk-taking behavior, sexual behaviors, disruptive and destructive behaviors, lying, stealing, sneaking, and hoarding—are common presenting complaints by adults who bring abused children to treatment (Cosentino et al., 1995). These behaviors have their origin in such a child's life experiences, but by the time a therapist sees the child there may be a complex overlay, including significant biological components (Ito et al., 1993; De Bellis and Putnam, 1994). Behavioral problems are built up over time in an interactive process with the child's environment, biology, and developmental history. The enormous complexities of the interaction between behavior and biology in a developing child are just beginning to be appreciated. The therapeutic possibilities of significant biological changes emerging from appropriate treatment have not yet been considered, except by a farsighted few.

The problem behaviors of traumatized children often relate directly to disturbances in the developmental themes traced in this book. Successful self-control of behavior involves regulation of affect, control of impulses, biological regulation, development of metacognitive functions, and integration of sense of self. Traumatic disruption of any of these processes produces developmentally cumulative effects, which give rise to problem behaviors that accrue over the life span. Disruption in one process (e.g., regulation of affect) has secondary, tertiary, and higher-level derivative impacts on other developmental processes, which in turn produce their own effects. Behavior alters biology (e.g., Wolpaw, Schmidt, and Vaughan, 1991). Biology influences behavior.

In helping children acquire "control" over their behavior, it is important to consider the flip side of control, "dyscontrol." In some instances, apparent dyscontrol of behavior actually represents a form of control for a child. By going "out of control," the child may in fact be "taking control." (It is important to state clearly that in other instances, the child is simply overwhelmed by acute internal and external stresses and triggers, and is unable to regulate his or her behavior.) When dyscontrol is a strategy for control, the child often tests the therapist with out-of-control behavior—either by directly challenging the rules and boundaries of the therapeutic space, or by playing out themes of dyscontrol with figures and stories. The therapist's task is not to take control back from the child (though this may be necessary temporarily), but to help the child gain self-control.

Victims of abuse, in particular, tend to struggle over some of the smallest points and rules. Herman (1992) cogently points out that this is one of the few areas of control available to victims of captivity—which, in some fashion, most abused children are. They may not be able to control the larger events of their lives, but they can channel their anger and their need for autonomy and control into opposing specific rules and regulations. In therapy, this often takes the form of challenges to the integrity of the therapeutic space. In other instances, challenges centering around control take the form of self-destructive and self-jeopardizing behaviors. Like prisoners who fight back with a hunger strike, abused children may be showing that they can hurt themselves worse than anyone else can—and therefore that they have more control than anyone else does.

The nature and sources of dyscontrol dictate the kinds of therapeutic interventions that may be employed. In instances where dyscontrol is serving a dynamic purpose (either by expressing a central conflict or by permitting the child an escape), apt psychodynamic interventions aimed at restoring appropriate control or symbolic reparative work with damaged self-concepts can produce rapid improvement. In instances where dyscontrol is long-standing, has a heavy overlay of meanings and behaviors, and is associated with biological dysregulation (e.g., disturbances of the HPA stress response axis), acquisition of control proceeds in slow increments, with intermittent relapses and regressions.

The art of therapy requires distinguishing among the reasons and sources of dyscontrol and formulating appropriate interventions. A particular tragedy is the failure to recognize when dynamic interventions aimed at restoring control, dispelling a sense of powerlessness, or correcting logical binds are indicated. The converse tragedy is the unrealistic expectation that complex, multilayered, dyscontrol behavioral problems can be resolved with simple, one-shot interventions such as "ventilating anger." And there are many times when it is hard to know what approach is called for.

Transformation of Trauma

Adult Treatment Models

Therapists working with traumatized people generally endorse the principle that traumatic experiences must be described, discussed, and "worked through" before the individual can achieve a satisfactory resolution. This approach is well established in the treatment of adults who have experienced natural disasters, rape, child abuse, torture, combat, and other traumas.

Adults may have difficulty recalling some memories of traumatic experiences, particularly chronic trauma such as child abuse. Traumatic memories may be nonverbal, iconic, verbal, or some complex combination thereof (see the discussion in Chapter Six). The therapist helps the patient recognize traumatic memories, and often may help the patient "recover" and "reconstruct" traumatic memories that are not consciously available at first. This is a tricky process fraught with potential for contamination. In the course of reconstruction of the trauma, sensations and affects are reexperienced and identified. It is generally accepted that the identification of powerful sensory and affective experiences is crucial to the therapeutic reconstruction process. The goal is to put these affective, somatic, and perceptual experiences into words—words that can be examined and understood.

Research employing functional brain imaging together with traumatic reminders to stimulate trauma responses (e.g., Rauch et al., 1996) finds increased activity in right-hemisphere limbic and paralimbic structures, consonant with affective arousal. The visual cortex also lights up, supporting the reports of victims that they often see powerfully vivid intrusive images of the traumatic experience. In contrast, left-hemisphere language areas are often hypoactive, suggesting that the difficulties in talking about trauma often reported by victims have a biological basis. The notion of "unspeakable acts of evil" may be more than a metaphor.

Reconstructive memory work requires the utmost attention to technique and to countertransference. The therapist must be prepared to respect and to endure the enormous uncertainty that accompanies such recalled and reconstructed material. Often the content is a complex and dynamic mixture of the real, the imagined, and the feared—and there are no good rules for discerning which is what. It is crucial to avoid suggesting events or experiences. When all is said and done, considerable ambiguity about what really happened will often remain.

As memories become available, they are sequenced and integrated with other material. In the therapy, they are reconsidered from new perspectives and reinterpreted so that new "meaning" emerges. The reported experiences are placed in a cognitive, emotional, and moral context that allows the individual new ways of conceptualizing them (Herman, 1992). The therapeutic process of reconstruction also plays a crucial role in validation of the experience: Finally, someone is "hearing" what happened. Testimony may be an essential part of the healing process. Treatments devised for torture victims and political prisoners frequently place great emphasis on a formal testimonial process that allows the survivors to tell their stories to the world (see, e.g., Krell, 1985).

Child Treatment Models

With children, particularly young children, the therapeutic approach to the transformation of trauma is not at all well understood. (As noted above, this is far from a simple and straightforward process with adults.) Children do not have the verbal capacities to articulate traumatic experiences in the manner of adults. Their ability to retrieve traumatic memories may be quite context- and behavioral-state-dependent. Memories are rarely directly available in the therapy setting, although they may figure strongly in a child's awareness in other settings. Children often express traumatic memories in behavior and play in ways that are difficult for adults to recognize.

Paradoxically, even when a therapist recognizes the connection between a given behavior and a past traumatic experience, attempting to give a child "insight" into this by having him or her verbalize the connection often dooms the intervention. Efforts to impose an adult model of therapeutic reconstruction and transformation of trauma on children and adolescents are misguided; they ignore the special needs and capacities of children. Making "meaning" with children often requires working with traumatic material implicitly rather than explicitly, as I have noted in Chapter Thirteen. Play therapy and art therapy are especially helpful in this process. Transforming traumatic experiences may also involve facilitating autonomy, control, and competence in ways that do not need to directly acknowledge the role of the trauma in constricting or distorting these functions. Clarifying cognitive confusions and undoing pathological identifications by means of symbolic play replace verbalization and insight.

Approaches to therapeutic transformation of trauma in adolescents fall somewhere between those employed with children and with adults. Some adolescents can verbalize trauma and examine its effects on their lives, but often this is not sufficient to produce meaningful changes in their behavior. As I describe later, play or art therapy and the use of rule-based games to structure interpersonal interactions may be helpful when traditional psychotherapy is going nowhere.

A comment on traumatic reminders or "triggers" is in order here. Such reminders can be remarkably ubiquitous, especially for children, with their enhanced perceptual plasticity. Child abuse usually occurs in home settings, and all manner of daily objects and routines may take on abuse-related meanings that are invisible to others. In school, pictures in textbooks or spelling words may act as triggers for affective or dissociative traumatic states, in ways that mimic disruptive or attention-disordered behaviors.

Children typically try to avoid traumatic reminders. Sometimes avoidance is manifested in stereotypic or ritualized behaviors; at other times it occurs through induction of dissociative states or through oppositional behaviors. Even when a therapist suspects that this may be happening, it can be difficult to determine exactly what a child is attempting to avoid. Children can be asked about things that they "don't like to look at" or that "bother" them.

JIMMY

When Jimmy was 6, his older brother was a bystander killed in a drive-by shooting. Before the ambulance came, Jimmy saw the brother dying on the sidewalk, bleeding profusely. Jimmy subsequently developed chronic sleep problems, including traumatic nightmares and refusal to sleep in his own bed. More than a year after his brother's death, he was brought in at the request of the school for evaluation of disruptive behavior. I asked him to imagine himself back in his room trying to go to sleep, and to tell me what he was seeing and thinking about. He said that there was a spot on the wall that frightened him; he could see it at night even with his eyes shut. His mother confirmed that there was a dark waterstain on the wall near where his brother's bed had been. Suspecting that this might remind him of his brother's blood, I suggested to the mother that she cover the stain with a picture and rearrange the furniture. She reported a marked improvement in Jimmy's sleeping with the new room arrangement.

Loss, Grief, and Mourning

Death of a primary caretaker is the prototypic example of loss, but there are many other kinds, such as separation or detachment that leaves a child destitute. (Loss may also take the form of things that should have been but never were.) Both the loss itself and the changes it imposes on a child's life are painful. A major loss generally marks a life transition point for a child. It causes pain, sadness, anxiety, and depression (though only numbness may be experienced immediately); also, familiar old ways end, and new worries, responsibilities, and problems must be faced.

Loss, grief, and mourning are all intertwined, and problems occur when these processes cannot run their natural course. Pain and anguish may be deferred for years, but such deferral exacts a psychological and physiological price. Research indicates that bereaved children are at higher risk for depression, anxiety, and somatization (Weller and Weller,

1991). Therapists have long noted that unresolved grief places traumatized individuals at higher risk for depression and self-destructive behavior, as well as "trapping" them in the traumatic process (e.g., Shatan, 1973; Lifton, 1980; Herman, 1992).

For maltreated children, the issues of loss, grief, and bereavement are complicated and often atypical. The universal need of a grieving child to idealize a missing parent (or other relative or friend) may conflict with memories of maltreatment. Indeed, the person is often not dead, just absent because of abandonment or the denial of visitation rights. There are few (if any) peers with similar experiences in whom the child can confide and with whom feelings can be shared. The missing person is often vilified by others (e.g., foster parents and caseworkers), who do not acknowledge the child's grief over the loss. Grief in a maltreated child also produces powerful countertransference feelings in therapists and caretakers.

Little is known about the nature and efficacy of interventions for grief and mourning in general. Much less is understood about the special circumstances of maltreated children. It appears that it is important to identify and acknowledge the loss, and to help children express their grief in a developmentally appropriate fashion. When the loss results from a death, attending the funeral and participating in the mourning processes is important; they should not be prohibited just because a child is "too young to understand." Nor should young children be told that death is like sleep. This leads to anxieties about going to sleep and instills the notion that the dead person will wake up someday.

The grief process can often be facilitated through symbolic or ritual acts. Of course, this is the essence of funerals. But memorials and testimonials are also important, as indicated by the spontaneous shrines and memorials that spring up at sites of tragedy. Flowers, candles, personal mementoes, and letters to the deceased help to express grief and sanctify such sites.

Guilt and Self-Blame

Therapists working with victims of abuse or other trauma inevitably encounter strong feelings of guilt, shame, and self-blame. These painful emotions contribute to the feelings of worthlessness and fraudulence expressed by many abuse victims. Unabsolved guilt produces feelings of malignant badness that infect all aspects of self. Feelings of guilt, self-blame, and shame are usually kept secret; they become sources of private torment that nullify positive accomplishments. When a therapist encounters a patient who cannot accept real successes, there is often a source of secret, all-contaminating guilt.

It is an ironic paradox that abused children suffer more guilt than their abusers. Therapists tend to view such guilt feelings as irrational—something that they should be able to talk their patients out of. To a small extent this is true. But feelings of guilt, self-blame, and shame have their basis in life experiences and cannot be absolved until their sources have been clearly identified. These are tenacious feelings—deeply internalized at the very core of self-representation—and they do not yield to mere logic alone.

There can be many contributions to a patient's sense of guilt. Abuse survivors are often forced into complicity with their abusers. Such complicity has both psychological and physiological aspects. "Cooperation" with the abuse (e.g., keeping it a secret or even initiating abuse episodes as a form of control) can leave a victim with a shameful sense of responsibility. Harsh judgments by others, especially family members who might be expected to be supportive, often reinforce feelings of guilt. When feelings of arousal are associated with sexual abuse experiences, these become a particularly strong source of guilt in later life. Sexual practices and masturbatory fantasies that contain themes reminiscent of abuse experiences and are sexually arousing to a survivor convince the victim that he or she must have "wanted" it.

Feelings of guilt often express the victim's strong sense of identification with the abuser. When an adult victim's abuser was a parent, guilt may be strongly embedded in the internalized parental model carried by the victim now acting as a parent. Another strong source of guilt is surviving when others have died, particularly if the victim has witnessed the deaths of others in shared circumstances. "Survivor guilt" haunts victims of disaster, war, and atrocities. If the victim has also been a victimizer, profound guilt occurs as the victim comes to recognize the damage done to him or her by the victimization—and thus the damage that he or she has done in turn to others.

When young children are abused, feelings of guilt take root in their strongly egocentric and self-referential nature. Because of the dissociated, compartmentalized nature of abusive experiences, a child's developmental stage at the time of the abuse influences his or her attributions of responsibility at a later point. Feelings of guilt may be expressed in ruminations or cleansing obsessions. Most therapists working with sexual abuse survivors have encountered preoccupations with washing and hygiene, which mask feelings of guilt, dirtiness, and contamination. Adolescent survivors in particular tend to act out feelings of guilt and shame with excess cleanliness. (See the case of Tina in Chapter Eleven.)

Specific feelings of guilt are treated with therapeutic clarification and sometimes with cleansing rituals. With adults, clarification comes from placing the survivors' experiences within the larger context of their lives at the time, and from articulating the realities of their limited power and responsibility as children. Clarification often takes this course: An intellectual insight is belatedly followed by an emotional insight, at which point a fundamental shift occurs in a survivor's sense of responsibility.

Cleansing rituals, a cornerstone of spiritual healing, may be useful for some adults following therapeutic clarification. For children, rituals may provide a powerful intervention even when the children do not verbalize problems of guilt and self-blame. The therapist should offer a clarification in a developmentally appropriate manner—for example, "If something is dangerous or bad for a child, it does not matter what the child 'wants' to do. Daddies should never do these things to their daughters." Rituals may involve putting the "bad" and "dirty" feelings into some psychologically displaced container (e.g., a picture of the experience) and destroying the container physically or symbolically.

Enhancing Self-Confidence

Social, academic, athletic, artistic, and all other kinds of performance are enhanced by self-confidence, regardless of an individual's level of skill or knowledge. Individuals with histories of maltreatment often have pathologically low levels of self-esteem and self-confidence. These are usually addressed with cognitive interventions aimed at correcting distortions in thinking, but the efficacy of such cognitive interventions is not known. Research on enhancing human performance suggests that other approaches to enhancing self-confidence and self-esteem may be helpful (see Druckman and Bjork, 1994). At least three other approaches appear fruitful: instructional strategies, goal setting, and modeling.

Self-confidence and performance can be facilitated by instructional strategies that break a skill or behavior down into smaller parts and guide the person through the acquisition of these subparts, step by step. Progress is made in small increments, with multiple intermediate successes to bolster self-esteem and confidence. Eventually the individual can perform the action fully and independently of the instructor.

Goal setting involves defining realistic performance standards that the individual strives to attain. A combination of short- and long-term goals appears to be optimal. Early in the learning process, goals should emphasize the learning process itself rather than actual performance. Attention, effort, form, and strategy can be rewarded, regardless of overall success. Later, success brings its own rewards.

When an individual has essentially no experience with a task or situation, watching others model the behavior is particularly important. Models need not be similar to the individual in terms of personal characteristics (e.g., age, race, gender); more important is the similarity between the model's situation and that of the individual. Models should articulate their feelings, concerns, and strategies for the observer. Research suggests that the more different types of people an observer sees performing a task, the stronger the observer's conviction that he or she can also meet the challenge will be.

These confidence-enhancing strategies, individually and in combination, appear helpful for working with older maltreated children and adolescents. In my experience, cognitive approaches—however theoretically elegant—inevitably degenerate into numbingly repetitive exhortations to "stop thinking like that; you *can* do it." Such attempts at cognitive correction rapidly become a focus for oppositional behavior in children and adolescents, who become stuck in the counterposition of "No, I can't." The three approaches described above sidestep much of this by directing the focus away from the "Yes, you can"–"No, I can't" deadlock, as well as by providing more specific information and illustrations of *how* a thing is done. These interventions are also more easily disguised, permitting them to be instituted in an implicit, background manner. (Again, see the discussion of explicit versus implicit techniques in Chapter Thirteen.)

ISSUES AND INTERVENTIONS FOR DISSOCIATIVE SYMPTOMS AND BEHAVIORS

As should be apparent by now, I conceptualize pathological dissociative behaviors as extreme examples of discrete behavioral states of consciousness. Treatments directed toward decreasing dissociative behaviors involve a few basic strategies—which, of course, must be tailored to a given child or adolescent. These include (1) facilitating the acquisition of self-modulation of behavioral and affective states; (2) facilitating the development of metacognitive self-monitoring and integrative functions; and (3) breaking down the discreteness of pathological dissociative states by therapeutically processing and integrating compartmentalized affects and memories. Before I discuss these strategies, however, I raise the questions of when and how to work directly with alter personalities and other dissociative states. In general, as will be seen, I advocate caution in such work.

Thoughts on Working Directly with Alter Personalities and Other Dissociative States

Sometimes treatment is best accomplished by working directly with pathological dissociative states, such as the alter personalities in MPD patients. More often in children, effective treatment involves working implicitly with dissociative divisions of self and behavior—that is, focusing on self-monitoring and integrative capacities.

Clinicians working with dissociative children and adolescents frequently face the question of when and when not to engage dissociative states directly and explicitly in treatment. Children, in particular, raise this issue with their more amorphous clinical presentations; it is not always clear when the various identity disturbances and vivid ICs characteristic of dissociative children qualify as separate and distinct alter personality states. As a rule of thumb, I suggest that whenever there is ambiguity or doubt, the therapist bide his or her time and refrain from explicitly engaging dissociative identity shifts as if they were discrete alter personality states. In particular, identity alterations should not be called by separate names or engaged in ways indicating that they are considered separate or different from the child as a whole. The overall emphasis of the therapy should be on enhancing self-control, affect and impulse modulation, behavioral integration, and unification of awareness and self-representation.

This is important in the early stages of therapy, especially when a child has recently been removed from a traumatic situation. As noted earlier, a fair percentage of young children who exhibit pathological dissociation when evaluated shortly after the termination of maltreatment will show significant resolution of their symptoms over a few months with general or supportive treatment. If pathological dissociative behaviors persist, however, then treatment should move to more active integrative and metacognitive work. This must be tailored to the age/developmental stage of the child. Therapeutic efforts should focus on creating a supportive home or placement environment that will help the child learn to modulate mood and behavioral states and to restrain impulsivity, and will provide plenty of consistency and supportive feedback about behaviors and expectations (see Chapter Fifteen). Every effort should be made to help the child integrate dissociative behaviors by providing nonthreatening feedback about dissociated actions. The centrality and continuity of self should be consistently emphasized.

Alter personality states should only be engaged directly as discrete psychological entities (e.g., called out by name) when it is clear that they are behaviorally distinct, express strongly held convictions of separateness, and play an identifiable role in a child's or adolescent's symptoms and behaviors across several domains or contexts. At this point, they are sufficiently crystallized that it is highly unlikely that they will remit spontaneously. Discrete alter personality states may be found in a few traumatized children as young as 3 years of age (e.g., Riley and Mead, 1988), but are most commonly encountered in older children and adolescents (Putnam et al., 1996b).

Even when a therapist is satisfied that a child's alter personality states are enduring and pathological, it is important not to encourage further differentiation or separation. Whenever possible, the therapist should talk to the child/alter personality system as a whole. When it is necessary to work with specific alter personality states, this should be framed within the larger tasks of therapy (e.g., "I need to talk with the part of you called Jamie that is cutting you").

Little else is known about therapeutic approaches toward crystallized alter personality states in children and adolescents. Adult treatment models have elaborated a number of psychotherapeutic techniques. These are covered in my book on adult treatment (Putnam, 1989a) and in writings by other experienced therapists (e.g., Chu, 1990; Loewenstein, 1993; Kluft, 1994). Below, I confine myself to more general approaches to dissociative states that are applicable to pathological dissociative states in children, many of which are not yet crystallized around a separate sense of identity.

Facilitating Self-Modulation of Behavioral States

As emphasized at many points throughout this book, a major goal in working with traumatized children is to help them to acquire self-control over their behavioral and affective states (dissociative and otherwise). A major component of self-control is self-monitoring, a metacognitive function discussed below. Other critical aspects of self-control include the ability to sustain a desired behavioral state volitionally in the face of disruptive and destabilizing stimuli; the ability to reinstate a desired state volitionally if it is destabilized; and the ability to activate an appropriate behavioral state congruent with the situational demands.

Behavioral regulation requires a number of critical components (Kopp and Wyer, 1994). The child must have the metacognitive structures available to monitor his or her own behavior. In addition, the child must be motivated to acquire and exercise self-control. Self-regulation of affect and behavior largely occurs in social settings; thus, the child must also have the interpersonal skills and relatedness to respond to social cues, and the ability to differentiate between his or her affective issues and problematic affects of others. Finally, the child must understand and largely accept the rules of social behavior.

At times, a therapist or caretaker must intervene to stabilize a child in an appropriate behavioral state. Children who tend to slip into dissociative states in the face of specific traumatic triggers or more general stresses can be helped to "hang in there" in various ways. If a child is clearly beginning to "space out," it is important for a caring adult to provide active orientation to time, place, and situation, and to help the child focus on the here and now, the environment, the people, or the activity. Explicit expectations, clearly defined rules, or other organizing structures are also helpful in refocusing a dissociative child on the present situation. This must be done gently, as too-intense interventions will only further destabilize the child's state. (See also the discussion of the management of spontaneous abreactions in Chapter Fifteen.)

Some traumatized adolescents make maladaptive responses to encroaching dissociative states. Aggressive or paranoid behaviors, self-inflicted pain, or the activation of an alternative dissociative state (e.g., a cultivated fantasy world) may reflect attempts to stave off dysphoric dissociative or affective states. Therapists, caretakers, and significant others can help such adolescents recognize *what* is happening. It is not always necessary, or useful, to focus on *why* it is happening. Recognition of *what* facilitates the substitution of more adaptive responses.

Developing Metacognitive Functions

As previously discussed, metacognitive capacities emerge over the course of development and are strongly influenced by the input of significant others. Initially, parents or primary caretakers help children to sequence and integrate life experiences and to access and generalize the pool of information and knowledge that they possess—especially under new circumstances. Parents provide children with pertinent feedback about their behavior and act as externalized "observing egos," reflecting back to the children how they are coming across. With psychological maturation, the children increasingly internalize these capacities and perspectives.

Metacognitive self-reflective and integrative capacities are often disrupted in traumatized individuals. This is not to say that they are not present; rather, the ability to evaluate and make use of metacognitive knowledge is impaired. Dissociative individuals tend to make metacognitive errors about the source and certainty of information (see Chapter Six). In particular, they may be inappropriately overconfident about what they believe they know (which they in fact don't know). Paradoxically, they may devalue the certainty of things that they do know.

Therapists, caretakers, and other adults working with dissociative/traumatized children can stimulate and sharpen metacognitive capacities by providing relevant feedback to the children in a nonthreatening manner. (This can be difficult to do, especially with adolescents.) Self-monitoring capacities must be nurtured over time. Change may be slow; developmental restitution in other areas may be required before derivative metacognitive capacities show meaningful change.

Children must learn to listen to themselves and to track their own behavior. Gentle questioning, supportive feedback, games, sports, and activities that require self-attention are helpful. As in many other areas of therapy, attempts to make this task too explicit tend to activate oppositional responses, especially in adolescents. (The techniques used by speech therapists and educators who help children learn to monitor their own performance can be useful here.) Self-monitoring can be facilitated by significant adults, who can model it for the children. Children can be encouraged to develop sharable self-narratives—that is, explicit or metaphoric stories of their lives and experiences. They can also be taught ways to express themselves verbally, artistically, and athletically. Self-monitoring involves an active inner dialogue among levels of self-awareness.

A therapist's constancy—cognitive, affective, and behavioral—is an important metacognitive intervention aimed at creating consistency and continuity for the child. Richard Kluft's often-quoted remark that he wants to "bore" his patients into health illustrates the importance of a nonreactive therapeutic stance in buffering the affective and dissociative swings such patients experience. It is important for a therapist not to change each time a child or adolescent changes behavioral state. Caretakers and therapists are more likely to be able to influence youngster's self-monitoring and evaluative metacognitive capacities than to alter self-control and affect regulation directly.

Self-control issues can be played out in rule-based games. To do this, it is necessary to find a tolerable stage upon which problematic behavior can be played out and examined. It may be displaced into dolls and action figures, or contained in metaphoric stories and drawings shared between child and adult. There are various opportunities for creative forms of self-examination and supportive feedback. Again, for some children and adolescents, videotaping suggests itself; diaries, journals, or autobiographical "novels" may be helpful for others.

It is important to carry forward the continuity of these activities. That is, the themes in a particular therapy session should be connected to the last one, and the one before it, and so on (e.g., "This picture reminds me of what happened to the girl doll in our session last week"). Content is not nearly as important as the continuity and integration of a child's life story. And, once again, content is not necessarily historically accurate.

Eroding and Diffusing Dissociative States

Traditional treatment of dissociative and traumatized individuals has stressed the discharge of affects and painful memories, often through such therapeutic techniques as emotional flooding and therapeutic abreaction. Clinical experience indicates that these are useful interventions for some individuals; it is also clear that they are far from sufficient by themselves and must be coupled with psychotherapeutic processing of emotional material (Putnam, 1989a, 1992). In adults, abreactive discharge of compartmentalized affects and painful memories, coupled with psychotherapeutic integration, does appear to break down dissociative compartmentalization. It can also desensitize an individual to traumatic cues that previously activated a given dissociative state.

Recently, cognitive therapy approaches have been added to the psychotherapeutic repertoire for dissociative disorders (e.g., Ross, 1990; Fine, 1992). These interventions seek to correct dissociative illogic, such as "delusions of separateness" among alter personality states in adult patients. To some extent, one can reason away such cognitive distortions, although patients readily revert to these modes of thinking under stress. Relaxation training can also help to decrease cumulative stress.

Short-term cognitive-behavioral treatments have been developed for sexually abused children (e.g., Deblinger, McLeer, and Henry, 1990; Cohen and Mannarino, 1996). These appear promising, as measured by broadly focused scales such as the CBCL. However, the efficacy of these treatments for dissociative symptoms in children needs to be established.

Laboratory research with MPD patients suggests that the sense of separateness and dissociative compartmentalization of affect, information, and behavior among discrete alter personality states can be eroded by repeatedly juxtaposing states in the same activity or task. The more alter personality states are cooperatively engaged for a common purpose, the greater the erosion of dissociative compartmentalization will be. Clinically, this need not require individually interacting with the alter personality states. Implicitly engaging the different parts of the individual in solving a common task or problem can also cut across internal dividedness.

PLAY THERAPY

Play in Normal and Maltreated Children

Play is central to the life of children. It is a means by which they learn to understand the world; it is also an arena in which they can restore control and find meaning in the face of hurtful experiences. Play, of course, changes over the course of development. It goes almost without saying that play differs for children of different ages, but there are marked differences even within the same age group in the developmental levels and modes of play. Indeed, a given child may move up and down a developmental continuum during the course of a single play session. This is particularly true of dissociative children, who frequently regress in the presence of threatening stimuli. Of course, significant gender and cultural differences also exist.

Maltreated children show developmental deficits in play. Their overall play patterns are less cognitively and socially mature than those of nonmaltreated children (Cicchetti and Lynch, 1995). On average, they also play less than nonmaltreated children, and they exhibit less symbolic play. They have constricted affective and thematic ranges and tend toward concrete reenactments of family roles and events. Superstitious play/behavior (e.g., "Step on a crack and break your mother's back") is probably more common in maltreated youngsters and may reflect their more ambiguous or externalized locus of control.

Basic Guidelines for Play Therapy

Play therapy involves entering into a child's play world, deciphering the meanings and issues expressed in the process and content of the play, and making appropriate interventions to facilitate change. Play is a complex activity, and play therapy is anything but "just playing." Having once been a kid is not sufficient expertise. Neophyte play therapists should seek supervision from an experienced mentor. The following discussion briefly summarizes the principles and techniques of play therapy with traumatized children.

Play therapy occurs within the therapeutic space. It is a special kind of play and should make full use of the symbolic potential of the play therapy situation. Children appreciate the ceremonial aspects of the therapeutic space and the play therapy interaction. They know that this is not just play as usual; they understand that this experience is an important, shared interaction that is focused on their problems and their lives. In a thoughtful review, Ablon (1996) identifies numerous therapeutic functions of play: synthesis and organization of affects; facilitation of cognitive development; modulation of aggression; promotion of bonding and affection; emergence of new comprehensions; and promotion of self-regulation.

Play therapists have different ways of characterizing the types of play that children display in therapy. Donovan and McIntyre (1990) draw a distinction between "ludic" play (playful but meaningless play) and "semic" play (meaningful, communicative play). Communicative play is necessary for successful play therapy. Communication occurs between a child and therapist and between the child and himself or herself, in an oscillating dance of meaning (Ablon, 1996). What the child chooses to do and say in early play therapy sessions offers clues (and cautions) about his or her capacity to use the therapy to make meaning and to effect change.

The art of play therapy is finding the meaning of the play, and, conversely, recognizing when there is none. At times, it may seem as if one therapist's meaning is another's gibberish. Some opine that it is all meaningful, and perhaps at some level it is; still, but I would caution that there are times when children's play is not meaningfully communicative about what is happening in their lives. A therapist can go very wrong attempting to make sense out of nonsense. The art, of course, is to know when something important is being communicated and when it is not.

Play therapy requires more than the mangled toy soldier held up to me as sufficient for any and all therapeutic interactions (see Chapter Thirteen). Different authorities have their lists, but the basic set begins with puppets; a stuffed animal or two; and a family of dolls in sufficient numbers, ages, genders and ethnic diversity (or ambiguity) to allow children to construct families that resemble their own. Crayons, pencils, and paper for drawing and writing are mandatory. Some monster and hero figures are also necessary; they are central to expressing fears and to overcoming those fears through action. At times, play therapy is a mythic journey for both child and therapist.

The child should be permitted to initiate the play themes. Within a short time, salient issues will emerge. The therapist watches the play process, sometimes commenting and occasionally participating. Interpretations are usually made in the form of descriptive narrations of the ongoing play, together with subtle background comments or speculations about the characters' thoughts, feelings, concerns, and motives. It is important for the therapist not to intrude upon or redirect the play without good reason.

Painful affects may emerge, inducing powerful countertransference wishes to avoid these feelings. The therapist must tolerate and empathically appreciate the child's painful feelings, such as anger, sadness, helplessness, humiliation, worthlessness, sadism, sexuality, and dependence (Ablon, 1996). Various dynamic defenses are likely to be manifested, such as inhibition, avoidance, displacement, and dissociation. Wishes and impulses are expressed in the play or in asides to the therapist. Transference phenomena increase as the child comes to know the therapist and develops an attachment. Vacations or other breaks in the therapy often highlight the transference process.

The horrible monster who frightens and hurts is a common theme, typically appearing within a few sessions. But there may be concurrent themes of rejection, loss, and loneliness for the monster (i.e., the abuser/maltreater), who may now be out of the home or denied visitation. "Am I a monster?" is another side of the question, as maltreated children struggle with why they were victimized and why they are now so angry and aggressive toward others. A therapist can help such a child to triumph over evil and to establish safety and fairness. The therapist also helps the child to stop being a monster and to become a valued person.

Traumatic Play

"Traumatic play," originally described by Lenore Terr (1981) and implicit in Freud's concept of the repetition compulsion, is the recreation of aspects of the traumatic experience in play, fantasy, or behavior. Some children repeatedly play out graphic reenactments of traumatic experiences, whereas others handle trauma more symbolically. Either concrete or symbolic traumatic reenactments may be repeatedly and perseveratively played out with a stereotypic fixity. Fixed or ritualized play sequences are a clue to a child's anxieties, conflicts, and painful affects (Ablon, 1996). When a child exhibits such sequences, a therapist must be more active in helping to create new endings and alternative scenarios.

When the therapist recognizes traumatic reenactments in the play, it is important *not* to make this explicit—at least not at first. These issues are best approached in a displaced fashion and commented on with respect to the situations that the play characters (e.g., dolls or figures in a drawing) find themselves in. The therapist explores the thoughts, feelings, and fears of the play characters, not the child. The child is free to own or disown the affects, and to act as is dynamically necessary. Often no comment is needed or productive. I share Ablon's (1996, p. 546) "controversial belief" that much therapeutic work occurs during play therapy in the absence of interpretations or verbalization.

Nurturance and caregiving are also important play themes with traumatized children. Taking care of, feeding, protecting, and rescuing younger, weaker, vulnerable figures are productive themes that generally bode well; sometimes such behavior signals a breakthrough to a new level. A therapist should not be surprised, however, when a protector/rescuer suddenly brutalizes a vulnerable character in a dissociated rage and then goes on as if nothing untoward just happened. But such an occurrence should not pass unnoticed.

Indeed, it is important not to gloss over the thematic breaks, inconsistencies, or apparently tangential sideshows that go on during a play therapy session. Interruptions in the continuity of play are important clues to thematic triggers, symptoms, and defenses. In dissociative children, they may often reflect significant shifts in behavioral states and may be accompanied by partial or complete amnesia for preceding material. Dissociative discontinuities may be manifested in confusion about what is happening or in sudden, angry rejection of the prior play theme. Discontinuities may also reflect nondissociative sources of psychopathology, such as anxiety attacks.

When significant disruptions occur, the therapist should gently take the child back to the preceding play to see what can be learned. If the child appears not to recall what has happened, the therapist can briefly summarize the events preceding the thematic break. Without pushing too hard, of course, the therapist should try to establish what the child does and does not remember.

Alter Personalities as Play Characters

When an MPD child feels comfortable with the therapist and the therapeutic space, the alter personalities may become externalized characters in the child's play. Their various traits and styles become attributed to specific toy figures who recurrently reappear in play sequences that express polarized internal conflicts (e.g., good vs. bad behavior, love vs. hate, fear vs. aggression). Sometimes a pair of figures will become identified as "twins," one good and one bad. Often the child adopts the same voice and demeanor for the play figure as he or she exhibits when the alter personality state is active.

This is a great arena in which to work with the child's alters without socializing the child as a "multiple." (It also underlines the need for those toy figures and props to be consistently available session after session, as noted in the discussion of the therapeutic space in Chapter Thirteen.) As an active observer, the therapist has opportunities to reflect on the nature of the feelings and conflicts expressed, and to offer thoughts about ways to resolve them.

Rule-Based Play Therapy

As children enter first or second grade, their play becomes increasingly dominated by rules. They begin to like rule-based activities, such as board games and team sports. They also begin spontaneously generating all sorts of rules to govern their free-form games—for example, making up rules about which action figures can do what, or how powerful certain weapons are. They use rules to guide themselves, to control the action of others, and to make the play world predictable. When children this age get into conflict while playing together, it is often over the rules (i.e., whose rules rule).

Rule-based games are useful in play therapy with dissociative older children and adolescents. Their structure and predictability are important anchors to the here and now and to the continuity of interaction.

REGINALD

Reginald, a 17-year-old black male with MPD (see Chapter Five and Putnam, 1993a), and I often played chess during his weekly therapy session. When he was "with it," Reginald had the ability to plan several moves ahead. He was especially clever at setting traps. However, at times one of his alter personalities (usually "Reggie") would take over and deliberately sacrifice pieces and positions. Reginald would then suddenly find himself in a changed game. At first he would accuse me of cheating somehow. Each time this happened, I held him to the situation as he found it; I also placed a clock prominently by the chessboard to make his time loss more apparent. Gradually he came to accept that he was responsible for his losses at chess.

As time passed, Reginald began to acknowledge experiences of disruption in the temporal continuity of the game. He also gained a measure of coawareness of "Reggie" and other alter personality states, and began to accept that their behavior was his behavior. The chessboard, ceremonially set between us, provided a displaced arena of interpersonal interaction that was both aggressive and lawful. The games produced plenty of here-and-now examples of unintegrated and self-sabotaging behavior that was detrimental to him. It was relatively easy to examine these dissociative experiences, whereas it had been difficult to get him to talk about what was occurring outside of treatment. For example, I might say, "I can't figure out why you moved your bishop there. You know that I am going to take it with my knight and put you in check. Don't you?"

SUMMARY

Little is known about the efficacy of psychological treatments for maltreated children and adolescents, and still less is known about treatment outcomes for dissociative youngsters in particular. Taken as a whole, research indicates beneficial effects for some maltreated children; however, many extrinsic factors, especially family environment, appear to affect outcomes powerfully. Because of "sleeper effects" and developmental changes, long-term follow-up will be required to establish treatment effects. The lack of an adequate research infrastructure has crippled research on these questions.

Individual treatments generally face common sets of issues. The first set has to do with development of an adequate therapeutic alliance. Trust (and other attachment derivatives) is a central theme. Trust, or at least enduring trust, is not a prize that can be won; it must be continually nurtured. Work with maltreated children raises many issues for therapists, not the least of which are the anxieties associated with being held responsible in some fashion for the behavior of a disturbed child or teenager. Sometimes a therapist has to be a "hardass" and take a "my way or the highway" stance. Most of the time, therapists just have to be patient and persistent.

Treatments for adult PTSD and dissociative disorders are predicated on the well-established principle that traumatic experiences must be processed in a deliberate and conscious manner. This involves remembering and openly discussing the experiences. It is not clear whether that this is necessary, or even desirable, for many children. Traumatic themes can be worked with more implicitly as they are expressed in play, in art, and in stories. Maltreated children also face complex issues of grief and loss, guilt and self-blame, and low self-esteem. Control of behavior is a major treatment theme, and is frequently the reason why dissociative and traumatized children are referred for treatment. Eventually more and more control must be turned over to these children as they grow up. This is a risky and stressful business for those who are held responsible.

The DBS model of dissociation prescribes a treatment approach focused on facilitating self-modulation of behavioral states; facilitating metacognitive self-monitoring and integrative functions; and eroding the dissociative state dependency of traumatic affects, memories, and behaviors. In children, dissociative alter personality states should only be directly engaged when they are behaviorally distinct, express strongly held convictions of separateness, and are identifiable across different domains (e.g., are independently witnessed by parents and teachers).

Play therapy is a major mode of psychotherapy for younger children. Play is central to the mental and emotional lives of children, and is the realm in which they can express and work through feelings and conflicts. Play therapy should take full advantage of the power of the therapeutic space to evoke communicative, meaningful play. The defenses mobilized in play can be observed and worked with in a displaced fashion that does not require insight on the part of a child. Rule-based games provide a useful arena in which to identify and work with pathological dissociation in older children and adolescents.

Chapter Fifteen

Dissociative Families and Out-of-Home Placements

To a much greater extent than adults, children must be treated within the context of their homes or living arrangements. This is especially true for dissociative and traumatized children. These homes/living arrangements are quite varied and, in the case of dissociative families, may contain considerable psychopathology apart from the children's problems. This chapter discusses approaches to working with the different living situations frequently encountered in the treatment of dissociative children and adolescents.

DISSOCIATIVE FAMILIES

A Personal Disclaimer

My appreciation of the importance of family dynamics in affecting the outcomes of traumatized/dissociative children was late in coming—and probably has not fully arrived. This awareness of family process emerges more from my research than from clinical experience. Frankly, I was more interested in individual work and regarded family-oriented approaches as a lesser adjunctive intervention. The broader view provided by research has helped me to see the powerful influences, for better or for worse, that families exert on children's outcomes.

I claim no expertise in family therapy. The following discussion is intended to identify general issues and themes as I see them, and to suggest approaches and resources. I avoid discussions of technique and theory entirely, as I know little about these. Much of what I mention is based on the work of Lynn and Robert Benjamin, who have written a well-integrated series of articles on family, couple, and group treatment approaches with dissociative families (Benjamin and Benjamin, 1992, 1994a, 1994b, 1994c, 1994d, 1994e, 1994f, 1994g).

What Is Known about Dissociative Families?

"Dissociative families" are families in which one or more nuclear family members has a dissociative disorder. Obviously they come in a number of configurations: One or both parents, one or more children, or frequently a combination thereof may have MPD or another dissociative disorder. Relatively little is known about the treatment of dissociative families. Somewhat more has been written about family treatment in cases of PTSD and in traumatized families (Rosenheck and Thomson, 1986; Harkness, 1993; Allen and Bloom, 1994).

During the 1980s, discussions of dissociative families focused on their abusive characteristics and were largely based on retrospective accounts by adult patients (e.g., Kluft, Braun, and Sachs, 1984; Braun, 1985). Clinical impressions of high rates of substance abuse, psychosis, and dissociative disorders suggested massive family psychopathology. A second look came from questionnaire studies of therapists treating adult MPD patients, which sometimes included the reported frequency of dissociative diagnoses in family members (e.g., Putnam et al., 1986; Ross et al., 1989f). A third source of information was the assessment of children of parents with MPD, exemplified by Coons's (1985) study.

These three lines of information all suggested that a substantial percentage of dissociative patients have one or more additional first-degree relatives with a dissociative disorder. Although informative, these reports were partly impressionistic, which naturally opens them to question. In all fairness, the study of dissociative families is extremely difficult and exemplifies the methodological problems inherent in studying abusive families (Cicchetti and Nurcombe, 1994).

Yeager and Lewis (1996) demonstrate that the study of the families of children with dissociative disorders provides an excellent window into dissociative families. In a seminal paper, they reported on the symptomatology and family characteristics of 11 children with dissociative disorders. They found that 11 of the 18 parents studied had extensive dissociative psychopathology. Of the 11 siblings evaluated, 7 had dissociative disorders, and only 1 was judged free of major pathology. This study is notable for its careful documentation of the psychiatric disturbance, maltreatment, and domestic violence that characterizes these families; it confirms earlier clinical impressions that these are traumatized and traumatizing families. Moreover, the prevalence of dissociative disorders in first-degree relatives supports the clinical observation that dissociative disorders are frequently transgenerational.

Recently, another line of evidence has been added: the correlation of dissociative measures with negative family process variables. Anderson (1992) studied family medicine outpatients with the DES and found that even after age, gender, race, marital status, employment status, education, and income were controlled for, higher DES scores were strongly associated with increased psychological distress, poorer family functioning, and more office visits. Berenbaum and James (1994) found that higher DES scores were associated with increased negative dominant communication in the family. Egeland and Susman-Stillman (1996) found that higher DES scores in mothers who had themselves been abused was associated with abuse of their children.

Family process and family pathology thus appear to make a sizeable contribution to the development and perpetuation of pathological dissociation. Therefore, family interventions must often be an integral part of treating dissociative children (Benjamin and Benjamin, 1992). Much of what has been written about therapy with dissociative families has focused on the spouses or nuclear families of adults with MPD. From this literature, I extract therapeutic themes and issues that apply to the families of children and adolescents with dissociative disorders.

Overview of Treatment with Dissociative Families

Family therapy was described in a number of older MPD case reports (e.g., Davis and Osherson, 1977; Beal, 1978; Levenson and Berry, 1983). More recently, overviews by Williams (1991), Benjamin and Benjamin (1992), and Chiappa (1994) have helped to organize a scattered literature. Williams emphasizes addressing the effects of the patient's MPD on the family (e.g., helping family members understand and deal with hostile alter personalities). The Benjamins focus on parenting and marital issues for adult MPD patients. Chiappa takes the MPD family therapy literature to task for the contradictions and unaddressed questions in what has been offered so far.

After a family member is diagnosed with a dissociative disorder, one of the first questions that arises for the family is "What does it mean?" Education about MPD and dissociation is an important part of family treatment (Williams, 1991). Some spouses may be shocked, but children are often aware of the behavioral state differences in a dissociative parent. Portrayals of MPD in the popular media conjure up frightening images that must be examined and corrected with the patient and family. This is often a good place to begin the educational process and to dispel fears that the patient is a freak or monster. For adults and adolescents, literature can be provided. The book *Multiple Personality Disorder from the Inside Out* (Cohen, Giller, and W., 1991) is useful in this regard.

Family Members' Interactions with a Patient's Alter Personality States

One of the crucial questions faced by a therapist involves the extent to which family members are expected to interact directly with an MPD patient's alter personalities. In some cases, there will already be a long-standing pattern of overt interaction. In other instances, this pattern may be more covert: Family members may intuitively recognize the patient's different behavioral states and adjust their behavior accordingly, but alter personalities are not directly acknowledged as such. Simple, hard-and-fast rules cannot cover the range of situations likely to be encountered, but I venture a few generalizations.

Children should not be encouraged to interact directly with their parents' alter personality states. I am of the old school that thinks that children should address their parents as "Mom" and "Dad," no matter how they happen to be behaving at the moment. To do otherwise can be confusing for both a child and a dissociative parent. It can also lead to the child's becoming a focus in the internal conflicts among the parent's alter personality states. When there is a long-standing pattern of individualized relationships between an adult's alter personalities and his or her child, this should be gradually deemphasized and supplanted by a relationship between the child and the dissociative parent as "parent." Frequently, the redrawing of generational boundaries is best achieved by focusing on parenting issues with the dissociative parent and his or her partner (see discussion below).

Parents may well have to interact with the specific alter personalities of a dissociative child or foster child. But, as much as possible, they should do so in a way that addresses the child as a whole. At times, parents' working individually with specific alter personalities may be important in helping an MPD child or adolescent to overcome problems and to control his or her behavior. In day-to-day family life, as in the therapy, the alter personalities offer access to different levels of the child's cognition and behavior. When it is necessary to work on the special problems and issues that the alters personify, they may be identified and engaged.

It is critical not to socialize a child as a "multiple." By this, I mean that parents should not reinforce the idea that MPD confers a special status or exempts the child from normal behavior and responsibilities. Occasionally I have encountered parents or foster parents who are so taken with the notion of MPD that they make it an issue at school and with friends and family. The children are expected to display their multiplicity. Obviously this augurs poorly. In addition, adolescents in particular may think that MPD is a nifty thing to have, and may seek to exploit the bizarreness or notoriety that comes with the diagnosis. Appropriately acknowledging the presence of MPD, while not focusing on it, is a delicate balance that requires healthy parents—rarely found in the nuclear families of MPD children, but more commonly encountered in foster and adoptive families.

Siblings should be discouraged from direct interactions with a child patient's specific alter personalities. Parents or foster parents should be alert for alter-focused sibling interactions and should intervene as necessary to prevent the establishment of a pattern. Similarly, extended family members, friends, and other significant people should be actively discouraged from interacting with individual alter personalities. The overall message should be that a person with MPD is expected to relate to the world at large as a unified person.

Although alters will probably emerge in family therapy sessions, the therapist should direct interventions to the person as a whole. Family therapy is not the place for individual work with alter personalities. There may be merit to including specific alters in marital therapy for certain issues, but a therapist should avoid working with a patient as a multiple in front of his or her family.

Again, I emphasize that it is important to avoid socialization of a patient as a "multiple." Multiplicity should be a private experience. I realize that this position is unpopular with those who promote multiplicity as a special way of being. However, my experience indicates that although the world at large is fascinated by multiplicity, it is not ready to relate to this condition as anything more than a bizarre mental disorder. MPD patients who reveal their status too publicly usually experience a lot of pain and humiliation.

Family Therapy

Family therapy is an essential element for most child/adolescent treatment programs. Those who regard family therapy as a minor adjunctive treatment often believe that the individual therapist can do a few sessions with the family and then get back to the "real" treatment. Experience makes it clear, however, that family therapy should be conducted by a second therapist trained in a standard model. There is no way that a patient's individual psychotherapist can double as an effective family therapist. The blurring of boundaries, loyalties, issues of confidentiality, and differences in focus and techniques will ultimately undermine both therapeutic efforts.

However, the creation of such a treatment team has its own problems. Effective communication between the individual and family therapists is absolutely critical, as MPD patients are masters at splitting those working with them (Putnam, 1989a). Family therapy sessions need not be held as frequently as individual sessions. Profitable family treatment can be conducted on a monthly basis.

Family therapy interventions should support the reorganization of the family system; develop appropriate generational boundaries; strengthen the marital dyad; and develop family members' skills in communication, negotiation, conflict resolution, and stress reduction (Chiappa, 1994). The family is the unit of treatment. The focus should not be on the identified patient or on the dissociative psychopathology per se. In fact, it is not even necessary for the family therapist to be an expert in dissociative disorders. Good family therapy involves paying attention to the systems issues, not the individual issues of the identified patient. I am not qualified to judge the superiority of one family therapy model over another, but the discussions by Benjamin and Benjamin (1994a) of a contextual approach and by Chiappa (1994) of a family systems approach are helpful.

Parenting in Dissociative Families

A deep concern about the impact of pathological dissociation on parental functioning is apparent throughout the writings of Benjamin and Benjamin (1994f, 1994g). Empathetically, they lay out a series of issues and problems produced or aggravated by a parent's pathological dissociation and history of childhood trauma (Benjamin and Benjamin, 1992). Supplementing the Benjamins' themes with my own experience, I group dissociative parenting issues into four basic problems.

The first problem consists of the parental absence and the inconsistencies produced by pathological dissociation. Amnesias, switching of alter personalities, trance states, behavioral regression, depersonalization/derealization, and various forms of social withdrawal disconnect dissociative parents from their children. Multiple hospitalizations and substance abuse also contribute to the unavailability of many MPD parents. MPD parents often cannot remember what they say and do with or to their children. They make contradictory statements and demands; they forget to do what they promise; and they cannot explain what they do. They may even fail to provide crucial care or place children in dangerous situations. At times they cannot respond to the most basic needs of their children. In some extreme alter personality states, they do not recognize their children as their own and vehemently deny that they are their parents.

The second issue involves the array of negative affects dissociative parents direct toward their children. Anger, depression, jealousy, resentment, guilt, shame, fear, disgust, and other disapproving and hurtful emotions poison the parent–child relationship. The parents' damaged self-esteem and unstable sense of self impedes the expression of loving and nurturing feelings. Often childlike themselves, parents may demand nurturing from their children and resent their children's independence and accomplishments. When asked to assess their competency as parents, many dissociative patients bitterly condemn themselves, expressing feelings of unfitness and the belief that their children would be better off with someone else. Yet the majority of dissociative parents I have encountered also describe strong feelings of love for their children, which they desperately want to be able to express in positive ways.

The third issue involves the interactions between dissociative parents' alter personalities and their children. In the privacy of the home, parental alter personality states come and go overtly. Most children are aware of the different behavioral states manifested by MPD parents. From early infancy on, normal children monitor these parents' emotional responses to their behavior and make adjustments accordingly. Thus, the children of MPD parents learn to relate differentially to the different alter personality states—although they may not understand what is happening. They recognize that when the parents behave in a certain way they can be frightening or abusive, and that they themselves should disappear for a while. When the parents behave in another fashion, they and the children can play together like children. And so on.

MPD parents try to control which alter personalities relate to their children, but their efforts are erratic, especially during times of stress and crisis. Unfortunately, children often evoke dissociative responses in their MPD parents. At first, as infants and toddlers, they do this simply by overwhelming the parents with needs and demands. As they grow older, they may learn to activate specific alter personality states deliberately. This is just another way of pushing a parent's buttons—and thus a part of the eternal child–parent struggle over duties and privileges.

The fourth issue involves the transgenerational themes in dissociative families. As many have observed, and Yeager and Lewis (1996) have clearly documented, multigenerational dissociative disorders can frequently be found in dissociative families. Dissociative parents produce dissociation in their own children, in big and little ways. Dissociative parents may be abusive and should be considered at increased risk for abusing their children (Kluft, 1987b). They also induce dissociation in their children through mechanisms such as imitation, wherein the children mimic the abrupt behavioral shifts of the parents (Benjamin and Benjamin, 1992). Dissociative parents have considerable difficulty helping their children to integrate behavior and feelings—a normal developmental task previously discussed in Chapter Eight. In addition, dissociative parents may harbor enormous resentment toward their own children because the children seem to have it so much easier than they themselves did as children. In regressed states, dissociative parents may reverse generational roles and force their children to parent them. Traditional parent–child boundaries are usually seriously blurred or violated in dissociative families.

Mrs. K.

Mrs. K. was a divorced, middle-aged woman with MPD. At age 7, her son was placed with a foster family because of her neglect and suspected physical abuse of him. Barely a year into treatment for MPD, Mrs. K. won back custody of her son, now aged 10. Although she had related appropriately to him during visitation, his continuous presence and obvious distress at being separated from his foster family, friends, and former school generated feelings of resentment and anger in her, which led to harsh and often inappropriate discipline. Mrs. K. was in the throes of initial MPD treatment, with an eruption of alter personalities angrily asserting their separateness. Her therapist—who had strongly recommended against the return of her son until treatment was farther along—faced the possibility that she was abusing him. He asked child protective services to evaluate the son, and informed Mrs. K. that he was required by law to report any suspicion of child abuse. After determining that the child was probably not being maltreated, the therapist began working with Mrs. K. on her parenting. This topic became a principal focus of treatment over the next year.

At first, Mrs. K. struggled with acknowledging her prior neglect of her son. Alter personalities blamed each other or now-"deceased" alters. The therapist took the position that Mrs. K. as a whole was responsible for the past and present treatment of her son. As she began to focus on her parenting, she voiced feelings of being inadequate and overwhelmed by her son's demands, and expressed great anger toward her own mother. She became aware of how starved she was for affection as a child, and in return became better at responding to her son's need for affection and attention. Her personality system was able to find common ground in the tasks of parenting; this led to more cooperation and harmony among the alters.

The Benjamins were the first to systematically identify the strategy of using parenting as a treatment focus in individual therapy for dissociative adults (Benjamin and Benjamin, 1994f, 1994g). They have recognized that parenting is a core therapeutic issue, both in the here and now and in the past, and that many of a patient's most difficult problems and behaviors can be addressed through the theme of parenting. Working with dissociative parents to improve their parenting serves a crucial role in preventing the transmission of dissociative and abusive behavior to the next generation (e.g., Egeland and Susman-Stillman, 1996).

Focusing on parenting often works because dissociative parents, like many dysfunctional parents, are more strongly motivated to improve their children's lives than their own. They may also be more willing to deal with their own painful childhood issues in this displaced fashion. Improvement in parenting provides positive feedback for a patient struggling in a painful individual therapy. A patient who can begin to "do it better" for his or her own children may be able to change the future and break free of the past.

Parenting can be addressed in individual psychotherapy. It can be addressed in couple therapy, and it can be a theme for support groups for spouses and partners of MPD patients. In a series of articles, Benjamin and Benjamin (1994b, 1994c, 1994d) detail the format, process, themes, and dynamics of a long-running group for spouses and partners of MPD patients and parents of MPD children. This series is worth reading, as it is by far the most detailed discussion of running a support group for dissociative families. Such support groups are important resources for therapists working with dissociative patients—and more are needed.

Couple Therapy

The need for concurrent marital or couple therapy is a well-accepted principle in the individual treatment of MPD patients (Kluft et al., 1984; Putnam, 1989a; Williams, 1991; Benjamin and Benjamin, 1992, 1994e). Experience dictates that couple therapy be linked to the progress and issues in individual therapy (Benjamin and Benjamin, 1994e). As the primary patient progresses in individual therapy, the partners have to rework their relationship to encompass the changes and to permit the patient to assume more responsibility in the relationship and family.

For patients' spouses or partners, couple therapy may be their only treatment and the forum for all of their personal issues, as well as the marital and family problems. Partners of MPD patients may have significant psychopathology themselves and often carry cumulative trauma loads that rival those of the identified patients. For instance, partners may have substance abuse problems, which must be addressed by appropriate treatment programs—giving the identified patients an opportunity to switch roles and become the supportive partners. Not infrequently, the partners also suffer from dissociative disorder and require a full-fledged treatment program.

Pathological dissociation causes many problems within a marriage. Amnesias, depersonalization, derealization, and hostile alter personalities all interfere with the empathetic reciprocity necessary for a healthy relationship. Problems with trust and the past history of traumatic family interactions that an MPD patient brings into a relationship can damage the partners' bond. The course of the relationship is usually rocky, and the partner usually builds up anger, resentment, and even hatred toward the patient. Codependency problems are rife. In this context, the therapist must address and work with the dynamics commonly found in dysfunctional relationships: issues of power and control; intimacy, trust, and fidelity; shared and nonshared values; communication; regulation of affect; approaches to coping; and boundaries. There is also the ever-present necessity of helping the couple to work out mechanisms for accomplishing the tasks of daily family life.

Out of this should emerge a "healthy couple" (Kaslow, 1982; Benjamin and Benjamin, 1994e), although a somewhat healthier couple is usually the best that can be expected. Marital health is marked by clear and proper boundaries, both within the couple and between the couple and their children and their own parents. Communication should be clear and direct; feedback should be given and accepted appropriately. Each partner should feel comfortable with his or her personal identity and role within the relationship. The partners should be able to negotiate from a position of empathy for each other's perspective, and they should share a value system that gives a larger meaning to their lives (Benjamin and Benjamin, 1994e).

FOSTER AND ADOPTIVE FAMILIES

Foster Care: Problems and Benefits

At least half a million children are currently in foster care in the United States (Rosenfeld et al., 1997). Indeed, foster care has largely replaced institutional care for children in need of an out-of-home living situation. The numbers are overwhelming. The beleaguered foster care system cannot cope with the escalating increases in the numbers of children who need placement, particularly when one remembers that foster children have far more physical and mental health problems than children living with their natural parents. There are many special-needs children in this group, including physically disabled children, children with chronic illnesses, children with developmental disabilities, minority and biracial children, sibling groups, and infants prenatally exposed to drugs.

In U.S. metropolitan areas, the need for foster care and related services far exceeds the system's capacity, and children are frequently placed in inappropriate or even dangerous situations. One need only examine the situation in the District of Columbia over the 5 years preceding the August 1995 court takeover of the foster care system to find one horror story after another—all too frequently resulting in a child's death. Individual caseworkers are usually blamed, but the real problem lies in the collapse of child protective and social service systems in the United States. Even in relatively prosperous regions, these critical services are badly underfunded, understaffed, and disorganized; they suffer from high rates of staff turnover and poor morale. This is by and large a silent crisis, but nonetheless one with enormous long-term consequences (Friedrich-Velsor, 1992).

Maltreated children typically stay in foster placements for 2–3 years before a permanent disposition is arranged. For various societal reasons, we know little about the efficacy and outcomes of foster and adoptive placements. Although foster care is often portrayed as harmful in the popular press, most research indicates that children benefit, especially in comparison with maltreated children remaining in their homes (Reddy and Pfeiffer, 1997). Studies suggest, however, that sexually abused children do more poorly in foster and adoptive placements than other children do (Smith and Howard, 1994). In particular, they have more externalizing behavior problems (e.g., lying, defiance, profanity, vandalism, tantrums, and sexualized acting out). They also have more difficulty forming attachments to foster and adoptive parents.

Some of the very best parents I have ever met are foster parents. Again, on average, children are better off in foster placements than in the situations from which they were removed. I have seen foster parents make enormous personal sacrifices for their foster children. Unfortunately, the deteriorating social services system often places foster parents in untenable situations by dumping severely mentally and physically ill children on them without adequate support or resources.

Experienced foster parents are a godsend when a therapist is working with a severely dissociative child. Frequently the foster family is healthy enough that most of the work can focus on the dissociative child; in these situations, the child's therapist may be directly involved with the family work without becoming hopelessly entangled in issues of confidentiality, transference, and blurred boundaries. Moreover, perhaps because they have been intimately involved with the care of a half-dozen or more children (usually including some of their own), experienced foster parents recognize dissociation better than the average person. They also tend to be more objective observers than natural parents. A dissociative foster child is not their own child, but a stranger's child whom they are attempting to include in their functional family. The child's failures of integration do not go unnoticed.

MARIA

Mrs. D. brought in Maria, aged 3 years and 10 months, who had three discrete alter personality states (the youngest case of clear-cut MPD I have seen). Mrs. D. had been a foster mother to over 20 children. She said that she had noticed Maria was "different" from the beginning, but was first cued to the possibility of MPD by the unique way in which Maria told on herself. She said that Maria would approach her, identify herself as "Mary" rather than Maria, and then describe Maria's misbehavior (which was often serious) in the third person—for example, "I saw Maria take your ring." Mrs. D. also observed arguments between Maria and "Mary" in which the child alternated rapidly between different voices and punched herself.

Coincidental follow-up 8 years later revealed that Maria, at age 11, was in a residential treatment program with a well-documented diagnosis of MPD (see Headly-Carter, Two-Bulls, Benoit, Putnam, and Peterson, 1996). Just prior to her program placement, she had twice been hospitalized for "psychosis." After 13 months of residential treatment, she was doing extremely well, although her alter personalities were not integrated. The staff members were sophisticated about dissociation and able to sustain an integrative milieu that emphasized continuity of self across Maria's changes in personality state. Direct work with the alters was confined to individual therapy and was not overly emphasized. Ironically, the biggest problem now was Mrs. D., who refused to invest emotionally in Maria or participate in family therapy, although she adhered to the basic responsibilities legally required of foster parents.

Foster placements evoke primal issues of attachment and insecurity for children. Foster children obsess about how long the current placement is going to last and whether they will return home again, for better or for worse. Some become caught in the throes of an ambivalent dance, alternately idealizing and vilifying their natural and foster parents in turn. Many children who are veterans of multiple placements become hardened and resentful. They put the current foster parents through hell to test their commitment—often creating self-fulfilling prophecies of rejection.

The primary task in working with foster parents is to help them to construct and maintain a home environment that reduces cues for pathological dissociation and switching, and promotes integration of self and behavior. The key words here are consistency, stability, and connection. Traumatized and dissociative children are hypersensitive to change and disorganization. They need a stable physical environment and clear-cut daily routines and expectations to provide external organization and security. This can be hard to achieve when such a child is seriously disrupting the family by creating multiple crises at home, school, and elsewhere.

The Need for Consistency and Stability

Foster parents and other caretakers need above all to be consistent and to provide stability. No matter how a child is switching, regressing, or otherwise changing, the parents/caretakers must be affectively well modulated and clear about the rules. And they must stick to them. This requires more than inflexible rigidity, which can be dissociogenic in its own right. The rules must be reasonable and appropriate, and they must be applied in a dispassionate and objective fashion by a concerned and involved adult. Both the child and the adult must follow the rules. Duties and expectations should be clear and consistently applied to all parties. Inevitable deviations from the rules should be honestly acknowledged and explained as much as is reasonable. This helps to create a caring holding structure, which is critical for the development of boundaries and behavioral organization in a dissociative child. All parts of a dissociative child must come to accept that the rules governing social behavior exist independently of the child's moment-to-moment experience of himself or herself.

Of course, no one can be consistent and stable all the time. All parents/caretakers experience significant changes in behavioral and mood states while interacting with their children; for example, a parent may suddenly become very angry in response to a child's behavior. These inevitable mood/state switches frequently trigger switches in behavioral states or alter personalities in children with pathological dissociation. Not uncommonly, the behavioral/alter personality states evoked in the child by the adult's emotional shifts are dissociated from (i.e., unaware of or detached from) the adult–child interactions that preceded them.

MRS. G. AND JAMIE

Mrs. G., a foster mother, described seeing a specific behavioral state emerge in her 9-year-old ward, Jamie, whenever there was a high-affect situation that demanded action. For example, when Jamie spilled cranberry juice on the couch, Mrs. G. yelled, "Run get some paper towels, quick!" When Jamie was slow to react, Mrs. G.—who had been dealing with the child's misbehavior all morning—angrily shouted the order. Jamie responded in a dazed fashion, picking up a magazine and wandering around looking at it. The more Mrs. G. shouted at her to get the paper towels, the more intently Jamie studied the magazine—seemingly oblivious to the situation. Feeling beside herself with frustration and anger, Mrs. G. suddenly realized that she was seeing a dissociated behavioral state repeatedly elicited by such urgent demands.

What is critical in a case like Jamie's is for parent/caretaker to monitor changes in his or her own state sufficiently well to track corresponding responses in the child. Of course, the very kinds of situations that provoke major affective state shifts in parental figures tend to distract them from examining the process. The therapist can help identify these interactions by going over examples and reconstructing situations. Obviously, the mental health, self-observing capacities, and psychological-mindedness of the parents/caretakers play a critical role. Children and adolescents are almost never aware of (able to articulate?) the dissociative behavioral shifts triggered in them by their caretakers.

The Need to Help Children Make Connections

In a stable and consistent environment, foster parents can help a dissociative child to connect with the world and to make connections between past and present, cause and effect, behavior and its consequences. Making connections, and reestablishing connections when they have been lost as a result of a dissociative shift, are major milieu interventions promoting integration of self.

First, the foster parents must themselves be connected to the child. They must have a relationship with the child that is meaningful. It may be turbulent; such children are stressful to live with and to be responsible for day in and day out. Nevertheless, there must be a significant connection between them, so that the foster child responds (if only inwardly at times) to the observations and interventions of the foster parents.

Foster parents must find a balance between being deeply involved and emotionally invested without being intrusive. They must nurture their relationship with a child during the bad times as well as the good. Such children are desperate for a parental relationship. They need to be loved, cared about, and believed in by a parental figure. If that emotional investment is not there—if a foster parent only sees a child as a job or a legal obligation—then much less can be accomplished.

Then foster parents must use this relationship to help the dissociative child to connect with the world, to maintain these connections when stressed, and to reestablish the connections when they have been broken by a dissociative reaction—perhaps in response to something a foster parent did or said. This is done more through grounding and guiding the child than through formal direction. The fostering of connections must be largely a background task, in which a caring adult helps a child fill in the missing information and make connections with what the child already knows but cannot access from where he or she is in mental state space. Attempts to do this in a direct or formal manner are often resisted and become points of conflict. Nobody likes to be told what to do, think, or feel. Well-meaning attempts to get a child to examine every aspect of his or her behavior usually backfire. The promotion of connections in dissociative children must be handled at an almost subliminal level if it is to be effective.

MRS. F. AND JAKE

Jake, a street-tough, off-putting adolescent, was trying to intimidate his newest foster parents with threats and foul language. Although she admitted to me that he did scare her, Mrs. F. was "hanging tough" and trying to stay with him. She had a quick wit and was good on the comeback. With my professional blessing, she began to banter with Jake in response to his threats. Banter requires a delicate touch. The banterer needs to get close to the mark without wounding deeply—just leaving a good-natured pinprick that makes the point. Mrs. F. was good at it. She had a firm grasp of Jake's issues and could weave in connections while making a funny comeback to an angry challenge. Even Jake had to laugh at times, in spite of himself. To a stranger, their continual sparring might have seemed unduly hostile, but once they settled into this mode of relating, Jake's behavior improved tremendously. Not everyone can banter successfully, and when a comment misses too widely or hits too close to home, it can be disruptive. But in the right situation, banter discharges anger, injects humor, and gets things said that need to be said in order to move forward.

Issues Related to the Dangerousness of Children

A major problem that comes up for foster families working with severely abused children is the dangerousness of these children to others. Foster parents often fear for the safety of other children in the home and for their own safety. Those who have not worked with these children cannot appreciate how dangerous they can be at times. Not infrequently, I find foster parents who lock themselves in their room or a child in his or her room at night because they fear being attacked while asleep. Traumatized children sometimes do weird things or act in weird ways at night: strange alter personality states, nightmares, night terrors, abreactions, hypnopompic phenomena, sleepwalking—and other nocturnal states. I have heard stories of nocturnal behaviors that would alarm anyone who has to sleep in the same house.

Maltreated children frequently destroy their foster families' property and personal effects. This damage, which is not reimbursed by social agencies, is one of those extra burdens that comes with foster parenting. Destruction of mementoes and family treasures is a personal wound that makes foster parents ask, "Why do we put up with it?" Severely abused children are understandably angry and distrustful. They lash out and struggle with anyone and everyone—and their foster families are the closest and safest targets. Foster parents usually agonize more over the effects of a disturbed child on their own children or other foster children in the home than on themselves.

Dangerousness should be taken seriously, regardless of a dissociative child's age or gender. The safety of younger children in the home must be insured—even at the cost of transferring the dissociative child to another placement. I know of several serious assaults made by dissociative children on younger children living in the same home. These included a 7-year-old girl's stabbing the 3-year-old daughter of the foster mother, and a 6-year-old girl's almost drowning a 2-year-old in a backyard wading pool. In the latter case, the foster mother returned from answering the phone to find the dissociative child sitting on the toddler, who was face down in the pool. Fortunately, the call was a wrong number, and the mother was only gone momentarily. Living with such possibilities is one of the gnawing anxieties of foster parents who take in dissociative children.

Issues Related to Parental Visitation

A central tenet of foster care is that the out-of-home placement is supposed to be temporary and that the child will eventually return to his or her biological parents. This is often patently unreasonable, but nonetheless the system proceeds as if it were true. Visitation by the biological parents is a required part of foster care. For the most part, foster parents dread such visits. They learn to expect behavioral problems, aggression, tantrums, oppositionality, regression, and worse from a child, both before and after a visit. Furthermore, the system expects that they will prepare the child for and support visitation at the same time that they are being asked to make a strong emotional investment in the child (Rosenfeld et al., 1997).

Maltreating biological parents often get into struggles with foster parents. They may encourage acting out to disrupt a child's relationship with the foster family. They may act inappropriately during a visit, and they often disappoint the child by not meeting their commitments. They may tell the child not to cooperate with foster parents or caseworkers, or make the child afraid of these figures by hinting darkly that "they" will never let the child come home again. Paradoxically, a child's behavior during the actual visit with a biological parent may be overcontrolled and passive, but there is usually hell to pay later. Not surprisingly, foster parents complain a lot about the effects of visitation on a child.

There is often little that can be done about visitation procedures until the accrued evidence is overwhelming. Foster parents can be helped to understand the painful double bind that they are placed in. Their efforts to nurture and rear this child must be integrated with their concerns about the child's potential reunion with his or her biological parents. Sometimes foster parents themselves act out before or after parental visits, and a counselor must help them do the right thing for the child.

When foster parents legally adopt a child, it is usually after they have lived together for years and after a lengthy judicial process to terminate the biological parents' rights has taken place. They have usually been through some very difficult times together, and the adoptive parents are aware of how difficult the child can be. Fortunately, things sometimes get much better when such an adoption is finalized and the child comes to believe in the permanence of the relationship. The dissociative symptoms of one child whom I followed for several years virtually disappeared overnight when she was formally adopted.

Alas, this is not always the case. Adoptive parents who do not know a severely abused child very well are likely to panic when they experience the full brunt of the child's posttraumatic and dissociative symptoms. This can become a tragic situation if the frightened adoptive parents seek to extricate themselves.

GROUP HOMES, RESIDENTIAL PLACEMENTS, AND INPATIENT SETTINGS

ADRIENNE

Almost nothing was known about Adrienne's early life. She had been in the system for over 10 years, and her trail had grown cold. At about age 4 years (her birth date is unknown), Adrienne became a ward of the District of Columbia. One Mrs. S. said that a woman claiming to be a distant cousin from North Carolina had arrived with Adrienne in tow and asked her to babysit for a few hours while she visited a sick friend in D.C. Mrs. S. reluctantly agreed when the woman broke into tears. The woman never returned, and Adrienne was sent to the first of a series of foster care and group home placements.

I met Adrienne in a religiously affiliated group home, where she had stayed for the last year (except for two hospitalizations). Tall and painfully thin, she hid behind a cloud of frizzy red-blond hair. At 15, she still had a strong childlike quality. Avoiding eye contact, she shot me suspicious glances on the sly. Open-ended questions led nowhere, and she deferred or denied virtually everything that I asked her. Even simple rapport-building inquiries went nowhere.

Adrienne was identified by the home's director as the most difficult child the home had ever tried to keep. Yet when I met with members of the staff prior to seeing her, I found them animated—a little angry, perhaps, but largely upbeat about her. There were knowing laughs and exasperated head nodding when I asked whether she had a sense of humor. Despite all of her problems and the chaos that she caused, the staff clearly loved her. This probably made a difference in her case compared with that of Reginald (see Chapters Five and Fourteen, and Putnam, 1993a), who shared a similar childhood of numerous temporary placements.

In contrast to Adrienne, who denied any and all experiences of dissociation, the staff provided unending examples of her major and minor amnesias associated with identity alterations. Among themselves, they used various names to designate different behavioral states that Adrienne could exhibit. "Mute," also known as "Baby," was an infantile state during which she would curl up in a fetal position and rock while mouthing silent cries. "Hyper" was a be-bopping, hip-hopping, tense, hyperaroused, street-talking, oppositional personality state given to sneaking out at night and visiting the boys' cottage. "Put-together" was mature and well groomed, liked to read, listened to classical music, and did her schoolwork. "Belligerent" was paranoid, could be aggressive, and accused the staff of controlling her and setting her up for problems and punishments. Several staff members described other states that they saw on occasion, including a "6- or 7-year-old child."

Although she endorsed many critical items on the DES, which was given to her during one hospitalization, Adrienne would rarely talk with me about dissociative experiences. Certain topics, such as time loss, were clearly upsetting for her. On one occasion she described "voices in my head," saying that they could become so loud that she couldn't think, and then she would "just go away." Everyone commented on her "blank spells," in which she would go into an unresponsive, trance-like state, staring into the distance. When asked later about what had happened, she usually gave one of two explanations: "The voices in my head got too loud for me to think," or "My mind had stopped."

Diagnosed as having a seizure disorder during one hospitalization, Adrienne was being treated with valproic acid. This diagnosis was based on an EEG with bitemporal slowing, without any spike or wave abnormalities. Over the years, she had undergone numerous contradictory medical examinations—including one neurological exam documenting extensive cranial nerve abnormalities, followed a few weeks later by a consultation noting "no abnormalities on careful examination." Adrienne suffered from frequent severe headaches that would come and go suddenly. Several staff members felt that this was attention-seeking behavior, but others protested that at times she really seemed to be hurting and was in tears from the pain.

The problems leading to my consultation included violent, uncontrollable temper tantrums during which Adrienne threw furniture and smashed things. On one occasion she had pulled a knife on her caseworker and threatened to kill her. From time to time, staff members found knives or similar weapons hidden in her room. She tended to deny recall of the violent outbursts and to protest that she was being punished for things she had not done. She intermittently refused to attend school, although in the "Put-together" mode she clearly enjoyed school, taking leadership roles in extracurricular activities such as the French club and the newspaper.

On the one hand, staff members were frightened of Adrienne, particularly after the knife-pulling episode. On the other, she was regarded as one of the brightest and most appealing kids in the home. The more I talked with the staffers, the clearer it became how invested they were in her—and how pained they were by her erratic, aggressive, and paranoid behaviors. Questions about the need to transfer Adrienne to a more structured therapeutic setting topped their agenda. From my perspective, they were doing most things right, and it was highly unlikely that the state residential facility for which she was eligible could do nearly as well. I saw my consultant's task as clarifying the dissociative components of her behavior, supporting the overall milieu approach that had already been adopted, and suggesting some additional interventions. Thus I sought to reinforce and fine-tune existing approaches. This is a much easier situation than having to try to change the staff's attitudes and behaviors.

In a group home/residential situation such as Adrienne's, treatment should emphasize the organizing and integrative role of the milieu. It is particularly important for the staff to relate to such a child as a whole person. Although the personnel at Adriennes's group home continued to discuss her behavior among themselves by the labels they had given her, I stressed that it was critical that they relate to her as Adrienne. Staff members should not relate to a child as a "multiple" or develop individualized relationships with alter personality states. The staff's fascination with multiplicity should be redirected to education about dissociation and the effects of maltreatment.

Staff Issues and Dynamics

A great deal could be said about the issues, dynamics, and strategies required to treat traumatized and dissociative children effectively in the context of a long-term group home or residential placement. Once again, my experience has sufficed to acquaint me with the complexity of the task, but not to claim expertise.

Traumatized and dissociative children and adolescents rarely arrive in such facilities already diagnosed and in appropriate treatment. Recognition of the traumatic nature of their symptoms is slow to emerge, usually well after there have been negative child–staff interactions. Thus these children have already acquired a bad reputation prior to receiving a dissociative or other trauma-related diagnosis, which is typically rejected by a percentage of the staff.

Success requires that the staff members accomplish a number of cooperative objectives: (1) agreeing on common goals for managing and treating such a child; (2) maintaining adequate communication among themselves about what is going on; (3) understanding and accepting their necessary interdependence in working effectively with the child; (4) maintaining consistency across staff members and over time; and (5) constructively managing the inevitable conflicts that arise. There must be effective leadership that can facilitate the negotiations among staff members, and between the staff and the child, that inevitably occur. It would be great if all personnel got the training they need, but that is not going to happen.

A lot of things can disrupt the cooperation and consistency of a group home or residential treatment staff. A primary factor is simply the all-too-frequent changes in team membership. As a consultant, I am dismayed by how often I return to a group home or residential facility and find new staffers, completely unfamiliar with the treatment plan, in key positions. It becomes a Sisyphean labor to take them through the ins and outs of pathological dissociative behavior, and to help them to reframe a child's perplexing behavioral discontinuities as demonstrative of a failure to integrate self and behavior rather than as premeditated oppositionality.

Among the signs that things are not going well are frequent staff meetings focused on a child, or successive meetings in which the subject of the child's behavior comes to monopolize the discussion. When the child is a ward of the state, these meetings can involve large numbers of people from different agencies. Then a consultant is really in trouble, because he or she is never going to get meaningful agreements on how to handle things. These meetings are temporizing affairs; they typically reach agreements that the responsible parties can never fulfill. It is better to express open disagreement respectfully than to accept plans and recommendations that cannot and will not be carried out. Working groups should be kept as small as feasible, and should be able to render and enforce decisions on the spot as necessary.

Outcome measures, both formal and informal, are helpful in tracking progress. It is also useful to have staff members track behavioral regression and discontinuities, perplexing forgetfulness, and posttraumatic symptoms. How many times did the staff have to go over this or that rule or contract tonight? Did the night shift report nightmares again? Was the child seen arguing with himself or herself again? By actively and objectively tracking symptoms, staff members become familiar with the ways in which pathological dissociation influences the child's behaviors. With this understanding, staffers often contribute creative interventions to vexing problems; they also become less involved in emotionally reacting to the child, and can see pathological dissociation for what it is.

Naideane

Naideane was an appealing child. At age 9½, she had curly black hair, a sweet face, and a chubby body showing signs of the teenager to come. This was her second hospitalization. After 6 months with a foster family, she was readmitted after telling the foster mother about vivid fantasies of killing her and the other foster children with a knife. Prior to the readmission, she had begun to talk about "another Naideane."

Naideane was removed from her natural home at age 8 after her mother brought her to a local emergency room and demanded that they take her because Naideane was out of control. A caseworker recalled that the first thing her mother said when they met was "Take her," to which Naideane screamed, "No, no, no." At that time, Naideane was described as assaultive, suicidal, stealing, lying, hoarding, and uncontrollably masturbating till she was raw and bleeding.

Little was documented about her childhood. Her mother was a known crack cocaine addict, and caseworkers suspected that she prostituted Naideane for drugs. Both the foster mother and the hospital staff had witnessed nightmare/abreaction episodes in which Naideane writhed in bed and screamed, "Get off me." She was extraordinarily hypersexualized and had to be continually monitored in groups. In the hospital, she masturbated herself to sleep, but no longer injured herself. Staff members were particularly upset by the heavy breathing and orgasmic moaning that accompanied this.

At first, Naideane was compliant but almost mute; this soon changed into an all-consuming struggle for control with the hospital staff. In individual therapy sessions, she regressed and crawled under furniture. Gradually she began to draw and to write, but would not allow her therapist to look at the paper until after she left the room. The drawings were filled with red and black figures, which some regarded as evidence of satanic abuse. The art therapist pointed out, however, that similar imagery is found in many disturbed children's drawings. After a few months, she allowed her therapist to look at the paper as she drew and wrote, but refused to discuss the contents. Eventually she would read her thoughts out loud as she wrote them down during therapy.

In the words of one staff member, "Naideane is a control freak"—meaning that she continually struggled with the staff for control over every little detail. However, the staff members had their act together and were comfortable sharing control with her when this was feasible. As Naideane acquired power over some aspects of her life, she relaxed the struggle in other areas—just a bit.

Control Issues

Naideane presented two problems often faced on child inpatient units—struggles for control, and hypersexuality. Struggles for control with traumatized individuals often tap into specific aspects of their past. I have previously discussed this dynamic in therapy with respect to traumatized adults (Putnam, 1989a). In children and adolescents, control struggles also reflect developmental issues related to the emergence of autonomy and independence. The drive toward autonomy and self-determination is normal and is a critical part of the development of self and social relatedness. Appropriate development of autonomy is critical in self-regulation and self-control. Disturbances in the development of autonomy result in problems with undercontrol, overcontrol, or some mixture of both (Ryan, Deci, and Grolnick, 1995).

Autonomy is a crucial part of the constructs of "authenticity" and "agency." Authentic actions emerge from the core of "true self" and are owned by the person (Ryan et al., 1995). The experience of autonomy also includes a sense of agency (i.e., the sense that one's actions are willful and intentional, and that one is at the center of their causation). Overcontrol problems may be reflected in rigidity of behavior, obsessive–compulsive behaviors, and self-disparagement. Undercontrol is manifested in behavioral impulsivity, emotional volatility, and lack of a stable self (Ryan et al., 1995).

Many trauma victims exhibit problems with both overcontrol and undercontrol. As I have previously discussed in Chapters Two and

Three, problems with the integration of self are a central developmental theme uniting different psychiatric outcomes of childhood maltreatment. Trauma-related disturbances in the normal development of autonomy contribute mightily to problems with integration of self and acquisition of self-control.

The problem for the staff of a treatment facility is how to help a traumatized child deal with both the healthy and the pathological aspects of his or her need to control self and others. In Naideane's case, the staff members' solidarity was sufficient to permit them to allow her increasing control over a number of areas of her life. This process was not explicitly understood or stated until months into the second hospitalization, by which time they would consider dealing with the latest control issue in terms of what had and had not worked previously. The recognition that Naideane responded positively to being given some control was helpful in the milieu and in her individual therapy.

Management of Hypersexuality

The eroticization of children who have been severely sexually abused is widely recognized by those who know and work with them. (See Chapter Two for a discussion of this symptom of sexual abuse.) Hypersexuality may be manifested in a variety of ways, but typically it is expressed by excessive and inappropriate masturbation, frequent insertion of objects into orifices, sexually aggressive actions toward other children, and sexual approaches toward adults (Cosentino et al., 1995). In my experience, hypersexuality results as often as aggression in the failure of a foster care or group home placement.

Little is known about how to reverse this process and how to restore age-appropriate sexual behavior. Attempts to punish and suppress hypersexualized behaviors are rarely successful; they generally only succeed in distorting them more and/or displacing these behaviors into school and other less monitored settings. Hypersexualized behaviors must be contained by clear limits, which should be enforced in a way that promotes the development of self-monitoring and self-regulation.

Education is an important intervention (Carrey and Adams, 1992). Children are afraid that they are going to be blamed, lectured, or punished. They feel relieved when age-appropriate information is conveyed in an open, nonjudgmental fashion. Preschoolers do not have to be taught about sexuality per se, but rather should be told about privacy and respect for their bodies and the bodies of others. Prepubertal and pubertal children can be told about dating patterns and behaviors to expect and demand from the opposite sex; they can also be given information on the male and female genitalia, the menstrual cycle, intercourse, conception, pregnancy, birth, and development. Simple illustrations are useful.

Individual therapy is an important place to address these problems. In many instances, a child will "test" a therapist with sexualized approaches and explicit statements. Without exception, strict limits on sexual behavior directed at the therapist must be maintained. This is, of course, complicated by the natural tendency of adults to touch and hug children in distress. Within strict limits, physical contact offered as comforting may be appropriate in public places, but should be avoided in private settings such as individual therapy.

The therapist should also help the child to develop self-monitoring skills with respect to his or her behavior. Sexualized and aggressive behavior should be made a focus of self-observation. Reflecting the child's behavior back to him or her, perhaps indirectly or in a displaced fashion, and suggesting alternative responses are important. In adolescents, self-monitoring skills may be improved by peer groups focused on such subjects as appropriate behavior with the opposite sex.

Basic self-discipline strategies can be helpful in controlling these behaviors. The long-term goal is to help the child or adolescent assume responsibility for his or her behavior. This often requires setting goals and designing consequences for misbehavior. The basic principles and rules are similar to those proven in the classroom (Sprick, 1985). That is, a therapist or staff member must establish clear behavioral expectations; establish consequences for misbehavior; reinforce appropriate behavior; provide feedback in a matter-of-fact fashion, with descriptive rather than judgmental statements; be consistent; and be persistent.

In long-term living situations (e.g., residential placement), teenagers who are interested in each other should be provided with opportunities to express affection appropriately. Members of "couples" can be given permission to hold hands in restricted public settings, such as the hallways. Girls in particular benefit from this intervention, because it satisfies their need for signs of affection and publicly reinforces the "couple" message that they wish to send to peers. It also permits them to establish firmer boundaries during the unobserved moments that every teenage couple finds embedded within an institutional routine (e.g., staff meetings during shift change).

These approaches helped Naideane. She continued to masturbate, but more privately and less compulsively. Her outward sexualized behavior came increasingly under self-control, but the sexual thoughts that she occasionally shared with her therapist contained grimly masochistic, submissive, and bondage themes. This is an even more difficult problem to address than externalized sexual behavior. Sexual fantasies are difficult to work with in psychotherapy, because the content is hard to talk about, and because the fantasies are conditioned to an altered state of consciousness (i.e., sexual arousal and orgasm). Behavioral techniques used in the treatment of sexual offenders, such as masturbatory reconditioning and covert sensitization, appear to be capable of modifying sexual fantasies (Leitenberg and Henning, 1995). Obviously, however, such extreme measures should only be used when there is clear indication that fantasy is driving predatory or coercive sexual behavior. Let us hope that we will become more adept at addressing this aspect of the hypersexuality that occurs in so many victims of early childhood sexual abuse.

Management of Spontaneous Abreactions

Spontaneous abreactions, especially those involving explicit sexual behaviors, are extremely upsetting to residential and hospital staffers. Abreactions may be triggered by interactions centering around apparently innocuous activities of daily living, such as bathing and dressing. The first impulse is often an attempt to interrupt or suppress the behavior with physical restraint or medication; usually, however, this does not work well. Restraint or confinement often exacerbates the immediate abreaction or leads to a subsequent cluster of abreactions. Doses of medication sufficient to suppress an abreaction will put a child into a stupor.

In most instances, as long as the child is not in physical danger, an abreaction should be permitted to run its course. Often it will end abruptly, leaving the child momentarily disoriented but cognitively clear. During the abreaction, a staff member should stay close by the child, gently talking to him or her and providing "grounding" information: "It's okay, Daisy. You are safe. You are in the Children's Home. It's me, Martha. What you are seeing and feeling happened a long time ago. You are safe here." Even when the child appears completely lost in the abreaction, there is a part of him or her that is hearing this reassurance and reorientation.

After an abreaction, the child should be gently reoriented and reintegrated into the ongoing activities. Other patients can be told that an abreaction is "kind of like a seizure" and that the child will be okay in a few minutes. Staff members may need to be debriefed if they are frightened or repulsed by what they have seen. I do not recommend the use of therapeutic abreactive treatments for children in the same manner as they are sometimes used with dissociative and traumatized adults.

SUMMARY

Treatment of pathological dissociation in children and adolescents must necessarily address the circumstances of their living situations. Some dissociative children continue living with their natural families, where they are often exposed to considerable parental, sibling, and extended family psychopathology. Most of these require intensive family therapy, together with individual treatment for other family members. Many other dissociative children are in out-of-home placements, where their considerable psychopathology disrupts the foster families, group homes, or residential placement programs responsible for their care.

Whatever their living situation, dissociative children and adolescents must be supported by an organizing and integrating milieu. They require firm but reassuring boundaries, as well as people who can help them make the psychological connections between past and present, cause and effect, and one sense of self and another. Socialization of a child as a "multiple" should be avoided. Dissociative symptoms should be tracked, but not held up to the child as proof of the disorder; rather, they should be framed as challenges to be mastered through self-control and self-awareness.

Dissociative and traumatized children present many problems, especially in the form of dangerous or socially inappropriate behaviors. These require active attention from caretakers; dangerousness to self or others should not be underestimated. A long-term approach to helping the children confront these problems and gain control of their behavior will be needed. Sustained milieu interventions are probably more important than individual treatment for many dissociative children, particularly for younger children.

Chapter Sixteen

Psychopharmacology

Medication is often the first and the last resort of clinicians working with child and adolescent posttraumatic and dissociative disorders. It is considered first because of the increasing (and unreasonable) demands for quick, cheap solutions to complex and difficult cases. It becomes the last resort when nothing else has worked.

Psychiatric medication of children and adolescents is an art that is as yet poorly informed by systematic studies. The lack of scientific data on psychoactive drug effects in children and adolescents results from several factors—most importantly, the very much smaller research base dedicated to child mental health problems. In addition, pharmaceutical companies are reluctant to investigate child and adolescent usages of their medications. Psychopharmacological research with children is difficult, expensive, and routinely fraught with thorny ethical issues. Possible delayed adverse effects put investigators at considerable long-term liability. Large-sample studies are likely to identify rare pediatric side effects that further limit sales in an already small market.

Despite these difficulties, pharmaceutical companies bet that desperate practitioners will give their medications a try with young patients anyway. The prescription of medications for uses not approved by the Food and Drug Administration (FDA)—so-called "off-label use"—constitutes much of the clinical knowledge of pediatric psychopharmacology. This does not mean that such uses are invalid; although not yet fully substantiated, many off-label uses are clinically warranted. It does mean that there is no substitute for clinical knowledge and experience.

Pediatric psychopharmacology is a job for the specialist. It should not be undertaken by physicians without proper training and experience. Consequently, this chapter is offered simply as a review of the principles, issues, indications, targets, and outcomes of psychopharmacology for pediatric posttraumatic and dissociative disorders. The intention is to inform child clinicians, most of whom are not trained in psychopharmacology, about potential medications and issues. The information contained in this chapter will become outdated with time, and readers should obtain the most current information before recommending pharmacotherapy in any particular case.

GUIDELINES AND SUGGESTIONS FOR USE OF PEDIATRIC PSYCHOACTIVE MEDICATIONS

General Principles

"When in doubt, don't" (Werry and Aman, 1993, p. 15) is probably the most basic principle of pediatric psychopharmacology. Even when medication is recommended, it should only be employed in conjunction with a comprehensive treatment plan; it should never be the only form of therapy. The treatment plan must be discussed with the legal guardian and with the child or adolescent to a degree appropriate to his or her age. The potential benefits and possible side effects should be reviewed with all parties. It is important to sound out the parents' or caretakers attitudes toward medication, to assess their reliability and likely cooperation with prescribed administration and side effect monitoring. A good therapeutic alliance in regard to this specific aspect of the treatment is critical. It is important that parents/caretakers not manipulate the dosage without clearly specified contingencies; for example, they should not withhold medication when a child is doing well or increase medication when the child is having a "bad day" (Green, 1991). Informed consent should be obtained, and the consent form should be included in the medical records.

Since no medications have as yet been approved by the FDA for pediatric posttraumatic and dissociative disorders, it is important to choose a drug that has efficacy for specific target symptoms (discussed below). Several medications—often belonging to different classes—may have reported success for a given symptom, and a prescriber has to choose among them. A comparative knowledge of the dosage, pharmacokinetics, and side effects of the medications is helpful in selecting the drug to be tried.

It is important to keep things as simple as possible. Whenever possible, no more than one medication should be prescribed at a time. Too often the complex symptom picture of dissociative and posttraumatic disorders evokes a knee-jerk polypharmacy response. In particular, the use of secondary medications to counteract the side effects of primary medications is to be avoided; this just generates iterative complexity, rarely helps, and usually overmedicates a child. Prescribers should avoid unsubstantiated uses of a medication and be leery of fads, particularly whenever a medication first comes on the market. It is wise to stick to the tried-and-true older medications, and to resist advertising-driven ploys to boost sales of newly released medications. Experience with adults should be allowed to accrue before a new drug is tried with children.

Baseline Assessments

Children and adolescents who are to receive psychoactive medications should have an evaluation that includes a comprehensive medical history, a review of systems, and a physical and neurological examination. (See Chapter Twelve for a discussion of the physical examination in maltreated children). The aims of this evaluation are to rule out organic factors contributing to the symptoms; to identify medical problems that might interact with the medication; and to establish a medical baseline for assessing side effects and therapeutic improvement. The medical history should include a record of immunizations, hospitalizations, trauma, transfusions, substance use, allergies, past and current medications, and any positive responses or side effects.

The laboratory tests listed in Table 16.1 are routinely recommended by pediatric psychopharmacology experts (Green, 1991; Werry and Aman, 1993). Other tests may be indicated to rule out organic causes for a child's problems (e.g., tumors, infections, neurological and vascular disorders, endocrinopathies, nutritional deficiencies, etc.). A preg-

TABLE 16.1. Premedication Laboratory Tests

Complete blood count (CBC) with hematocrit and differential

Serum electrolytes—sodium (Na), potassium (K), chloride (Cl), carbon dioxide (CO_2), calcium (Ca), and phosphate (PO_4)

Liver function tests—aspartate aminotransferase (AST) or serum glutamic oxaloacetic transminase (SGOT), alanine aminotransferase (ALT) or serum glutamic pyruvic transaminase (SGPT), alkaline phosphatase, lactic dehydrogenase (LDH), and bilirubin (total and direct)

Serum lead levels

Thyroid function tests—triiodothyronine resin uptake (T_3RU), thyroxine (T_4), and thyroid-stimulating hormone (TSH)

Complete urinalysis

Baseline electrocardiogram (EKG)—especially when antipsychotics, lithium, or tricyclic antidepressants are prescribed

nancy test should be included for any adolescent girl who might be pregnant. A toxicology screen for drugs of abuse may be indicated.

Again, baselines should be established in two broad areas: side effects (discussed below) and therapeutic improvement. Measuring therapeutic effects requires clear thinking about the specific symptoms being targeted and allied symptoms also likely to change for better or worse. Baseline evaluation should include a careful clinical evaluation with good documentation. However, many times a clinical impression still remains the most sensitive early monitoring system.

Baseline assessments should include scales and measures pertinent to the symptoms being targeted. These are periodically completed by the parents/guardians, teachers, and the child or adolescent. In some instances, formally administered structured interviews or neuropsychological tests are warranted. Generally, there should be one or two broadly based measures focusing on general behavioral problems, and a couple of selected measures more tightly focused on specific clinical issues (e.g., dissociation, hyperactivity, depression, anxiety, conduct problems, etc.).

The most commonly used general measure is the Child Behavior Checklist (CBCL; Achenbach, 1991a). A parent report checklist (response options include "very true," "sometimes or somewhat true," and "never") with 20 Social Competence items and 112 Behavior Problem items, the CBCL provides two broad-band constructs (Externalizing and Internalizing Behaviors) and eight derived subscales (Aggressive Behavior, Anxious/Depressed, Attention Problems, Delinquent Behavior, Social Problems, Somatic Complaints, Thought Problems, and Withdrawn). The Teacher Report Form (TRF) is closely related and contains overlapping as well as school-specific items (Achenbach, 1991b). The time frame for the CBCL is the prior year, so a clinician must get a baseline and then instruct the informants to fill out subsequent forms for the specific periods (e.g., after a change in medication dosage).

A systematic review of the numerous child and adolescent scales focusing on specific problems is beyond the scope of this chapter. However, I identify some of the more solidly established instruments. The Conners Parent and Teacher Rating Scales are the standard measures for documenting attentional and hyperactivity problems (Conners, 1990). These instruments (for which abbreviated versions are available) are also informative about oppositional, conduct, and aggressive problems. A number of validated depression scales exist (Aman, 1993). I have found the Children's Depression Inventory valuable both clinically and for research (Kovacs, 1991). The State–Trait Anxiety Inventory for Children has also proven useful (Spielberger, 1973); it measures both transient stressor-related anxiety and the more stable personality anxiety traits. The self-report Leyton Obsessional Inventory—Child Version comes in both a long and a short form (Berg, Rapoport, and Flament, 1986). It is more useful for monitoring drug response than for diagnosis or screening. The PTSD Reaction Index, a semistructured interview, is the most widely used diagnostic and research measure of posttraumatic symptoms, but its sensitivity to therapeutic drug effects is not well established (Putnam, 1996b). Of course, I strongly recommend that pathological dissociation be documented and followed with the CDC, A-DES, and DES as age-appropriate.

Developmental Pharmacokinetics, Pharmacodynamics, and Choice of Drug

Pharmacokinetics (the metabolic fate of administered drugs) and pharmacodynamics (the mechanisms by which drugs produce their effects) are subjects well beyond the scope of this book. However, a few basic principles related to children and adolescents are in order. Little is known about the factors that influence drug metabolism and action during early development. In general, rates of drug absorption in children and adolescents are roughly equivalent to those in adults (Riddle, 1991; Paxton and Dragunow, 1993); however, drug distribution is influenced by age-related factors, such as body size and percentage of fat. Therefore, body size and pubertal status are important considerations in titrating dose.

The liver and the kidneys are the two major organs for clearing drugs from the body. Hepatic function develops during the first year of life, with different microsomal enzyme systems maturing at different rates. Hepatic function is highest at about 1–2 years of age, and then declines over childhood until puberty, when a marked decrease in hepatic activity occurs (Paxton and Dragunow, 1993). During adolescence, hepatic function further declines to adult levels, paralleling increases in gonadal steroid hormone production.

It is believed that elevated hepatic function is responsible for the short half-life of some benzodiazepines (BZs) in children, and for the higher doses of tricyclic antidepressants (TCAs) and neuroleptics required to achieve therapeutic blood levels (Riddle, 1991). However, certain BZs (e.g., oxazepam and lorazepam) are not metabolized in the liver prior to conjugation and may have somewhat different pharmacokinetics (Riddle, 1991). Renal filtration increases rapidly in the neonate and approaches adult levels by 6 months of age (Paxton and Dragunow, 1993). Tubular excretion and reabsorption reach adult levels by 1 year of age. In general, children will clear drugs from their systems faster than adults will. This is particularly apparent with such drugs as lithium.

Regulation and Monitoring of Medication

Whenever possible, a trial of medication should begin with a drug approved by the FDA for the patient's age and target symptoms. Information about prior medication responses in the child or effects on parents or siblings may be helpful in selecting a drug. In general, a trial begins with a very low dose, which is gradually increased to a therapeutic level or until significant or persistent side-effects have developed. Although this cautious approach may seem too prolonged, it minimizes a number of problems. First, it avoids overdosing children who are extremely sensitive to medication for genetic, medical, or developmental reasons. Second, for some drugs (e.g., methylphenidate), clinical response is not related to blood levels (Green, 1991). Initial low doses with gradual increases prevent "behavioral toxicity," particularly in younger children. Behavioral toxicity includes worsening of target symptoms, changes in activity level, and affective lability, and may precede appearance of more classic side effects (Green, 1991). Finally, an excessive initial dose may induce side effects that do not occur if the dose is gradually increased to the same level.

The art and science of pediatric psychopharmacotherapy lie in determining the lowest possible dose that produces the desired clinical effects. Generally this requires first determining the upper level of the therapeutic range and then systematically backing down a bit. The upper level of the therapeutic range is established by gradually increasing the dose until an entirely satisfactory therapeutic response is obtained, until the upper limit of the FDA-recommended dosage has been reached, until significant side effects have appeared, or until no further improvement occurs or symptoms worsen.

Dosing of a medication should be based on a knowledge of the pharmacokinetics of the drug (i.e., the rate of absorption and half-life) and the time(s) when the maximum effects are desired (e.g., during the school day, at nighttime). Administration may also have to be timed to minimize side effects (e.g., stimulants may need to be given with meals, or neuroleptics at bedtime). Dose increases should be based on a knowledge of the expected response time; TCAs frequently take months to manifest a clinical effect, whereas stimulant efficacy can be observed shortly after the first dose. In general, pediatric psychopharmacology should be considered a slow-motion process, with long-term goals deliberately carried out in small steps.

Serum levels may or may not be helpful in establishing therapeutic levels. When they are known to be correlated with clinical response (e.g., imipramine), serum levels provide an objective index with which to titrate dosage. In other instances, serum levels may bear no significant relationship to clinical efficacy and are not worth the effort or expense. Lithium serum levels are considered mandatory (Green, 1991).

Side Effects

When an optimal dosage has been determined, the child should be followed and reassessed on a regular basis. Side effects should be inquired about at each visit. For children on medications, I routinely record vital signs at every office visit. Twice a year, the medication and its costs and benefits should be reviewed in depth. An explicit list of possible side effects should be periodically reviewed with caretakers. Many child psychiatry clinics have useful informational handouts discussing medication benefits and listing side effects for commonly prescribed medications. Parents in the throes of trying to decide whether a child is having a medication side effect or is just coming down with the flu find such handouts helpful. Complaints and symptoms can be extremely intermittent and ambiguous, even for normal children.

Length of Treatment

Because the long-term effects of medications on the development of children and adolescents are not well understood, drugs should be used for as short a time as clinically possible. Some experts recommend discontinuing psychotropic medications every 6 months to 1 year (Green, 1991); in many instances, however, is not clinically possible. When medication is being withdrawn, it is important to taper dosage gradually. Children seem to be especially sensitive to withdrawal effects caused by too-rapid decreases in dose. When possible, "drug holidays" are useful to decrease total medication exposures. Drug holidays should be timed to avoid life changes or stressful periods (e.g., the start of a new school year).

In some cases children will not require the reinstatement of medication. Behavioral measures collected while a child is on therapeutic levels of a drug can be compared with measures completed off medication. If the child shows little or no change, the medication can be discontinued. In many instances, however, it will be obvious that it is necessary to restart the medication. Sometimes after a drug has been withdrawn and is then reinstated, it is difficult to reestablish therapeutic effect. This risk of loss of efficacy creates one of those "between a rock and a hard place" dilemmas.

TARGET SYMPTOMS IN POSTTRAUMATIC AND DISSOCIATIVE DISORDERS

The use of medication for a traumatized or dissociative patient must be considered within the context of treatment of the whole individual. Medication should not be given merely to "do something" or to "treat" other members of the treatment team. A therapist must make a careful clinical assessment and determine which symptoms are likely to be medication-responsive and which are not. Among the indications for pharmacotherapy are posttraumatic, affective, and anxiety symptoms that impair an individual's ability to make use of environmental supports and treatment, or that significantly impair daily functioning, particularly at work or at school.

High rates of comorbid psychiatric disorders are commonly noted in patients with posttraumatic and dissociative disorders. Most commonly these include depression, anxiety, substance abuse, eating disorders, and somatization. Some of these, especially depression and anxiety, are often medication-responsive. This section reviews the effects of medication on symptoms and behaviors commonly seen in these patients. It should be reiterated that most of what is known about medication effects comes from clinical experience with adults.

Posttraumatic Symptoms

Intrusive symptoms, such as traumatic nightmares, flashbacks, and trauma-related intrusive thoughts and images, may be among the most pharmacologically responsive posttraumatic symptoms. Virtually all classes of medication found to be of benefit to adult PTSD patients improve intrusive symptoms.

By contrast, avoidant and emotional numbing symptoms are the most difficult to treat. Most studies find little or no improvement in such symptoms as avoidance of traumatic cues, affective constriction, depersonalization, and emotional numbing. However, more recent reports from open trials with selective serotonin reuptake inhibitors (SSRIs), together with a double-blind, placebo-controlled study of fluoxetine by van der Kolk et al. (1994), indicate that avoidant symptoms may be at least partially medication-responsive.

Posttraumatic symptoms reflecting autonomic hyperarousal, such as hypervigilance, exaggerated startle responses, irritability, and insomnia, are responsive to a range of medications. These include TCAs, SSRIs, BZs, buspirone, phenelzine, clonidine, and propranolol.

Dissociative Symptoms

With the exception of depersonalization, dissociative symptoms (e.g., the functional amnesias, passive influence/interference experiences, and identity alterations) are not responsive to medication. To date, few treatment studies of PTSD in adults have included measures of dissociation, so little is known. In the only systematic assessment to date, van der Kolk et al. (1994) did not find any change in DES scores with fluoxetine.

However, there is reason to believe that pathological dissociation may be responsive to medication. Good (1989) notes that there are psychoactive substances affecting cholinergic, beta-adrenergic, dopaminergic, and serotonergic neurotransmitter systems that produce subsets of dissociative symptoms (e.g., fugues, amnesias, and depersonalization). Our efforts to model dissociative memory disturbances in the laboratory also support this observation (Weingartner et al., 1995). Theoretically if dissociative symptoms can be induced with drugs, it may well be possible to treat them with medication also.

Depersonalization, particularly when it appears as an isolated symptom or in conjunction with panic disorder, may respond to a variety of medications, including desipramine, fluoxetine, and clonazepam (Steinberg, 1991). However, chronic depersonalization is notoriously medication-resistant, and most patients report little or no sustained benefit.

Problems with Impulse Control

A few medications, notably lithium and carbamazepine, are clinically regarded as being relatively specific for problems with impulse control (Campbell et al., 1995; Campbell and Cueva, 1995b). In my experience, this efficacy remains to be convincingly demonstrated. In general, impulse control can often be improved by medications that dampen hyperarousal and intrusive symptoms. In dissociative patients, impulse control problems often reflect the acting out of internal psychological conflicts in dissociated behavioral states. In such instances, direct and indirect psychotherapeutic/milieu interventions should be put into place before drugs are tried. However, carbamazepine (discussed below) has been reported to be helpful in controlling episodic violence in dissociative patients (Fichner, Kuhlman, Gruenfeld, and Hughes, 1990; Coons, 1992).

Affective Symptoms

Affective symptoms, particularly depression, are among the more pharmacologically responsive symptoms in traumatized and dissociative patients. However, response to antidepressants is often incomplete, and a combination of approaches (e.g., psychotherapy and medication) is necessary. Antidepressants, particularly the TCAs, are generally the first drug of choice in treating chronic PTSD in adults. In MPD patients, pharmacotherapy of depression should be limited to those instances in which depressive symptoms are persistent and widely distributed across contexts and dissociated behavioral states (Loewenstein, 1991c).

Anxiety Symptoms and Panic Attacks

Anxiety and panic symptoms in patients with posttraumatic and dissociative disorders frequently show improvement with conventional anxiolytic medications. As is the case with affective symptoms, improvement is often less than complete. Medications that dampen adrenergic hyperarousal usually improve anxiety symptoms. Anxiolytics also help dissociative patients. BZs are commonly prescribed for this purpose, but concerns about their addiction potential and long-term withdrawal effects are curtailing the use of these medications. They are seldom appropriate for prolonged treatment of children or adolescents (Coffey, 1993).

Sleep Disturbances

Sleep disturbances (difficulty falling asleep, nocturnal awakenings) and recurrent nightmares are common symptoms in traumatized children, as in adults. There are no systematic studies of treatment, but clinical experience suggests that clonidine at bedtime may be helpful. Horrigan (1996) has reported sustained improvement in posttraumatic nightmares with guanfacine in a single case.

Somatoform Symptoms

Somatic symptoms and psychogenic pain are particularly troublesome in dissociative patients, and to a lesser extent in patients with posttraumatic disorders. Usually these symptoms reflect underlying psychodynamic processes, such as reliving of abusive experiences (Lindy et al.,

1992). They are often best dealt with through psychotherapeutic and related interventions. However, it is important not to overlook actual physical components, which are amplified by psychological factors. Our research on differentiating psychogenic and neurogenic dysphonias indicates that some patients have an organic basis for their physical complaints, which becomes heavily overlaid with psychogenic features.

Hallucinations

Hallucinations are common in dissociative disorders. Nor are they infrequent in PTSD if therapists systematically look for them. As discussed in Chapter Five, dissociative hallucinations can frequently be differentiated from schizophreniform hallucinations by their internalization, vividness, and specific personality attributes. In most instances, traumatized and dissociative patients recognize the hallucinatory nature of their experience and show good general reality testing. In contrast to schizophreniform hallucinations, posttraumatic/dissociative hallucinations are rarely medication-responsive.

MEDICATION CLASSES

Antidepressants

Antidepressants are the best-studied class of medications in adult PTSD. The TCAs, monoamine oxidase inhibitors (MAOIs), and SSRIs are effective for certain posttraumatic symptoms (Solomon et al., 1992; Sutherland and Davidson, 1994). Controlled studies of two TCAs, amitriptyline and imipramine, demonstrate significant improvement in intrusive symptoms that is independent of antidepressant and antianxiety effects (Frank, Kosten, Giller, and Dan, 1988; Davidson et al., 1990; Kosten, Frank, Dan, McDougle, and Giller, 1991). Phenelzine, an MAOI, has been shown to be beneficial for intrusive symptoms (e.g., nightmares and flashbacks) and slightly superior to imipramine for anxiety in adult PTSD patients (Frank et al., 1988). However, the need for severe restrictions in diet and for prohibition of alcohol and some over-the-counter drugs limits the utility of MAOIs.

The SSRIs show great promise for the treatment of adult PTSD (Davidson, Roth, and Newman, 1991; Sutherland and Davidson, 1994; van der Kolk et al., 1994). Fluoxetine has been shown to reduce overall posttraumatic symptomatology, with notable improvement in numbing and avoidant symptoms relative to TCAs (Davidson et al., 1990; van der Kolk et al., 1994). Fluoxetine also shows promise for some dissociative symptoms, particularly depersonalization (Hollander et al., 1990). In our survey of MPD treatment practices (Putnam and Loewenstein, 1993), we found that fluoxetine was the most commonly prescribed drug for adult MPD patients, receiving a mean rating of "moderately effective" in overall symptom reduction.

TCAs are used to treat depression, ADHD, enuresis, school phobia, and anxiety disorders in children and adolescents. Imipramine is the TCA most widely used in children. Manufacturers recommend that the dose should not exceed 2.5 mg/kg. In low doses, TCAs often have "stimulant-like" effects; that is, they decrease hyperactivity, improve attention, and increase cooperativeness much as stimulant medications do. Sedation is a common side effect that can interfere with school performance. Dry mouth, dizziness, nausea, constipation, palpitations, chest pain, blurred vision, and stomachaches often occur during early phases of treatment.

There have been a few cases of sudden death in children attributed to the cardiovascular effects of the TCAs, especially desipramine (Werry and Aman, 1993; Campbell and Cueva, 1995a). The electrocardiogram (EKG) should be periodically monitored, and medication should be decreased or discontinued if the PR interval is ≥ 0.21 seconds, the QRS interval is ≥ 0.12 seconds, heart rate is >130 beats per minute, or blood pressure is >130/85 (Werry and Aman, 1993).

The MAOIs have not been studied in children. The most dangerous side effect is hypertensive crisis, induced by tyramine-containing foods or over-the-counter cold medicines containing ephedrine or related stimulants. A hypermetabolic crisis resulting in seizures or death can occur if food or drugs high in serotonin are ingested. Common side effects include significant hypotension, insomnia, afternoon sedation, dry mouth, nocturnal myoclonic jerking, and constipation. The MAOIs should be considered medications of last resort in children and adolescents.

The SSRIs, fluoxetine and clomipramine, have been used in children and adolescents for obsessive–compulsive disorder. They are generally well tolerated. Clomipramine is FDA-approved for children 10 years and older; its most significant side effect appears to be a small, cumulative increase in risk of seizures. Open trials of fluoxetine suggest efficacy for obsessive–compulsive disorder in children. It is generally less sedating than the TCAs. The most frequently reported side effects are nausea, weight loss, insomnia, and excessive perspiration (Green, 1991).

Anxiolytics

Anxiolytics, particularly BZs, are widely prescribed in adult PTSD treatment, although there are few empirical data on their efficacy (Solomon et al., 1992). Generally these medications are used to target sleep disturbances and anxiety. The single placebo-controlled trial to date (whose *n* was small) showed that alprazolam, a triazolo-BZ, reduced anxiety symptoms but did not improve posttraumatic symptoms (Braun, Greenberg, Dasberg, and Lerer, 1990). Nonetheless, open trials of clonazepam suggest some improvement in hyperarousal symptoms in adult MPD patients (Loewenstein, Hornstein, and Farber, 1988). In our MPD treatment practices survey (Putnam and Loewenstein, 1993), clonazepam received the highest overall rating of efficacy. A single-case report by Stein and Uhde (1989) describes improvement in depersonalization symptoms in a 27-year-old woman.

Abuse and dependence are serious concerns with prolonged BZ use (Solomon et al., 1992; Sutherland and Davidson, 1994). The high rates of substance abuse in traumatized and dissociative patients heighten these concerns. A characteristic BZ withdrawal syndrome, consisting of excitation, anxiety, agitation, autonomic hyperactivity, and tremor, has been described (Miller, Gold, and Stennie, 1995). BZ use has not been well studied in children. Although FDA pediatric guidelines exist for some BZs, their use should be regarded as experimental. Long-term BZ use is rarely indicated in children. Behavioral toxicity and paradoxical increases in aggression have been reported when BZs were used to manage agitation in children and adolescents with conduct disorder and delinquency (Campbell, Gonzalez, and Silva, 1992).

Anticonvulsants

The anticonvulsants carbamazepine, clonazepam, and valproate have been tried for both posttraumatic and dissociative disorders. Clonazepam, a BZ, is described above. Valproate has been used in open trials for combat-related PTSD, which suggested some improvement in hyperarousal and avoidant symptoms (Fesler, 1991). Valproate's main clinical effect is antiepileptic, but quieting, antiagitation, and sedating responses have been noted in children. Fatal liver toxicity can occur, particularly in young children, and neutropenia is not uncommon—so extreme caution is required.

A few uncontrolled studies suggest that carbamazepine is helpful in combat-related PTSD (Lipper, Davidson, Grady, Edinger, and Cavenar, 1986; Wolf, Alavi, and Mosnam, 1988; Lipper, 1990; Li and Spiegel, 1992). Hostility and impulsivity show the greatest improvement. Case studies suggest that carbamazepine exerts similar effects in some adult MPD patients (Fichner et al., 1990; Coons, 1992). There is no evidence to date that carbamazepine improves dissociative symptoms, but it may also be helpful for affective symptoms in some MPD patients (Devinsky et al., 1989). Carbamazepine has been found helpful in the management of self-mutilation in adult BPD and PTSD (Cowdry and Gardner, 1988; Saporta and Case, 1993).

Little is known about the efficacy of carbamazepine in children and adolescents for psychiatric disorders. It is widely used in Europe for behavioral dyscontrol and hyperactivity. A double-blind, placebo-controlled study in a modest sample (n = 22) of aggressive children with conduct disorder found that it was no more effective than placebo and was associated with untoward side effects, primarily leukopenia, which fortunately was transient (Cueva et al., 1996).

A preliminary report describes carbamazepine's use for children and adolescents with a formal diagnosis of PTSD (Looff, Grimley, and Kuller, 1995a; Looff, Grimley, Kuller, Martin, and Shonfield, 1995b). Following pretreatment medical assessment, children aged 6–12 years were started at 100 mg twice a day and those aged 13 and older were begun at 200 mg twice a day. The drug was administered with meals, and dosage was increased every 4–7 days until a serum level of 10–11.5 μg/ml was reached. A high percentage of subjects (78.5%) reportedly became asymptomatic at this level. The remainder were reported to be improved, especially in regard to intrusive symptoms. No significant side effects were noted; however, carbamazepine can have life-threatening side effects, notably aplastic anemia. Proper precautions and serial blood work are thus mandatory when this drug is prescribed.

Lithium

Lithium is widely prescribed for the management of aggression in children. This use is supported by a number of open trials and controlled studies by Campbell et al. (1995). Since the major route of elimination is renal, kidney function tests are indicated. Cardiovascular disease and concurrent use of medications that alter sodium regulation are contraindications. In the Campbell et al. (1995) study, the optimal daily dose ranged from 600 mg to 1,800 mg (mean = 1,248 mg) with a mean serum level of 1.12 mEq/liter. GI distress and polyuria were the most common side effects. There were moderately positive effects on aggression measures, notably decreased bullying, fighting, and temper outbursts. Lithium has a narrow therapeutic range, and lethal toxicity can occur in younger children at relatively low serum levels (Green, 1991). Serum level is sensitive to physical illness, vigorous exercise, and hot weather—situations commonly encountered by active children. I have been underwhelmed by lithium's effects on aggression in traumatized children I have treated, but a few colleagues do report beneficial effects.

Propranolol

Propranolol, a nonselective beta-blocker, has been used in open trials for PTSD in combat veterans (Kolb, Burris, and Griffiths, 1984). It reportedly decreased explosiveness, nightmares, startle responses, intrusive thoughts, and sleep problems. Famularo et al. (1988) used propranolol in an off–on–off design to treat 11 children (mean age 8.5 years) diagnosed with acute PTSD. Subjects had significantly fewer posttraumatic symptoms on medication. No serious side effects were encountered, but lowered blood pressure and pulse rate limited the dosage for several subjects.

Beta-blockers have also been used with mentally retarded children for control of aggression, self-injurious behavior, and impulsivity. A review of this literature suggests positive responses in about three-quarters of cases, but results from such uncontrolled studies are usually overly optimistic (Arnold and Aman, 1991). Beta-blockers interact with a large number of over-the-counter medications and are contraindicated in the presence of asthma or cardiorespiratory disease. Side effects include hypotension, bradycardia, bronchoconstriction, depression, hallucinations, nausea, and vomiting.

Clonidine

Clonidine, an alpha-2-adrenergic agonist, stimulates presynaptic autoreceptors producing inhibition of noradrenergic activity. Open trials with adult PTSD patients reported some significant improvements, primarily in intrusive symptoms (Kolb et al., 1984; Kinzie and Leung, 1989). Clonidine is often the second drug of choice for ADHD and Tourette's syndrome, and considerable experience has accrued with children. It has also been used to treat sleep disturbances in ADHD children (Wilens, Biederman, and Spencer, 1994) and in adults with PTSD (Kinzie, Sack, and Riley, 1994).

Sedation and hypotension are the two primary side effects and are usually not severe. Clonidine has been administered prophylactically to acutely traumatized children in an attempt to reduce hyperarousal, which is thought to contribute to the subsequent development of PTSD (B. Perry, personal communication, November 1994). Clinical experience with this intervention is positive, but at present such use must be considered experimental.

A small-scale, open trial by Harmon and Riggs (1996) for preschoolers formally diagnosed with PTSD in a preschool/day hospital setting found moderate to great improvement in aggression, impulsivity, emotional outbursts/mood lability, hyperarousal, insomnia, and night-mares. They also noted a marked decrease in traumatic play in one boy and a decrease in dissociative episodes in a girl, both associated with stabilization on the clonidine. Treatment was initiated with an oral dose of 0.05 mg in the morning while each child was observed in the day hos-pital. If this was tolerated, the dose was increased with 0.05 mg at bed-time. Children frequently experienced transient sedation during the first week. After cessation of sedation, maintenance doses averaged 0.1 mg at bedtime. Blood pressure decreases averaged less than 10% of base-line. A clonidine patch, replaced every 5 days, proved successful with several children; it enhanced compliance without loss of efficacy.

Concerns have been raised about clonidine's effects on the EKG, so baseline and follow-up EKGs are warranted (Harmon and Riggs, 1996). Particular caution should be exercised in combining clonidine with methylphenidate or other drugs commonly prescribed for ADHD. Cantwell and colleagues (Cantwell, Swanson, and Connor, 1997) report serious cardiac side effects in three such cases. As discussed above for pediatric psychotropic medications in general, the dose of clonidine must be tapered gradually to avoid dangerous withdrawal side effects, for example, rebound noradrenergic hyperactivity (Cantwell et al., 1997).

Opiate Antagonists

There is interest in the use of opiate antagonists in the treatment of post-traumatic and dissociative disorders. Anecdotal accounts suggest that certain patients (particularly those with a propensity toward self-injuri-ous behavior) respond positively to naltrexone, a potent, long-acting opiate antagonist. This lore remains to be confirmed by controlled tri-als. According to van der Kolk's "addiction to trauma" hypothesis, the endogenous opiate system may play a reinforcing role in perpetuating self-mutilation and risk-taking behaviors; this theory has also spurred interest in the use of these medications (Pitman et al., 1990).

Naltrexone and naloxone have been used investigationally in chil-dren to treat self-injurious behavior in mental retardation and autism (Green, 1991; Werry and Aman, 1993). A review of open-trial studies suggests that approximately half of the retarded and autistic young sub-jects showed improvement (Werry and Aman, 1993); response was highly variable, however. Optimum doses appear to be in the range of 0.5–2.0 mg/kg. Common side effects include insomnia, anxiety, lethar-gy, nausea, stomachaches, and joint pains. Contraindications include opioid use or dependence and liver disease.

Stimulants

Questions about the use of stimulant medications, such as methylphenidate, quickly arise in clinical discussions. Many traumatized children exhibit agitation, motoric restlessness, hyperactivity, and difficulties with attention, concentration, and memory. Diagnoses of ADHD are significantly more common in maltreated children in than the general population (De Bellis et al., 1994b; Merry and Andrews, 1994; Glod and Teicher, 1996).

At present there are no controlled trials of stimulant medications in traumatized children. Clinical impressions suggest that in comparison with nontraumatized children diagnosed with ADHD, traumatized children derive no particular benefit from stimulant medications. De Bellis et al. (1994b) speculate that stimulants may even be contraindicated in traumatized children, whose attentional and activity problems may arise from sympathetic nervous system hyperarousal, as evidenced by increased urinary catecholamine levels. The field desperately needs a well-done study of this question to guide our treatment of hyperactivity and attentional problems in traumatized children.

Neuroleptics

There was a time when the use of neuroleptics was considered contraindicated in dissociative disorders (Putnam, 1989a). In part, this position represented a reaction to the misdiagnosis of MPD patients as schizophrenic. As experience has accrued, it has become apparent that there is a role for low-dose neuroleptics in dissociative and posttraumatic disorders. Our treatment practices survey (Putnam and Loewenstein, 1993) found that neuroleptics, primarily thioridazine, were used and received positive ratings in about a third of all medication-treated adult MPD cases. Low-dose neuroleptics are often used to target nocturnal agitation and sleep difficulties, and to treat subtle "cognitive slippage" that falls short of a formal thought disorder.

Neuroleptic medications have been used in children for a variety of disorders—generally nonpsychotic conditions, such as Tourette's syndrome, aggression, and conduct problems. These drugs can have numerous serious and even lethal side effects. Irreversible tardive dyskinesia is a serious concern. Sedation and cognitive dulling can also be expected and usually interfere with school and social activities. A comparison study of haloperidol and lithium for treatment of aggressive conduct disorder found both to be superior to placebo, but haloperidol interfered more with the children's daily routine (Campbell, Small, and

Green, 1984). Chronic use is to be avoided if possible, but low-dose neuroleptics may be warranted in some difficult cases.

SUMMARY

The prescription of medication for posttraumatic and dissociative disorders is often approached with unrealistic expectations that there are definitive pharmacological treatments. The cumulative experience with the pharmacological treatment of adult PTSD is that medications are best considered as important adjunctive interventions. There are, however, a number of medications that have at least partial efficacy for some posttraumatic symptoms (e.g., hyperarousal and intrusive thoughts) as well as depression and anxiety. Posttraumatic avoidant symptoms are less medication-sensitive, as are aggression and impulsivity, but nonetheless may still respond in some patients. Dissociative symptoms, posttraumatic/dissociative hallucinations, and somatoform symptoms appear to be especially resistant to medication, although there is reason to believe that they too are potentially treatable. A number of classes of medications have been found effective, but surprisingly few well-done research studies are available. Antidepressants are the best-studied medications in adult PTSD and probably should be the drug of first choice in most cases.

Pediatric psychopharmacology is an art that is best left to an experienced practitioner, although experts are few and far between, and front-line clinicians must often shoulder these responsibilities. A good baseline assessment is critical and should include a thorough medical workup and behavioral scales that cover both general problems and mediation target symptoms and behaviors. Special attention should be paid to titration of dose, possible side effects, and effects on general and target symptoms. Whenever possible, drug holidays should be used to minimize cumulative dosage and to check for remission of symptoms.

Dissociative Experiences Scale–II (DES-II)

Eve Bernstein Carlson, PhD
Frank W. Putnam, MD

DIRECTIONS

This questionnaire consists of twenty-eight questions about experiences that you may have in your daily life. We are interested in how often you have these experiences. It is important, however, that your answers show how often these experiences happen to you when you **are not** under the influence of alcohol or drugs.

To answer the questions, please determine to what degree the experience described in the question applies to you, and circle the number to show what percentage of the time you have the experience.

Example:

0% ⑩ 20 30 40 50 60 70 80 90 100%
(never)   (always)

Date: _____   Age: _____   Sex: M   F

1. Some people have the experience of driving or riding in a car or bus or subway and suddenly realizing that they don't remember what has happened during all or part of the trip. Circle a number to show what percentage of the time this happens to you.

   0%   10   20   30   40   50   60   70   80   90   100%

2. Some people find that sometimes they are listening to someone talk and they suddenly realize that they did not hear part or all of what was said. Circle a number to show what percentage of the time this happens to you.

   0%   10   20   30   40   50   60   70   80   90   100%

3. Some people have the experience of finding themselves in a place and having no idea how they got there. Circle a number to show what percentage of the time this happens to you.

   0%   10   20   30   40   50   60   70   80   90   100%

4. Some people have the experience of finding themselves dressed in clothes that they don't remember putting on. Circle a number to show what percentage of the time this happens to you.

   0%   10   20   30   40   50   60   70   80   90   100%

5. Some people have the experience of finding new things among their belongings that they do not remember buying. Circle a number to show what percentage of the time this happens to you.

   0%   10   20   30   40   50   60   70   80   90   100%

6. Some people sometimes find that they are approached by people that they do not know, who call them by another name or insist that they have met them before. Circle a number to show what percentage of the time this happens to you.

   0%   10   20   30   40   50   60   70   80   90   100%

7. Some people sometimes have the experience of feeling as though they are standing next to themselves or watching themselves do something and they actually see themselves as if they were looking at another person. Circle a number to show what percentage of the time this happens to you.

   0%   10   20   30   40   50   60   70   80   90   100%

8. Some people are told that they sometimes do not recognize friends or family members. Circle a number to show what percentage of the time this happens to you.

   0%   10   20   30   40   50   60   70   80   90   100%

9. Some people find that they have no memory for some important events in their lives (for example, a wedding or graduation). Circle a number to show what percentage of the time this happens to you.

0%   10   20   30   40   50   60   70   80   90   100%

10. Some people have the experience of being accused of lying when they do not think that they have lied. Circle a number to show what percentage of the time this happens to you.

0%   10   20   30   40   50   60   70   80   90   100%

11. Some people have the experience of looking in a mirror and not recognizing themselves. Circle a number to show what percentage of the time this happens to you.

0%   10   20   30   40   50   60   70   80   90   100%

12. Some people have the experience of feeling that other people, objects, and the world around them are not real. Circle a number to show what percentage of the time this happens to you.

0%   10   20   30   40   50   60   70   80   90   100%

13. Some people have the experience of feeling that their body does not seem to belong to them. Circle a number to show what percentage of the time this happens to you.

0%   10   20   30   40   50   60   70   80   90   100%

14. Some people have the experience of sometimes remembering a past event so vividly that they feel as if they were reliving that event. Circle a number to show what percentage of the time this happens to you.

0%   10   20   30   40   50   60   70   80   90   100%

15. Some people have the experience of not being sure whether things that they remember happening really did happen or whether they just dreamed them. Circle a number to show what percentage of the time this happens to you.

0%   10   20   30   40   50   60   70   80   90   100%

16. Some people have the experience of being in a familiar place but finding it strange and unfamiliar. Circle a number to show what percentage of the time this happens to you.

0%   10   20   30   40   50   60   70   80   90   100%

17. Some people find that when they are watching television or a movie they become so absorbed in the story that they are unaware of other events happening around them. Circle a number to show what percentage of the time this happens to you.

0%   10   20   30   40   50   60   70   80   90   100%

18. Some people find that they become so involved in a fantasy or daydream that it feels as though it were really happening to them. Circle a number to show what percentage of the time this happens to you.

    0%   10   20   30   40   50   60   70   80   90   100%

19. Some people find that they sometimes are able to ignore pain. Circle a number to show what percentage of the time this happens to you.

    0%   10   20   30   40   50   60   70   80   90   100%

20. Some people find that they sometimes sit staring off into space, thinking of nothing, and are not aware of the passage of time. Circle a number to show what percentage of the time this happens to you.

    0%   10   20   30   40   50   60   70   80   90   100%

21. Some people sometimes find that when they are alone they talk out loud to themselves. Circle a number to show what percentage of the time this happens to you.

    0%   10   20   30   40   50   60   70   80   90   100%

22. Some people find that in one situation they may act so differently compared with another situation that they feel almost as if they were two different people. Circle a number to show what percentage of the time this happens to you.

    0%   10   20   30   40   50   60   70   80   90   100%

23. Some people sometimes find that in certain situations they are able to do things with amazing ease and spontaneity that would usually be difficult for them (for example, sports, work, social situations, etc.). Circle a number to show what percentage of the time this happens to you.

    0%   10   20   30   40   50   60   70   80   90   100%

24. Some people sometimes find that they cannot remember whether they have done something or have just thought about doing that thing (for example, not knowing whether they have just mailed a letter or have just thought about mailing it). Circle a number to show what percentage of the time this happens to you.

    0%   10   20   30   40   50   60   70   80   90   100%

25. Some people find evidence that they have done things that they do not remember doing. Circle a number to show what percentage of the time this happens to you.

    0%   10   20   30   40   50   60   70   80   90   100%

26. Some people sometimes find writings, drawings, or notes among their belongings that they must have done but cannot remember doing. Circle a number to show what percentage of the time this happens to you.

    0%   10   20   30   40   50   60   70   80   90   100%

27. Some people sometimes find that they hear voices inside their head that tell them to do things or comment on things that they are doing. Circle a number to show what percentage of the time this happens to you.

    0%   10   20   30   40   50   60   70   80   90   100%

28. Some people sometimes feel as if they are looking at the world through a fog, so that people and objects appear far away or unclear. Circle a number to show what percentage of the time this happens to you.

    0%   10   20   30   40   50   60   70   80   90   100%

Child Dissociative Checklist (CDC), Version 3.0

Frank W. Putnam, MD
Unit on Developmental Traumatology, NIMH

Date: _____ Age: _____ Sex: M F Identification: _____

Below is a list of behaviors that describe children. For each item that describes your child NOW or WITHIN THE PAST 12 MONTHS, please circle 2 if the item is VERY TRUE of your child. Circle 1 if the item is SOMEWHAT or SOMETIMES TRUE of your child. If the item is NOT TRUE of your child, circle 0.

0 1 2   1. Child does not remember or denies traumatic or painful experiences that are known to have occurred.

0 1 2   2. Child goes into a daze or trance-like state at times or often appears "spaced out." Teachers may report that he or she "daydreams" frequently in school.

0 1 2   3. Child shows rapid changes in personality. He or she may go from being shy to being outgoing, from feminine to masculine, from timid to aggressive.

0 1 2   4. Child is unusually forgetful or confused about things that he or she should know, e.g. may forget the names of friends, teachers or other important people, loses possessions or gets lost easily.

0 1 2   5. Child has a very poor sense of time. He or she loses track of time, may think that it is morning when it is actually afternoon, gets confused about what day it is, or becomes confused about when something happened.

0 1 2   6. Child shows marked day-to-day or even hour-to-hour variations in his or her skills, knowledge, food preferences, athletic abilities, e.g. changes in handwriting, memory for previously learned information such as multiplication tables, spelling, use of tools or artistic ability.

0 1 2   7. Child shows rapid regressions in age-level of behavior, e.g. a twelve-year-old starts to use baby-talk, sucks thumb or draws like a four-year-old.

0 1 2   8. Child has a difficult time learning from experience, e.g. explanations, normal discipline or punishment do not change his or her behavior.

0 1 2   9. Child continues to lie or deny misbehavior even when the evidence is obvious.

0 1 2   10. Child refers to him or herself in the third person (e.g. as she or her) when talking about self, or at times **insists** on being called by a different name. He or she may also claim that things that he or she did actually happened to another person.

0 1 2   11. Child has rapidly changing physical complaints such as headache or upset stomach. For example, he or she may complain of a headache one minute and seem to forget all about it the next.

0 1 2   12. Child is unusually sexually precocious and may attempt age-inappropriate sexual behavior with other children or adults.

0 1 2   13. Child suffers from unexplained injuries or may even deliberately injure self at times.

0 1 2   14. Child reports hearing voices that talk to him or her. The voices may be friendly or angry and may come from "imaginary companions" or sound like the voices of parents, friends or teachers.

0 1 2   15. Child has a vivid imaginary companion or companions. Child may insist that the imaginary companion(s) is responsible for things that he or she has done.

0   1   2   16. Child has intense outbursts of anger, often without apparent cause and may display unusual physical strength during these episodes.

0   1   2   17. Child sleepwalks frequently.

0   1   2   18. Child has unusual nighttime experiences, e.g. may report seeing "ghosts" or that things happen at night that he or she can't acount for (e.g. broken toys, unexplained injuries).

0   1   2   19. Child frequently talks to him or herself, may use a different voice or argue with self at times.

0   1   2   20. Child has two or more distinct and separate personalities that take control over the child's behavior.

Adolescent Dissociative Experiences Scale (A-DES), Version 1.0

Judith Armstrong, PhD
Frank W. Putnam, MD
Eve Bernstein Carlson, PhD

DIRECTIONS

These questions ask about different kinds of experiences that happen to people. For each question, circle the number that tells how much that experience happens to you. Circle a "0" if it never happens to you, circle a "10" if it is always happening to you. If it happens sometimes but not all of the time, circle a number between 1 and 9 that best describes how often it happens to you. When you answer, only tell how much these things happen when you HAVE NOT had any alcohol or drugs.

Example:

0	①	2	3	4	5	6	7	8	9	10
(never)										(always)

1. I get so wrapped up in watching TV, reading, or playing video games that I don't have any idea what's going on around me.

   0   1   2   3   4   5   6   7   8   9   10
   (never)   (always)

2. I get back tests or homework that I don't remember doing.

   0   1   2   3   4   5   6   7   8   9   10
   (never)   (always)

3. I have strong feelings that don't seem like they are mine.

   0   1   2   3   4   5   6   7   8   9   10
   (never)   (always)

4. I can do something really well one time and then I can't do it at all another time.

   0   1   2   3   4   5   6   7   8   9   10
   (never)   (always)

5. People tell me I do or say things that I don't remember doing or saying.

   0   1   2   3   4   5   6   7   8   9   10
   (never)   (always)

6. I feel like I'm in a fog or spaced out and things around me seem unreal.

   0   1   2   3   4   5   6   7   8   9   10
   (never)   (always)

7. I get confused about whether I have done something or only thought about doing it.

   0   1   2   3   4   5   6   7   8   9   10
   (never)   (always)

8. I look at the clock and realize that time has gone by and I can't remember what has happened.

   0   1   2   3   4   5   6   7   8   9   10
   (never)   (always)

9. I hear voices in my head that are not mine.

   0   1   2   3   4   5   6   7   8   9   10
   (never)   (always)

10. When I am somewhere that I don't want to be, I can go away in my mind.

    0   1   2   3   4   5   6   7   8   9   10
    (never)   (always)

11. I am so good at lying and acting that I believe it myself.

    0   1   2   3   4   5   6   7   8   9   10
    (never)   (always)

12. I catch myself "waking up" in the middle of doing something.

    0   1   2   3   4   5   6   7   8   9   10
    (never)   (always)

13. I don't recognize myself in the mirror.

    0   1   2   3   4   5   6   7   8   9   10
    (never)   (always)

14. I find myself going somewhere or doing something and I don't know why.

    0   1   2   3   4   5   6   7   8   9   10
    (never)   (always)

15. I find myself someplace and don't remember how I got there.

    0   1   2   3   4   5   6   7   8   9   10
    (never)   (always)

16. I have thoughts that don't really seem to belong to me.

    0   1   2   3   4   5   6   7   8   9   10
    (never)   (always)

17. I find that I can make physical pain go away.

    0   1   2   3   4   5   6   7   8   9   10
    (never)   (always)

18. I can't figure out if things really happened or if I only dreamed or thought about them.

    0   1   2   3   4   5   6   7   8   9   10
    (never)   (always)

19. I find myself doing something that I know is wrong, even when I really don't want to do it.

    0   1   2   3   4   5   6   7   8   9   10
    (never)   (always)

20. People tell me that I sometimes act so differently that I seem like a different person.

    0   1   2   3   4   5   6   7   8   9   10
    (never)   (always)

21. It feels like there are walls inside of my mind.

    0   1   2   3   4   5   6   7   8   9   10
    (never)   (always)

22. I find writings, drawings or letters that I must have done but I can't remember doing.

    0   1   2   3   4   5   6   7   8   9   10
    (never)   (always)

23. Something inside of me seems to make me do things that I don't want to do.

    0   1   2   3   4   5   6   7   8   9   10
    (never)   (always)

24. I find that I can't tell whether I am just remembering something or if it is actually happening to me.

    0   1   2   3   4   5   6   7   8   9   10
    (never)   (always)

25. I find myself standing outside of my body, watching myself as if I were another person.

    0   1   2   3   4   5   6   7   8   9   10
    (never)   (always)

26. My relationships with my family and friends change suddenly and I don't know why.

    0   1   2   3   4   5   6   7   8   9   10
    (never)   (always)

27. I feel like my past is a puzzle and some of the pieces are missing.

    0   1   2   3   4   5   6   7   8   9   10
    (never)   (always)

28. I get so wrapped up in my toys or stuffed animals that they seem alive.

    0   1   2   3   4   5   6   7   8   9   10
    (never)   (always)

29. I feel like there are different people inside of me.

    0   1   2   3   4   5   6   7   8   9   10
    (never)   (always)

30. My body feels as if it doesn't belong to me.

    0   1   2   3   4   5   6   7   8   9   10
    (never)   (always)

References

Abeles, M., and P. Schilder (1935). Psychogenic loss of personal identity. *Archives of Neurology and Psychiatry* **34**: 587–604.

Aber, J. L., J. P. Allen, V. Carlson, and D. Cicchetti (1989). The effects of maltreatment on development during early childhood: Recent studies and their theoretical, clinical, and policy implications. In D. Cicchetti and V. Carlson (Eds.), *Child maltreatment: Theory and research on the causes and consequences of child abuse and neglect*. Cambridge, UK, Cambridge University Press. 579–619.

Ablon, S. (1996). The therapeutic action of play. *Journal of the American Academy of Child and Adolescent Psychiatry* **35**: 545–547.

Achenbach, T. M. (1991a). *Manual for the CBCL/4–18 and 1991 Profile*. Burlington, University of Vermont, Department of Psychiatry.

Achenbach, T. M. (1991b). *Manual for the TRF and 1991 Profile*. Burlington, University of Vermont, Department of Psychiatry.

Aggleton, J. P., Ed. (1992). *The amygdala: Neurobiological aspects of emotion, memory and mental dysfunction*. New York, Wiley–Liss.

Ahern, G. L., A. M. Herring, J. Tackenberg, J. F. Seeger, K. J. Oommen, D. M. Labiner, and M. E. Weinand (1993). The association of multiple personality and temporolimbic epilepsy: Intracarotid amobarbital test observations. *Archives of Neurology* **50**(10): 1020–1025.

Aldrich, M. S. (1992). Narcolepsy. *Neurology* **42**(Suppl. 6): 34–43.

Alessandri, S. M. (1991). Play and social behavior in maltreated preschoolers. *Development and Psychopathology* **3**: 191–205.

Alexander, P. C., and C. M. Schaeffer (1994). A typology of incestuous families based on cluster analysis. *Journal of Family Process* **8**: 458–470.

Allen, D. S., and K. J. Tarnowski (1989). Depressive characteristics of physically abused children. *Journal of Abnormal Child Psychology* **17**: 1–11.

Allen, S. N., and S. L. Bloom (1994). Group and family treatment of post-traumatic stress disorder. *Psychiatric Clinics of North America* **17**: 425–437.

Aman, M. G. (1993). Monitoring and measuring drug effects: II. Behavioral, emotional and cognitive effects. In J. S. Werry and M. G. Aman (Eds.),

Practitioner's guide to psychoactive drugs for children and adolescents. New York, Plenum Press. 99–161.

Amaya-Jackson, L., and J. S. March (1993). Post-traumatic stress disorder in children and adolescents. *Child and Adolescents Psychiatric Clinics of North America* 2: 639–654.

American Academy of Child and Adolescent Psychiatry (1995). Practice parameters for the psychiatric assessment of children and adolescents. *Journal of the American Academy of Child and Adolescent Psychiatry* 34: 1386–1402.

American Medical Association (1993). American Medical Association diagnostic and treatment guidelines on child sexual abuse. *Archives of Family Medicine* 2: 19–27.

American Psychiatric Association (1952). *Diagnostic and statistical manual of mental disorders.* Washington, DC, American Psychiatric Association.

American Psychiatric Association (1968). *Diagnostic and statistical manual of mental disorders, second edition.* Washington, DC, American Psychiatric Association.

American Psychiatric Association (1980). *Diagnostic and statistical manual of mental disorders, third edition.* Washington, DC, American Psychiatric Association.

American Psychiatric Association (1987). *Diagnostic and statistical manual of mental disorders, third edition, revised.* Washington, DC, American Psychiatric Association.

American Psychiatric Association (1993). Practice guidelines for eating disorders. *American Journal of Psychiatry* 150: 212–228.

American Psychiatric Association (1994). *Diagnostic and statistical manual of mental disorders, fourth edition.* Washington, DC, American Psychiatric Association.

Anderson, G. L. (1992). Dissociation, distress and family function. *Dissociation* 5: 210–215.

Anderson, G., L. Yasenik, and C. A. Ross (1993). Dissociative experiences and disorders among women who identify themselves as sexual abuse survivors. *Child Abuse and Neglect* 17(5): 677–686.

Andorfer, J. C. (1985). Multiple personality in the human information-processor: A case history and theoretical formulation. *Journal of Clinical Psychology* 41(3): 309–324.

Andreasen, N. C. (1995). The validity of psychiatric diagnosis: New models and approaches [Editorial]. *American Journal of Psychiatry* 152: 161–162.

Andrews, B. (1995). Bodily shame as a mediator between abusive experiences and depression. *Journal of Abnormal Psychology* 104: 277–285.

Andrews, B. (1997). Can a survey of British False Memory Society members reliably inform the recovered memory debate? *Applied Cognitive Psychology* 11: 19–23.

Andrews, B., J. Morton, D. A. Bekerian, C. R. Brewin, G. M. Davies, and P. Mollon (1995). The recovery of memories in clinical practice: Experiences and beliefs of British Psychological Society practitioners. *The Psychologist* 8: 209–214.

Armstrong, J. (1991). The psychological organization of multiple personality disordered patients as revealed in psychological testing. *Psychiatric Clinics of North America* 14(3): 533–546.

Armstrong, J. (1996). Psychological assessment. *Treating dissociative identity disorder*. San Francisco, Jossey-Bass. 3–38.

Armstrong, J., M. Laurenti, and R. Loewenstein (1990). *Dissociative Behaviors Checklist—II*. Baltimore, Sheppard Pratt Hospital.

Armstrong, J., and R. Loewenstein (1990). Characteristics of patients with multiple personality and dissociative disorders on psychological testing. *Journal of Nervous and Mental Disease* 178: 448–454.

Armstrong, J., F. W. Putnam, and E. B. Carlson (in press). Development and validation of a measure of adolescent dissociation: The Adolescent Dissociative Experiences Scale (A-DES). *Journal of Nervous and Mental Disease*.

Armsworth, M. W., and M. Holaday (1993). The effects of psychological trauma on children and adolescents. *Journal of Counseling and Development* 72: 49–56.

Arnold, L. E., and M. G. Aman (1991). Beta blockers in mental retardation and developmental disorders. *Journal of Child and Adolescent Psychopharmacology* 1: 361–373.

Arnow, B., J. Kenardy, and W. S. Agras (1995). The Emotional Eating Scale: The development of a measure to assess coping with negative affect by eating. *International Journal of Eating Disorders* 18(1): 79–90.

Arroyo, W., and S. Eth (1985). Children traumatized by Central American warfare. *Post-traumatic stress disorder in children*. Washington, DC, American Psychiatric Press. 101–120.

Attie, I., and J. Brooks-Gunn (1995). The development of eating regulation across the life span. In D. Cicchetti and D. Cohen (Eds.), *Developmental psychopathology: Vol. 2. Risk, disorder and adaptation*. New York, Wiley–Interscience. 332–368.

Bagley, C., and R. Ramsay (1986). Sexual abuse in childhood: Psychosocial outcomes and implications for social work practice. *Journal of Social Work and Human Sexuality* 4: 33–47.

Balthazard, C., and E. Woody (1989). Bimodality, dimensionality, and the notion of hypnotic types. *International Journal of Clinical and Experimental Hypnosis* 37: 70–89.

Barach, P. M. (1991). Multiple personality disorder as an attachment disorder. *Dissociation* 4: 117–123.

Barnett, D., J. T. Manly, and D. Cicchetti (1991). Continuing toward an operational definition of psychological maltreatment. *Development and Psychopathology* 3: 19–29.

Barton, S. (1994). Chaos, self-organization, and psychology. *American Psychologist* 49: 5–14.

Beal, E. W. (1978). Use of the extended family in the treatment of multiple personality. *American Journal of Psychiatry* 135: 539–542.

Beitchman, J. E., K. J. Zucker, J. E. Hood, G. A. DaCosta, D. Akman, and E. Cassavia (1992). A review of the long-term effects of child sexual abuse. *Child Abuse and Neglect* 16: 101–118.

Bell, C. C., and E. J. Jenkins (1993). Community violence and children on Chicago's south side. *Psychiatry* 56: 46–54.

Belter, R. W., and M. P. Shannon (1993). Impact of natural disasters on children and families. *Children and disaster*. New York, Plenum Press. 85–103.

Benedek, E. P. (1985). Children and psychic trauma: A brief review of contemporary thinking. In S. Eth and R. S. Pynoos (Eds.), *Post-traumatic stress disorder in children*. Washington, DC, American Psychiatric Press. 1–16.

Benjamin, L. R., and R. Benjamin (1992). An overview of family treatment in dissociative disorders. *Dissociation* 5: 236–241.

Benjamin, L. R., and R. Benjamin (1994a). Application of contextual therapy to the treatment of MPD. *Dissociation* 7: 12–22.

Benjamin, L. R., and R. Benjamin (1994b). A group for partners and parents of MPD clients: Part I. Process and format. *Dissociation* 7: 35–43.

Benjamin, L. R., and R. Benjamin (1994c). A group for partners and parents of MPD clients: Part II. Themes and responses. *Dissociation* 7: 104–111.

Benjamin, L. R., and R. Benjamin (1994d). A group for partners and parents of MPD clients: Part III. Marital types and dynamics. *Dissociation* 7: 191–196.

Benjamin, L. R., and R. Benjamin (1994e). Issues in the treatment of dissociative couples. *Dissociation* 7: 229–238.

Benjamin, L. R., and R. Benjamin (1994f). Utilizing parenting as a clinical focus in the treatment of dissociative disorders. *Dissociation* 7: 239–245.

Benjamin, L. R., and R. Benjamin (1994g). Various perspectives on parenting and their implications for the treatment of dissociative disorders. *Dissociation* 7: 246–260.

Benner, D. G., and B. Joscelyne (1984). Multiple personality as a borderline disorder. *Journal of Nervous and Mental Disease* 172(2): 98–104.

Benson, D. F. (1986). Interictal behavior disorders in epilepsy. *Psychiatric Clinics of North America* 9(2): 283–292.

Benward, J., and J. Densen-Gerber (1975). Incest as a causative factor in antisocial behavior: An exploratory study. *Contemporary Drug Problems* 4: 32–35.

Berenbaum, H., and T. James (1994). Correlates and retrospectively reported antecedents of alexithymia. *Psychosomatic Medicine* 56: 353–359.

Berg, C. J., J. L. Rapoport, and M. Flament (1986). The Leyton Obsessional Inventory—Child Version. *Journal of the American Academy of Child and Adolescent Psychiatry* 25: 84–91.

Berger, D., Y. Onon, K. Nakajima, and H. Suematsu (1994). Dissociative symptoms in Japan. *American Journal of Psychiatry* 151: 148–149.

Berman, R. J. (1978). Psychogenic visual disorders in an abused child: A case report. *American Journal of Optometry and Physiological Optics* 5: 735–738.

Bernstein, E., and F. W. Putnam (1986). Development, reliability and validity of a dissociation scale. *Journal of Nervous and Mental Disease* 174: 727–735.

Bidell, T. R., and K. W. Fischer (1992). Beyond the stage debate: Action, structure, and variability in Piagetian theory and research. In R. Steinberg and

C. Berg (Eds.), *Intellectual development*. New York, Cambridge University Press. 100–140.

Bisson, J. I. (1993). Automatism and post-traumatic stress disorder. *British Journal of Psychiatry* **163**: 830–2.

Black, M., H. Dubowitz, and D. Harrington (1994). Sexual abuse: Developmental differences in children's behavior and self-perception. *Child Abuse and Neglect* **18**: 85–95.

Bliss, E. L. (1983). Multiple personalities, related disorders and hypnosis. *American Journal of Clinical Hypnosis* **226**: 114–123.

Blumberg, M. J. (1981). Depression in abused and neglected children. *American Journal of Psychotherapy* **35**: 342–355.

Boon, S., and N. Draijer (1993). *Multiple personality disorder in the Netherlands*. Amsterdam, Swets & Zeitlinger.

Boor, M. (1982). The multiple personality epidemic. *Journal of Nervous and Mental Disease* **170**(5): 302–304.

Boudewyn, A. C., and J. H. Liem (1995). Childhood sexual abuse as a precursor to depression and self-destructive behavior in adulthood. *Journal of Traumatic Stress* **8**: 445–459.

Boustany, N., and D. Priest (1992, February 23). Pain has not gone away. *The Washington Post* 1A, 18A.

Bower, G. (1994). Temporary emotional states act like multiple personalities. *Psychological concepts and dissociative disorders*. Hillsdale, NJ, Erlbaum. 207–234.

Bowlby, J. (1958). The nature of the child's tie to his mother. *International Journal of Psycho-Analysis* **39**: 350–373.

Bowlby, J. (1973). *Attachment and loss: Vol. 2. Separation: Anxiety and anger*. New York, Basic Books.

Bowlby, J. (1982). *Attachment and loss: Vol. 1. Attachment, second edition*. New York, Basic Books.

Bowman, E. S. (1990). Adolescent multiple personality disorder in the nineteenth and early twentieth centuries. *Dissociation* **3**: 179–187.

Bowman, E. S. (1993). Etiology and clinical course of pseudoseizures: Relationship to trauma, depression, and dissociation. *Psychosomatics* **34**(4): 333–342.

Bowman, E. S., S. Blix, and P. M. Coons (1985). Multiple personality in adolescence: Relationship to incestual experiences. *Journal of the American Academy of Child Psychiatry* **24**(1): 109–114.

Brain, P. F., S. Parmigiani, R. J. Blanchard, and D. Mainardi (Eds.). (1990). *Fear and defense*. London, Harwood Academic.

Brainerd, C., and P. A. Ornstein (1991). Children's memory for witnessed events: The developmental backdrop. In J. Doris (Ed.), *The suggestibility of children's recollections*. Washington, DC, American Psychological Association. 10–20.

Branscomb, L. (1991). Dissociation in combat-related post-traumatic stress disorder. *Dissociation* **4**(1): 13–20.

Braun, B. G. (1985). The transgenerational incidence of dissociation and multiple personality disorder: A preliminary report. *Childhood antecedents of multiple personality*. Washington, DC, American Psychiatric Press. 127–150.

Braun, B. G., and R. G. Sachs (1985). The development of multiple personality disorder: Predisposing, precipitating and perpetuating factors. *Childhood antecedents of multiple personality*. Washington, DC, American Psychiatric Press. 37–64.

Braun, P., D. Greenberg, H. Dasberg, and B. Lerer (1990). Core symptoms of posttraumatic stress disorder unimproved by alprazolam treatment. *Journal of Clinical Psychiatry* 51: 236–238.

Bremner, J. D., J. H. Krystal, S. M. Southwick, and D. S. Charney (1995a). Functional neuroanatomical correlates of the effects of stress on memory. *Journal of Traumatic Stress* 8: 527–553.

Bremner, J. D., P. Randall, T. M. Scott, R. A. Bronen, J. P. Seibyl, S. M. Southwick, R. C. Delaney, M. G., D. S. Charney, and R. B. Innis (1995b). MRI-based measurement of hippocampal volume in combat-related posttraumatic stress disorder. *American Journal of Psychiatry* 152: 973–981.

Bremner, J. D., P. Randall, E. Vermetten, L. Staid, R. A. Bronen, C. Mazure, S. Capelli, G. McCarthy, R. B. Innis, and D. S. Charney (1997). Magnetic resonance imaging-based measurement of hippocampal volume in posttraumatic stress disorder related to childhood physical and sexual abuse: A preliminary report. *Biological Psychiatry* 41: 23–32.

Bremner, J. D., T. M. Scott, R. C. Delaney, S. M. Southwick, J. W. Mason, D. Johnson, R. B. Innis, M. G., and D. S. Charney (1993a). Deficits in short-term memory in post-traumatic stress disorder. *American Journal of Psychiatry* 149: 328–332.

Bremner, J. D., S. M. Southwick, E. Brett, A. Fontana, R. Rosenheck, and D. S. Charney (1992). Dissociation and posttraumatic stress disorder in Vietnam combat veterans. *American Journal of Psychiatry* 149(3): 328–332.

Bremner, D. J., S. M. Southwick, D. R. Johnson, R. Yehuda, and D. S. Charney (1993b). Childhood physical abuse and combat-related posttraumatic stress disorder in Vietnam veterans. *American Journal of Psychiatry* 150: 235–239.

Brende, J. O. (1984). The psychophysiologic manifestations of dissociation: Electrodermal responses in a multiple personality patient. *Psychiatric Clinics of North America* 7(1): 41–50.

Breslau, N., G. C. Davis, P. Andreski, and E. Peterson (1991). Traumatic events and posttraumatic stress disorder in an urban population of young adults. *Archives of General Psychiatry* 48: 216–222.

Bretherton, I. (1989). Pretense: The form and function of make-believe play. *Developmental Review* 9: 383–401.

Brett, E. (1996). The classification of posttraumatic stress disorder. In B. A. van der Kolk, A. C. McFarlane, and L. Weisaeth (Eds.), *Traumatic stress: The effects of overwhelming experience on mind, body, and society*. New York, Guilford Press. 117–128.

Brewerton, T. D., E. J. Stellefson, N. Hibbs, E. L. Hodges, and C. E. Cochrane (1995). Comparison of eating disorder patients with and without compulsive exercising. *International Journal of Eating Disorders* 17(4): 413–416.

Briere, J., and J. Conte (1993). Self-reported amnesia for abuse in adults molested as children. *Journal of Traumatic Stress* **6**: 21–31.

Briere, J., and M. Runtz (1986). Suicidal thoughts and behaviours in former sexual abuse victims. *Canadian Journal of Behavioural Science* **18**: 413–423.

Briere, J., K. Smiljanich, and D. Henschel (1994). Sexual fantasies, gender, and molestation history. *Child Abuse and Neglect* **18**: 131–137.

Bronfenbrenner Life Course Center (1996). Who are the victims? *Bronfenbrenner Life Course Center Issue Brief* **1**: 1–4.

Brown, G. R., and B. Anderson (1991). Psychiatric morbidity in adult inpatients with histories of sexual and physical abuse. *American Journal of Psychiatry* **148**: 55–61.

Brown, G. W. (1983). Multiple personality disorder, perpetrator of child abuse. *Child Abuse and Neglect* **7**(1): 123–126.

Brown, R., and J. Kulik (1977). Flashbulb memories. *Cognition* **5**: 73–99.

Browne, A., and D. Finkelhor (1986). Impact of child sexual abuse: A review of the research. *Psychological Bulletin* **99**: 66–77.

Bruce, J. W., and J. Coid (1992). Identity diffusion presenting as multiple personality disorder in a female psychopath. *British Journal of Psychiatry* **160**: 541–544.

Bryant, R. A. (1995). Autobiographical memory across personalities in dissociative identity disorder: A case report. *Journal of Abnormal Psychology* **104**: 625–631.

Bryer, J. B., B. A. Nelson, J. B. Miller, and P. Krol (1987). Childhood sexual and physical abuse as factors in adult psychiatric illness. *American Journal of Psychiatry* **144**: 1426–1430.

Buck, O. D. (1983). Multiple personality as a borderline state. *Journal of Nervous and Mental Disease* **171**(1): 62–65.

Bunney, W., T. Wehr, J. Gillin, R. Post, F. Goodwin, and D. van Kammen (1977). The switch process in manic–depressive psychosis. *Annals of Internal Medicine* **87**: 319–355.

Burnam, M. A., J. A. Stein, J. M. Golding, J. M. Siegel, S. B. Sorenson, A. B. Forsythe, and C. A. Telles (1988). Sexual assault and mental disorders in a community population. *Journal of Consulting and Clinical Psychology* **56**: 843–850.

Burton, L. (1968). *Vulnerable children*. London, Routledge and Kegan Paul.

Bye, A. M., and S. Foo (1994). Complex partial seizures in young children. *Epilepsia* **35**(3): 482–488.

Byram, V., H. Wagner, and G. Waller (1995). Sexual abuse and body image distortion. *Child Abuse and Neglect* **19**: 507–510.

Caffey, J. (1972). On the theory and practice of shaking infants: Its potential residual effects of permanent brain damage and mental retardation. *American Journal of Diseases of Children* **124**: 161–169.

Calverley, R., K. Fischer, and C. Ayoub (1994). Complex splitting of self-representations in sexually abused adolescent girls. *Development and Psychopathology* **6**: 195–213.

Campbell, M., P. B. Adams, A. M. Small, V. Kafantaris, R. R. Silva, J. Shell, R. Perry, and J. E. Overall (1995). Lithium in hospitalized aggressive children with conduct disorder: A double-blind and placebo-controlled study. *Journal of the American Academy of Child and Adolescent Psychiatry* **34**: 445–453.

Campbell, M., and J. Cueva (1995a). Psychopharmacology in child and adolescent psychiatry: A review of the past seven years. Part I. *Journal of the American Academy of Child and Adolescent Psychiatry* **34**: 1124–1132.

Campbell, M., and J. Cueva (1995b). Psychopharmacology in child and adolescent psychiatry: A review of the past seven years. Part II. *Journal of the American Academy of Child and Adolescent Psychiatry* **34**: 1262–1272.

Campbell, M., N. M. Gonzalez, and R. R. Silva (1992). The pharmacologic treatment of conduct disorder and rage outbursts. *Psychiatric Clinics of North America* **15**: 69–85.

Campbell, M., A. M. Small, and W. H. Green (1984). Behavioral efficacy of haloperidol and lithium carbonate: A comparison in hospitalized aggressive children with conduct disorder. *Archives of General Psychiatry* **41**: 650–656.

Cantwell, D. P., J. Swanson, and D. F. Connor (1997). Case study: Adverse response to clonidine. *Journal of the American Academy of Child and Adolescent Psychiatry* **36**: 539–544.

Cardeña, E., and D. Spiegel (1993). Dissociative reactions to the San Francisco Bay Area earthquake of 1989. *American Journal of Psychiatry* **150**(3): 474–478.

Carlson, E. B., and J. Armstrong (1994). The diagnosis and assessment of dissociative disorders. *Dissociation: Clinical and research perspectives.* New York, Guilford Press. 159–174.

Carlson, E. B., and F. W. Putnam (1993). An update on the Dissociative Experiences Scale. *Dissociation* **6**: 16–27.

Carlson, E. B., F. W. Putnam, C. A. Ross, M. Torem, P. M. Coons, D. L. Dill, R. J. Loewenstein, and B. G. Braun (1993). Validity of the Dissociative Experiences Scale in screening for multiple personality disorder: A multicenter study. *American Journal of Psychiatry* **150**: 1030–1036.

Carlson, E. B., and R. Rosser-Hogan (1991). Trauma experiences, posttraumatic stress, dissociation, and depression in Cambodian refugees. *American Journal of Psychiatry* **148**: 1548–1551.

Carlson, E. T. (1981). The history of multiple personality disorder in the United States: I. The beginnings. *American Journal of Psychiatry* **138**: 666–668.

Carrey, N. J., and L. Adams (1992). How to deal with sexual acting-out on the child psychiatric inpatient ward. *Journal of Psychosocial Nursing* **30**: 19–23.

Carrey, N. J., H. J. Butter, M. A. Persinger, and R. J. Bialik (1995). Physiological and cognitive correlates of child abuse. *Journal of the American Academy of Child and Adolescent Psychiatry* **34**: 1067–1075.

Castillo, R. (1990). Depersonalization and meditation. *Psychiatry* **53**: 158–168.

Caul, D., and C. A. Wilbur (1978, May). *General Amnesia Profile (G.A.P.).* Paper presented at the annual meeting of the American Psychiatric Association, Atlanta.

Ceci, S. J., D. F. Ross, and M. P. Toglia (1991). *Perspectives on children's testimony.* New York, Springer-Verlag.

Cerezo, M., and D. Frias (1994). Emotional and cognitive adjustment in abused children. *Child Abuse and Neglect* 18: 923–932.

Cervantes, R. (1994). DSM-IV: Implications for Hispanic children and adolescents. *Hispanic Journal of Behavioral Sciences* 16: 8–27.

Charney, D. S., A. Y. Deutch, J. H. Krystal, S. M. Southwick, and M. Davis (1993). Psychobiological mechanisms of posttraumatic stress disorder. *Archives of General Psychiatry* 50: 294–305.

Chess, S. (1989). Defying the voice of doom. *The child in our times.* New York, Brunner/Mazel. 179–199.

Chiappa, F. (1994). Effective management of family and individual interventions in the treatment of dissociative disorders. *Dissociation* 7: 185–190.

Choe, B., and R. Kluft (1995). The use of the DES in studying treatment outcome with dissociative identity disorder: A pilot study. *Dissociation* 8: 160–174.

Chu, J. A. (1990). Some aspects of resistance in the treatment of multiple personality disorder. *Dissociation* 1: 34–38.

Chu, J. A., and D. L. Dill (1990). Dissociative symptoms in relation to childhood physical and sexual abuse. *American Journal of Psychiatry* 147: 887–892.

Cicchetti, D. (1989). How research on child maltreatment has informed the study of child development: Perspectives from developmental psychopathology. In D. Cicchetti and V. Carlson (Eds.), *Child maltreatment: Theory and research on the causes and consequences of child abuse and neglect.* Cambridge, UK, Cambridge University Press. 377–431.

Cicchetti, D. (1993). Developmental psychopathology: Reactions, reflections, projections. *Developmental Review* 13: 471–502.

Cicchetti, D., and M. Beeghly (1987). Symbolic development in maltreated youngsters: An organizational perspective. In D. Cicchetti and M. Beeghly (Eds.), *Atypical symbolic development.* San Francisco, Jossey-Bass. 31–55.

Cicchetti, D., and V. Carlson, Eds. (1989). *Child maltreatment: Theory and research on the causes and consequences of child abuse and neglect.* Cambridge, UK, Cambridge University Press.

Cicchetti, D., and D. J. Cohen, Eds. (1995a). *Developmental psychopathology.* 2 vols. New York, Wiley–Interscience.

Cicchetti, D., and D. J. Cohen (1995b). Perspectives on developmental psychopathology. In D. Cicchetti and D. Cohen (Eds.), *Developmental psychopathology: Vol. 1.* New York, Wiley–Interscience. 3–20.

Cicchetti, D., and M. Lynch (1995). Failures in the expectable environment and their impact on individual development: The case of child maltreatment. In D. Cicchetti and D. Cohn (Eds.), *Developmental psychopathology: Vol. 2.* New York, Wiley–Interscience. 32–71.

Cicchetti, D., and B. Nurcombe (1994). Advances and challenges in the study of sequelae of child maltreatment. In D. Cicchetti (Ed.), *Development and psychopathology: Vol. 6.* New York, Cambridge University Press. 1–3.

Clary, W. F., K. J. Burstin, and J. S. Carpenter (1984). Multiple personality and borderline personality disorder. *Psychiatric Clinics of North America* 7(1): 89–99.

Cloitre, M., K. Tardiff, P. Marzuk, A. Leon, and L. Portera (1996). Childhood abuse and subsequent sexual assault among female inpatients. *Journal of Traumatic Stress* 9: 473–482.

Cochrane, C. E., T. D. Brewerton, D. B. Wilson, and E. L. Hodges (1993). Alexithymia in the eating disorders. *International Journal of Eating Disorders* 14(2): 219–222.

Cocker, K. I., G. A. Edwards, J. W. Anderson, and R. A. Meares (1994). Electrophysiological changes under hypnosis in multiple personality disorder: A two-case exploratory study. *Australian Journal of Clinical and Experimental Hypnosis* 22: 165–176.

Coffey, B. (1993). Review and update: Benzodiazepines in childhood and adolescence. *Psychiatric Annals* 23: 332–339.

Cohen, B., E. Giller, and L. W., Eds. (1991). *Multiple personality disorder from the inside out.* Lutherville, MD, Sidran Press.

Cohen, B. A., P. Honig, and E. Androphy (1990). Anogenital warts in children: Clinical and virologic evaluation for sexual abuse. *Archives of Dermatology* 126: 1575–1580.

Cohen, J., and A. Mannarino (1996). A treatment outcome study for sexually abused preschool children: Initial findings. *Journal of the American Academy of Child and Adolescent Psychiatry* 35: 42–50.

Cohn, E. (1979). An evaluation of three demonstration child abuse and neglect treatment programs. *Journal of Child Psychiatry* 18: 283–291.

Cole, P. M., K. C. Barrett, and C. Zahn-Waxler (1992). Emotion display in two-year-olds during mishaps. *Child Development* 63: 314–324.

Cole, P. M., and F. W. Putnam (1992). The effect of incest on self and social functioning: A developmental psychopathological perspective. *Journal of Consulting and Clinical Psychology* 60: 174–184.

Condon, W. S., W. D. Ogston, and L. V. Pacoe (1969). Three faces of Eve revisited: A study of transient microstrabismus. *Journal of Abnormal Psychology,* 74: 618–620.

Congdon, M. H., J. Hain, and I. Stevenson (1961). A case of multiple personality illustrating the transition from role-playing. *Journal of Nervous and Mental Disease* 132: 497–504.

Conners, C. K. (1990). *Conners Rating Scales manual: Instruments for use with children and adolescents.* North Tonawanda, NY, Multi-Health Systems.

Conners, M. W., and W. Morse (1993). Sexual abuse and eating disorders: A review. *International Journal of Eating Disorders* 13: 1–11.

Coons, P. M. (1984). The differential diagnosis of multiple personality. *Psychiatric Clinics of North America* 7: 51–69.

Coons, P. M. (1985). Children of parents with multiple personality disorder. In R. P. Kluft (Ed.), *Childhood antecedents of multiple personality disorder.* Washington, DC, American Psychiatric Press. 152–165.

Coons, P. M. (1986). Treatment progress in 20 patients with multiple personality disorder. *Journal of Nervous and Mental Disease* 174(12): 715–721.

Coons, P. M. (1992). The use of carbamazepine for episodic violence in multiple personality disorder and dissociative disorder not otherwise specified: Two additional cases. *Biological Psychiatry* **32**: 717–720.

Coons, P. M. (1994a). Confirmation of childhood abuse in child and adolescent cases of multiple personality disorder and dissociative disorder not otherwise specified. *Journal of Nervous and Mental Disease* **182**(8): 461–464.

Coons, P. M. (1994b). Reports of satanic ritual abuse: Further implications about pseudomemories. *Perceptual and Motor Skills* **78**: 1376–1378.

Coons, P. M. (1996). Clinical phenomenology of 25 children and adolescents with dissociative disorders. *Child and Adolescent Psychiatric Clinics of North America* **5**: 361–374.

Coons, P. M., E. S. Bowman, R. Kluft, and V. Milstein (1991). The cross-cultural occurrence of MPD: Additional cases from a recent survey. *Dissociation* **4**: 124–128.

Coons, P. M., E. S. Bowman, and V. Milstein (1988). Multiple personality disorder: A clinical investigation of 50 cases. *Journal of Nervous and Mental Diease* **176**: 519–527.

Coons, P. M., and C. G. Fine (1990). Accuracy of the MMPI in identifying multiple personality disorder. *Psychological Reports* **66**: 831–834.

Coons, P. M., and V. Milstein (1992). Psychogenic amnesia: A clinical investigation of 25 cases. *Dissociation* **5**: 73–79.

Coons, P. M., V. Milstein, and C. Marley (1982). EEG studies of two multiple personalities and a control. *Archives of General Psychiatry* **39**: 823–825.

Cooper, L. M., and P. London (1971). The development of hypnotic susceptibility: A longitudinal (convergence) study. *Child Development* **42**: 487–503.

Cosentino, C. E., H. F. I. Meyer-Bahlburg, J. L. Alpert, and R. Gaines (1993). Cross-gender behavior and gender conflict in sexually abused girls. *Journal of the American Academy of Child and Adolescent Psychiatry* **32**: 940–947.

Cosentino, C. E., H. F. I. Meyer-Bahlburg, J. L. Alpert, S. L. Weinberg, and R. Gaines (1995). Sexual behavior problems and psychopathology symptoms in sexually abused girls. *Journal of the American Academy of Child and Adolescent Psychiatry* **34**: 1033–1042.

Courtouis, C. (1979). The incest experience and its aftermath. *Victimology* **4**: 337–347.

Cowdry, R. W., and D. L. Gardner (1988). Pharmacotherapy of borderline personality disorder: Alprazolam, carbamazepine, trifluoperazine and tranylcypromine. *Archives of General Psychiatry* **45**: 111–119.

Crabtree, A. (1988). *Animal magnetism, early hypnotism and psychical research, 1766–1925.* White Plains, NY, Kraus International.

Cueva, J., J. Overall, A. Small, J. Armenteros, R. Perry, and M. Campbell (1996). Carbamazepine in aggressive children with conduct disorder: A double-blind and placebo-controlled study. *Journal of the American Academy of Child and Adolescent Psychiatry* **35**: 480–490.

Cuffe, S., J. Waller, M. Cuccaro, A. Pumariega, and C. Garrison (1995). Race and gender differences in the treatment of psychiatric disorders in young adolescents. *Journal of the American Academy of Child and Adolescent Psychiatry* 34: 1536–1543.

Curran, T., and D. L. Hintzman (1995). Violations of the independence assumption in process dissociation. *Journal of Experimental Psychology: Learning, Memory, and Cognition* 21(3): 531–547.

Dahl, R. E., J. Holttum, and L. Trubnick (1994). A clinical picture of child and adolescent narcolepsy. *Journal of the American Academy of Child and Adolescent Psychiatry* 33: 834–841.

Darves-Bornoz, J., A. Degiovanni, and P. Gaillard (1995). Why is dissociative identity disorder infrequent in France? [Letter]. *American Journal of Psychiatry* 152: 1530–1531.

Davidson, J., H. Kudler, R. Smith, J. L. Mahoney, S. Lipper, E. Mannett, W. B. Saunders, and J. O. Cavenar (1990). Treatment of posttraumatic stress disorder with amitriptyline and placebo. *Archives of General Psychiatry* 47: 259–266.

Davidson, J., S. Roth, and E. Newman (1991). Fluoxetine in post-traumatic stress disorder. *Journal of Traumatic Stress* 4: 419–423.

Davis, P. H., and A. Osherson (1977). The concurrent treatment of a multiple-personality woman and her son. *American Journal of Psychotherapy* 31: 504–515.

De Bellis, M., L. Burke, P. Trickett, and F. W. Putnam (1996). Antinuclear antibodies and thyroid function in sexually abused girls. *Journal of Traumatic Stress* 9: 369–378.

De Bellis, M. D., G. P. Chrousos, L. D. Dorn, L. Burke, K. Helmers, M. A. Kling, P. K. Trickett, and F. W. Putnam (1994a). Hypothalamic–pituitary–adrenal axis dysregulation in sexually abused girls. *Journal of Clinical Endocrinology and Metabolism* 78: 249–255.

De Bellis, M. D., L. Lefter, P. K. Trickett, and F. W. Putnam (1994b). Urinary catecholamine excretion in sexually abused girls. *Journal of the American Academy of Child and Adolescent Psychiatry* 33: 320–327.

De Bellis, M. D., and F. W. Putnam (1994). The psychobiology of childhood maltreatment. *Child and Adolescent Psychiatric Clinics of North America* 3: 1–16.

Deblinger, E., S. McLeer, and D. Henry (1990). Cognitive behavioral treatment for sexually abused children suffering post-traumatic stress: Preliminary findings. *Journal of the American Academy of Child and Adolescent Psychiatry* 29: 747–752.

de Groot, J. M., G. Rodin, and M. P. Olmsted (1995). Alexithymia, depression, and treatment outcome in bulimia nervosa. *Comprehensive Psychiatry* 36(1): 53–60.

Delignieres, D., and J. Brisswalter (1994). Influence of an added perceptual motor task on perceived exertion: A test of the dissociation effect. *Perceptual and Motor Skills* 78(3, Pt. 1): 855–858.

Dell, P. F., and J. W. Eisenhower (1990). Adolescent multiple personality disorder. *Journal of the American Academy of Child and Adolescent Psychiatry* 29: 359–366.

Dembo, R., M. Dertke, L. La Voie, S. Borders, M. Washburn, and J. Schmeidler

(1987). Physical abuse, sexual victimization and illicit drug use: A structural analysis among high risk adolescents. *Journal of Adolescence* 10: 13–33.

Dembo, R., L. Williams, L. La Voie, J. Schmeidler, J. Kern, A. Getreu, E. Berry, L. Genung, and E. D. Wish (1990). A longitudinal study of the relationship among alcohol use, marijuana/hashish use, cocaine use, and emotional/psychological functioning problems in a cohort of high-risk youths. *International Journal of the Addictions* 25: 1341–1382.

Demitrack, M. A., F. W. Putnam, T. D. Brewerton, H. A. Brandt, and P. W. Gold (1990). Relation of clinical variables to dissociative phenomena in eating disorders. *American Journal of Psychiatry* 147: 1184–1188.

Demitrack, M. A., F. W. Putnam, D. R. Rubinow, T. A. Pigott, M. Altemus, D. D. Krahn, and P. M. Gold (1993). Relation of dissociative phenomena to levels of cerebrospinal fluid monoamines metabolities and beta-endorphin in patients with eating disorders: A pilot study. *Psychiatry Research* 49: 1–10.

Demos, E. V. (1989). Resiliency in infancy. In T. F. Dugan and R. Coles (Ed.), *The child in our times*. New York, Brunner/Mazel. 2–22.

Denny, K. (1995). Russian roulette: A case of questions not asked. *Journal of the American Academy of Child and Adolescent Psychiatry* 34: 1682–1683.

de Paul, J., and M. Arruabarrena (1995). Behavior problems in school-aged physically abused and neglected children in Spain. *Child Abuse and Neglect* 19: 409–418.

Despine, A. (1840). *De l'emploi du magnétisme animal et des eaux minérales dans le traitement des maladies nerveuses, suivi d'une observation tres curieuse de nevropathie*. Paris, Baillière.

Devinsky, O., K. Kelley, E. M. Yacubian, S. Sato, C. V. Kufta, W. H. Theodore, and R. J. Porter (1994). Postictal behavior: A clinical and subdural electroencephalographic study. *Archives of Neurology* 51(3): 254–259.

Devinsky, O., F. W. Putnam, J. Grafman, E. Bromfield, and W. H. Theodore (1989). Dissociative states and epilepsy. *Neurology* 39: 835–840.

de Vries, J. I. P., G. H. A. Visser, and H. F. R. Prechtl (1988). The emergence of fetal behavior: III. Individual differences and consistencies. *Early Human Development* 16: 85–103.

Deykin, E. Y., J. J. Alpert, and J. J. McNamara (1985). A pilot study of the effect of exposure to child abuse or neglect on adolescent suicidal behavior. *American Journal of Psychiatry* 142: 1299–1303.

Dick-Barnes, M., R. O. Nelson, and C. J. Aine (1987). Behavioral measures of multiple personality: The case of Margaret. *Journal of Behavior Therapy and Experimental Psychiatry* 18: 229–239.

DiLalla, L. F., and M. W. Watson (1988). Differentiation of fantasy and reality: Preschoolers reactions to interruptions in their play. *Developmental Psychology* 24: 286–291.

Donovan, D. M., and D. McIntyre (1990). *Healing the hurt child*. New York, Norton.

Draijer, N., and S. Boon (1993). The validation of the Dissociative Experiences

Scale against the criterion of the SCID-D using receiver operating characteristics (ROC) analysis. *Dissociation* **6**: 28–37.

Druckman, D., and R. Bjork, Eds. (1994). *Learning, remembering, believing: Enhancing human performance*. Washington, DC, National Academy Press.

Dubowitz, H., M. Black, D. Harrington, and A. Verschoore (1993). A follow-up study of behavior problems associated with child sexual abuse. *Child Abuse and Neglect* **17**: 743–754.

Dulit, R. A., M. R. Fyer, A. C. Leon, B. S. Brodsky, and A. J. Frances (1994). Clinical correlates of self-mutilation in borderline personality disorder. *American Journal of Psychiatry* **151**(9): 1305–1311.

Dunn, G. E., A. M. Paolo, J. J. Ryan, and J. V. Fleet (1993). Dissociative symptoms in a substance abuse population. *American Journal of Psychiatry* **150**(7): 1043–1047.

Egeland, B., and A. Susman-Stillman (1996). Dissociation as a mediator of child abuse across generations. *Child Abuse and Neglect* **20**: 1123–1132.

Ehlers, C. L. (1995). Chaos and complexity: Can it help us understand mood and behavior? *Archives of General Psychiatry* **52**: 960–964.

Einbender, A. J., and W. N. Friedrich (1989). Psychological functioning and behavior of sexually abused girls. *Journal of Consulting and Clinical Psychology* **57**: 155–157.

Ekman, P., R. W. Levenson, and W. V. Friesen (1983). Autonomic nervous system activity distinguishes among emotions. *Science* **221**: 1208–1210.

Elbert, T., C. Panev, C. Wienbruch, B. Rocksroh, and E. Taub (1995). Increased cortical representation of the fingers of the left hand in string players. *Science* **270**: 305–307.

Ellason, J. W., and C. A. Ross (1995). Positive and negative symptoms in dissociative identity disorder and schizophrenia: A comparative analysis. *Journal of Nervous and Mental Disease* **183**(4): 236–241.

Ellason, J. W., C. A. Ross, and D. Fuchs (1995). Assessment of dissociative identity disorder with the Millon Clinical Multiaxial Inventory—II. *Psychological Reports* **76**: 895–905.

Ellason, J. W., C. A. Ross, L. Mayran, and K. Sainton (1994). Convergent validity of the new form of the DES. *Dissociation* **7**: 101–103.

Ellenberger, H. F. (1970). *The discovery of the unconscious: The history and evolution of dynamic psychiatry*. New York, Basic Books.

Elliot, D. (1982). State intervention and childhood multiple personality disorder. *Journal of Psychiatry and the Law* **10**: 441–456.

Elliott, D. M., and J. Briere (1995). Posttraumatic stress associated with delayed recall of sexual abuse: A general population study. *Journal of Traumatic Stress* **8**: 629–647.

Engel, C. C., A. L. Engel, S. J. Campbell, M. E. McFall, J. Russo, and W. Katon (1993). Posttraumatic stress disorder symptoms and precombat sexual and physical abuse in Desert Storm veterans. *Journal of Nervous and Mental Disease* **181**: 683–688.

Ensink, B. J., and D. van Otterloo (1989). A validation of the Dissociative Experiences Scale in the Netherlands. *Dissociation* **2**: 221–224.

Erdreich, M. (1994). Sectorial automatism: A further development. *Medicine and Law* 13(1–2): 167–175.

Escorihuela, R. M., A. Tobena, and A. Fernandez-Teruel (1994). Environmental enrichment reverses the detrimental action of early inconsistent stimulation and increases the beneficial effects of postnatal handling on shuttlebox learning in adult rats. *Behavioral Brain Research* 61: 169–173.

Evers-Szostak, M., and S. Sanders (1992). The Children's Perceptual Alteration Scale (CPAS). *Dissociation* 5: 87–97.

Everson, M., and B. Boat (1990). Sexualized doll play among young children: Implications for use of anatomical dolls in sexual abuse evaluation. *Journal of the American Academy of Child and Adolescent Psychiatry* 29: 736–742.

Fagan, J., and P. P. McMahon (1984). Incipent multiple personality in children: Four cases. *Journal of Nervous and Mental Disease* 172(1): 26–36.

Fahy, T., and I. Eisler (1993). Impulsivity and eating disorders. *British Journal of Psychiatry* 162: 193–197.

Faith, M., and W. J. Ray (1994). Hypnotizability and dissociation in a college age population: Orthogonal individual differences. *Personality and Individual Differences* 17: 211–216.

Famularo, R., R. Kinscherff, and T. Fenton (1988). Propranolol treatment of childhood posttraumatic stress disorder, acute type. *American Journal of Diseases of Children* 142: 1244–1247.

Famularo, R., K. Stone, R. Barnum, and R. Wharton (1986). Alcoholism and severe child maltreatment. *American Journal of Orthopsychiatry* 56: 481–485.

Farah, M. J., R. C. O'Reilly, and S. P. Vecera (1993). Dissociated overt and covert recognition as an emergent property of a lesioned neural network. *Psychological Review* 100(4): 571–588.

Fast, I. (1974). Multiple identities in borderline personality organization. *British Journal of Medical Psychology* 47(4): 291–300.

Fein, G. G. (1981). Pretend play in childhood: An integrative review. *Child Development* 52: 1095–1118.

Feldman-Summers, S., and K. S. Pope (1994). The experience of "forgetting" childhood abuse: A national survey of psychologists. *Journal of Consulting and Clinical Psychology* 62: 636–639.

Fesler, F. A. (1991). Valproate in combat-related posttraumatic stress disorder. *Journal of Clinical Psychiatry* 52: 361–364.

Fichner, C. G., D. T. Kuhlman, M. J. Gruenfeld, and J. R. Hughes (1990). Decreased episodic violence and increased control of dissociation in a carbamazepine-treated case of multiple personality. *Biological Psychiatry* 27: 1045–1052.

Field, T. (1985). Attachment as psychobiological attunement: Being on the same wavelength. In M. Reite and T. Field (Eds.), *The psychobiology of attachment and separation.* New York, Academic Press. 415–454.

Field, T. (1994). The effects of mother's physical and emotional unavailability on emotion regulation. *Monographs of the Society for Research in Child Development* 59: 208–227.

Field, T., P. Greenwald, C. Morrow, B. Healy, T. Foster, M. Guthertz, and P. Frost (1992). Behavioral state matching during interactions of preadolescent friends versus acquaintances. *Developmental Psychology* 28: 242–250.

Fine, C. G. (1988). The work of Antoine Despine: The first scientific report on the diagnosis and treatment of a child with multiple personality disorder. *American Journal of Clinical Hypnosis* 31(1): 33–39.

Fine, C. G. (1992). The cognitive therapy of multiple personality disorder. *Comprehensive casebook of cognitive-behavior therapy*. New York, Plenum Press. 347–360.

Fink, D. (1991). The comorbidity of multiple personality disorder and DSM-III-R Axis II disorders. *Psychiatric Clinics of North America* 14(3): 547–566.

Finkelhor, D. (1979). *Sexually victimized children*. New York, Free Press.

Finkelhor, D. (1988). The trauma of sexual abuse: Two models. In G. E. Wyatt and G. J. Powell (Eds.), *Lasting effects of child sexual abuse*. Newbury Park, CA, Sage. 61–82.

Finkelhor, D. (1990). Early and long-term effects of child sexual abuse: An update. *Professional Psychology: Research and Practice* 21: 325–330.

Finkelhor, D., and L. Berliner (1995). Research on the treatment of sexually abused children: A review and recommendations. *Journal of the American Academy of Child and Adolescent Psychiatry* 34: 1408–1423.

Finkelhor, D., and J. Dziuba-Leatherman (1994). Children as victims of violence: A national survey. *Pediatrics* 94: 413–420.

Fischer, K. W., and C. Ayoub (1994). Affective splitting and dissociation in normal and maltreated children: Developmental pathways for self in relationships. In D. Cicchetti and S. L. Toth (Eds.), *Disorders and dysfunctions of the self: Vol. 5. Rochester Symposium on Developmental Psychopathology*. Rochester, NY, University of Rochester Press. 149–222.

Fivush, R., and A. Schwarzmueller (1995). Say it once again: Effects of repeated questions on children's event recall. *Journal of Traumatic Stress* 8: 555–580.

Flavell, J. H. (1989). The development of children's knowledge about the mind: From cognitive connections to mental representations. In J. W. Astington, P. L. Harris, and D. R. Olson (Eds.), *Developing theories of mind*. Cambridge, UK, Cambridge University Press. 244–267.

Fleischer, W., and G. Anderson (1995). Dissociative disorders in adolescence. *Adolescent Psychiatry* 20: 203–215.

Fletcher, K. E. (1996). Childhood posttraumatic stress disorder. In E. J. Mash and R. A. Barkley (Eds.), *Child psychopathology*. New York, Guilford Press. 242–276.

Flor-Henry, R., R. Tomer, I. Kumpula, Z. J. Koles, and L. T. Yeudall (1990). Neurophysiological and neuropsychological study of two cases of multiple personality syndrome and comparison with chronic hysteria. *International Journal of Psychophysiology* 10: 151–161.

Foa, E. B., C. Molnar, and L. Cashman (1995). Change in rape narratives during exposure therapy for posttraumatic stress disorder. *Journal of Traumatic Stress* 8: 675–690.

Foa, E. B., G. Steketee, and B. O. Rothbaum (1989). Behavioral/cognitive conceptualizations of post-traumatic stress disorder. *Behavior Therapy* **20:** 155–176.

Frank, J. B., T. R. Kosten, E. L. Giller, and E. Dan (1988). A randomized clinical trial of phenelzine and imipramine for posttraumatic stress disorder. *American Journal of Psychiatry* **145:** 1289–1291.

Frankel, F. H. (1990). Hypnotizability and dissociation. *American Journal of Psychiatry* **147:** 823–829.

Frankel, F. H. (1993). Adult reconstruction of childhood events in the multiple personality literature. *American Journal of Psychiatry* **150**(6): 954–958.

Frankel, F. H. (1994). The concept of flashbacks in historical perspective. *International Journal of Clinical and Experimental Hypnosis* **42:** 321–336.

Freud, A., and D. T. Burlingham (1943). *War and children.* London, Medical War Books.

Friedrich, W. N. (1993). Sexual victimization and sexual behavior in children: A review of the recent literature. *Child Abuse and Neglect* **17:** 59–66.

Friedrich, W. N., A. J. Einbender, and W. J. Luecke (1983). Psychological functioning and behavior of sexually abused girls. *Journal of Consulting and Clinical Psychology* **51:** 313–314.

Friedrich, W. N., P. Grambsch, and L. Damon (1992). Child Sexual Behavior Inventory: Normative and clinical comparisons. *Psychological Assessment* **4:** 303–311.

Friedrich-Velsor, B. (1992). Family foster care. *Journal of Pediatric Nursing* **7:** 216–217.

Frischholz, E. J., L. S. Lipman, B. G. Braun, and R. G. Sachs (1992). Psychopathology, hypnotizability and dissociation. *American Journal of Psychiatry* **149:** 1521–1525.

Fromuth, M. E., and B. R. Burkhart (1989). Long-term psychological correlates of childhood sexual abuse in two samples of college men. *Child Abuse and Neglect* **13:** 533–542.

Gardner, G. G., and K. Olness (1981). *Hypnosis and hypnotherapy with children.* Orlando, FL, Grune & Stratton.

Gardner, H. (1983). *Frames of mind: The theory of multiple intelligences.* New York, Basic Books.

Garrison, C. Z., E. S. Bryant, C. L. Addy, P. G. Spurrier, J. R. Freedy, and D. G. Kilpatrick (1995). Posttraumatic stress disorder in adolescents after Hurricane Andrew. *Journal of the American Academy of Child and Adolescent Psychiatry* **34:** 1193–1201.

Giovannoni, J. (1989). Definitional issues in child maltreatment. In D. Cicchetti and V. Carlson (Eds.), *Child maltreatment: Theory and research on the causes and consequences of child abuse and neglect.* Cambridge, UK, Cambridge University Press. 3–37.

Gjessing, L. (1974). A review of periodic catatonia. In N. Kline (Ed.), *Factors in depression.* New York, Raven Press. 227–249.

Gleaves, D. H., and K. P. Eberenz (1994). Sexual abuse histories among treatment-resistant bulimia nervosa patients. *International Journal of Eating Disorders* **15**(3): 227–231.

Gleick, J. (1987). *Chaos: Making of a new science.* New York, Penguin Books.

Glod, C., and M. Teicher (1996). Relationship between early abuse, posttraumatic stress disorder, and activity levels in prepubertal children. *American Journal of the American Academy of Child and Adolescent Psychiatry* **34**: 1384–1393.

Goff, D. C., and C. A. Simms (1993). Has multiple personality disorder remained consistent over time?: A comparison of past and recent cases. *Journal of Nervous and Mental Disease* **181**: 595–600.

Gold, P. W., H. Gwirtsman, P. C. Avgerions, L. K. Nieman, W. T. Gallucci, W. Kaye, D. Jimerson, M. Ebert, R. Rittmaster, D. L. Loriaux, and G. P. Chrousos (1986). Abnormal hypothalamic–pituitary–adrenal function in anorexia nervosa. *New England Journal of Medicine* **314**: 1335–1342.

Good, M. I. (1989). Substance-induced dissociative disorders and psychiatric nosology. *Journal of Clinical Psychopharmacology* **9**(2): 88–93.

Goodman, G. S., J. Hirschman, D. Hepps, and L. Rudy (1991). Children's memory for stressful events. *Merrill–Palmer Quarterly* **37**: 109–158.

Gopnik, A., and V. Slaughter (1991). Young children's understanding of changes in their mental states. *Child Development* **62**: 98–110.

Gott, P. S., C. H. Everett, and K. Whipple (1984). Voluntary control of two lateralized conscious states: Validation by electrical and behavioral studies. *Neurophysiologia* **22**(1): 65–72.

Gottschalk, A., M. S. Bauer, and P. C. Whybrow (1995). Evidence of chaotic mood variation in bipolar disorder. *Archives of General Psychiatry* **52**: 947–959.

Gralinski, J. H., A. W. Safyer, S. T. Hauser, and J. P. Allen (1995). Self-cognitions and expressed negative emotions during midadolescence: Contributions to young adult psychological adjustment. *Development and Psychopathology* **7**: 193–216.

Green, A. H. (1967). Self-mutilation in schizophrenic children. *Archives of General Psychiatry* **17**: 234–244.

Green, A. H. (1968). Self-destructive behavior in physically abused schizophrenic children. *Archives of General Psychiatry* **19**: 171–179.

Green, A. H. (1978). Self-destructive behavior in battered children. *American Journal of Psychiatry* **135**: 579–582.

Green, A. H. (1994). Impact of sexual trauma on gender identity and sexual object choice. *Journal of the American Academy of Psychoanalysis* **22**: 283–297.

Green, A. H., K. Voeller, R. Gaines, and J. Kubie (1981). Neurological impairment in maltreated children. *Child Abuse and Neglect* **5**: 129–134.

Green, B. L. (1993). Disasters and posttraumatic stress disorder. In J. R. Davidson and B. Foa (Eds.), *Posttraumatic stress disorder: DSM-IV and beyond*. Washington, DC, American Psychiatric Press. 75–97.

Green, W. H. (1991). Principles of psychopharmacology and specific drug treatments. In M. Lewis (Ed.), *Child and adolescent psychiatry*. Baltimore, Williams and Wilkins. 770–795.

Greenspan, G. S., and S. E. Samuel (1989). Self-cutting after rape. *American Journal of Psychiatry* **146**: 789–790.

Gross, R. J., H. Doerr, D. Caldirola, G. M. Guzinski, and H. S. Ripley

(1980–1981). Borderline syndrome and incest in chronic pelvic pain patients. *International Journal of Psychiatry in Medicine* 10: 79–96.

Groves, B., B. Zuckerman, S. Marans, and D. Cohen (1993). Silent victims: Children who witness violence. *Journal of the American Medical Association* 269: 262–263.

Gunderson, J. G., and A. N. Sabo (1993). The phenomenological and conceptual interface between borderline personality disorder and PTSD. *American Journal of Psychiatry* 150: 19–27.

Gutman, L. T., M. E. Herman-Giddens, and W. C. Phelps (1993). Transmission of human genital papillomavirus disease: Comparison of data from adults and children. *Pediatrics* 91: 31–38.

Hacking, I. (1991). Double consciousness in Britain 1815–1875. *Dissociation* 4: 134–146.

Hacking, I. (1995). *Rewriting the soul*. Princeton, NJ, Princeton University Press.

Handford, H., S. Mayes, R. Mattison, F. Humphrey, S. Bagnato, E. Bixler, and J. Kales (1986). Child and parental responses to the Three Mile Island nuclear accident. *Journal of the American Academy of Child and Adolescent Psychiatry* 25: 346–356.

Harkness, L. L. (1993). Transgenerational transmission of war-related trauma. *International handbook of traumatic stress syndromes*. New York, Plenum. 635–643.

Harmon, R., and P. Riggs (1996). Clonidine for posttraumatic stress disorder in preschool children. *Journal of the American Academy of Child and Adolescent Psychiatry* 35: 1247–1249.

Harris, P. L., E. Brown, C. Marriott, S. Whittall, and S. Harmer (1991). Monsters, ghosts and witches: Testing the limits of the fantasy–reality distinction in young children. *British Journal of Developmental Psychology* 9: 105–123.

Harrison, P. A., N. G. Hoffman, and G. E. Edwall (1989). Differential drug use patterns among sexually abused adolescent girls in treatment for chemical dependency. *International Journal of the Addictions* 24: 499–514.

Hart, B. (1926). The concept of dissociation. *British Journal of Medical Psychology* 10: 241–263.

Haule, J. (1986). Pierre Janet and dissociation: The first transference theory and its origins in hypnosis. *American Journal of Clinical Hypnosis* 29: 86–94.

Haviland, M. G., J. L. Sonne, and L. R. Woods (1995). Beyond posttraumatic stress disorder: Object relations and reality testing disturbances in physically and sexually abused adolescents. *Journal of the American Academy of Child and Adolescent Psychiatry* 34: 1054–1059.

Headly-Carter, M., R. Two-Bulls, M. Benoit, F. Putnam, and G. Peterson (1996). *A case of dissociative identity disorder in an eleven year old girl*. Paper presented at the 43rd Annual Meeting of the American Academy of Child and Adolescent Psychiatry, Philadelphia.

Hembrooke, H., and S. Ceci (1995). Traumatic memories: Do we need special mechanisms? *Consciousness and Cognition* 4: 75–82.

Hennig, C. W., W. P. Dunlap, and G. C. Gallup (1976). The effect of distance between predator and prey and the opportunity to escape on tonic immobility. *Psychological Record* **26**: 313–320.

Henninger, P. (1992). Conditional handedness: Handedness changes in multiple personality disorder subjects reflect shifts in hemispheric dominance. *Consciousness and Cognition* **1**: 265–287.

Herman, J. L. (1981). *Father–daughter incest.* Cambridge, MA, Harvard University Press.

Herman, J. L. (1992). *Trauma and recovery.* New York, Basic Books.

Herman, J. L., J. C. Perry, and B. A. van der Kolk (1989). Childhood trauma in borderline personality disorder. *American Journal of Psychiatry* **146**: 490–495.

Herman, J. L., and E. Schatzow (1987). Recovery and verification of memories of childhood sexual trauma. *Psychoanalytic Psychology* **4**: 1–14.

Herman-Giddens, M. E. (1994). Vaginal foreign bodies and child sexual abuse. *Archives of Pediatric and Adolescent Medicine* **148**: 195–200.

Herndon, D. N., R. L. Rutan, and T. C. Rutan (1993). Management of the pediatric patient with burns. *Journal of Burn Care and Rehabilitation* **14**: 3–8.

Herpertz, S. (1995). Self-injurious behaviour: Psychopathological and nosological characteristics in subtypes of self-injurers. *Acta Psychiatrica Scandinavica* **91**(1): 57–68.

Herrenkohl, E., R. Herrenkohl, L. Rupert, B. Egolf, and J. Lutz (1995). Risk factors for behavioral dysfunction: The relative impact of maltreatment, SES, physical health problems, cognitive ability, and quality of parent–child interaction. *Child Abuse and Neglect* **19**: 191–203.

Hibbard, R. A., K. Roghmann, and R. A. Hoekelman (1987). Genitalia in children's drawings: An association with sexual abuse. *Pediatrics* **79**: 129–137.

Hicks, R. (1993). *Failure to scream.* Nashville, TN, Thomas Nelson.

Hilgard, E. R. (1984). The hidden observer and mutiple personality. *International Journal of Clinical and Experimental Hypnosis* **32**: 248–253.

Hilgard, E. R. (1986). *Divided consciousness: Multiple controls in human thought and action, expanded edition.* New York, Wiley.

Hillary, B. E., and M. L. Schare (1993). Sexually and physically abused adolescents: An empirical search for PTSD. *Journal of Clinical Psychology* **49**: 161–165.

Hoffman, R., and T. McGlashan (1994). Corticocortical connectivity, autonomous networks, and schizophrenia. *Schizophrenia Bulletin* **20**: 257–261.

Holderness, C. C., J. Brooks-Gunn, and M. P. Warren (1994). Co-morbidity of eating disorders and substance abuse: Review of the literature. *International Journal of Eating Disorders* **16**(1): 1–34.

Hollander, E., J. L. Carrasco, L. S. Mullen, S. Trungold, C. M. DeCaria, and J. Towey (1992). Left hemispheric activation in depersonalization disorder: A case report. *Biological Psychiatry* **31**(11): 1157–1162.

Hollander, E., M. R. Liebowitz, C. DeCaria, J. Fairbanks, B. Fallon, and D. F. Klein (1990). Treatment of depersonalization with serotonin reuptake blockers. *Journal of Clinical Psychopharmacology* **10**: 200–203.

Hollander, E., D. J. Stein, C. M. DeCaria, L. Cohen, J. B. Saoud, A. E. Skodol,

D. Kellman, L. Rosnick, and J. M. Oldham (1994). Serotonergic sensitivity in borderline personality disorder: Preliminary findings. *American Journal of Psychiatry* **151**(2): 277–280.

Horen, S. A., P. P. Leichner, and J. S. Lawson (1995). Prevalence of dissociative symptoms and disorders in an adult psychiatric inpatient population in Canada. *Canadian Journal of Psychiatry* **40**(4): 185–191.

Horevitz, R. P., and B. G. Braun (1984). Are multiple personalities borderline? An analysis of 33 cases. *Psychiatric Clinics of North America* **7**(1): 69–87.

Hornstein, N. L. (1993). Recognition and differential diagnosis of dissociative disorders in children and adolescents. *Dissociation* **6**: 136–144.

Hornstein, N. L., and F. W. Putnam (1992). Clinical phenomenology of child and adolescent dissociative disorders. *Journal of the American Academy of Child and Adolescent Psychiatry* **31**: 1077–1085.

Hornstein, N. L., and S. Tyson (1991). Inpatient treatment of children with multiple personality/dissociative disorders and their families. *Psychiatric Clinics of North America* **14**: 631–648.

Horowitz, L., and F. W. Putnam (1996). *The revictimization of child sexual abuse survivors: An empirical and theoretical review.* Unpublished manuscript.

Horowitz, L., F. W. Putnam, J. Noll, and P. Trickett (1997). Factors affecting the utilization of treatment services by sexually abused girls. *Child Abuse and Neglect* **21**: 35–48.

Horrigan, J. (1996). Guanfacine for PTSD nightmares. *Journal of the American Academy of Child and Adolescent Psychiatry* **35**: 975–976.

Hubbard, J., G. M. Realmuto, A. K. Northwood, and A. S. Masten (1995). Comorbidity of psychiatric diagnoses with posttraumatic stress disorder in survivors of childhood trauma. *Journal of the American Academy of Child and Adolescent Psychiatry* **34**: 1167–1173.

Hughes, J. R., D. T. Kuhlman, C. G. Fichtner, and M. J. Gruenfeld (1990). Brain mapping in a case of multiple personality. *Clinical Electroencephalography* **21**: 200–209.

Hulbert, D. F., C. Apt, and L. C. White (1992). An empirical examination into the sexuality of women with borderline personality disorder. *Journal of Sex and Marital Therapy* **18**: 231–242.

Hull, J. W., J. F. Clarkin, and F. Yeomans (1993). Borderline personality disorder and impulsive sexual behavior. *Hospital and Community Psychiatry* **44**(10): 1000–1002.

Huxley, A. (1954). *The Doors of Perception.* New York, Harper & Row.

Irwin, H. J. (1994). Proneness to dissociation and traumatic childhood events. *Journal of Nervous and Mental Disease* **182**: 456–460.

Ito, Y., M. Teicher, C. Gold, D. Harper, E. Magnus, and H. Gelbard (1993). Increased prevalence of electrophysiological abnormalities in children with psychological, physical, and sexual abuse. *Journal of Neuropsychiatry and Clinical Neuroscience* **5**: 401–408.

Jackson, J. L., K. S. Calhoun, A. A. Amick, H. M. Maddever, and V. L. Habif (1990). Young adult women who report childhood intrafamilial sexual abuse. *Archives of Sexual Behavior* **19**: 211–221.

Jacobsen, T. (1995). Case study: Is selective mutism a manifestation of dissociative identity disorder? *Journal of the American Academy of Child and Adolescent Psychiatry* **34**: 863–866.

James, W. (1902). *The varieties of religious experience: A study in human nature.* New York, Signet, 1958.

Jampole, L., and M. K. Weber (1987). An assessment of behavior of sexually abused and nonabused children with anatomically correct dolls. *Child Abuse and Neglect* **11**: 187–192.

Janet, P. (1901). *The mental state of hystericals: A study of mental stigmata and mental accidents.* 2 vols. in 1. C. R. Corson, Trans. New York, Putnam.

Janet, P. (1930). Pierre Janet. In M. Murchison (Ed.), *History of psychology in autobiography, Vol. 1.* Worcester, MA, Clark University Press. 119–134.

Janus, M., F. Archambault, S. Brown, and L. Welsh (1995). Physical abuse in Canadian runaway adolescents. *Child Abuse and Neglect* **19**: 433–447.

Jensen, P. S., and J. Shaw (1993). Children as victims of war: Current knowledge and future research needs. *Journal of the American Academy of Child and Adolescent Psychiatry* **32**: 697–708.

Jessee, S. A. (1995). Orofacial manifestations of child abuse and neglect. *American Family Physician* **52**: 1829–1834.

Jimerson, D. C., B. E. Wolfe, D. L. Franko, N. A. Covino, and P. E. Sifneos (1994). Alexithymia ratings in bulimia nervosa: Clinical correlates. *Psychosomatic Medicine* **56**(2): 90–93.

Jonas, J., M. Gold, D. Sweeney, and A. Pottash (1987). Eating disorders and cocaine abuse: A survey of 259 cocaine abusers. *Journal of Clinical Psychiatry* **48**: 47–50.

Jungjohann, E. E. (1990). Symptom as a message: Psychosomatic reactions as signals in sexual exploitation of the child. *Acta Paedopsychiatrica* **53**: 54–61.

Kalichman, S. C. (1993). *Mandated reporting of suspected child abuse: Ethics, law and policy.* Washington, DC, American Psychological Association.

Kanzer, M. (1939). Amnesia: A statistical study. *American Journal of Psychiatry* **96**: 711–716.

Kaplan, H. I., and B. J. Sadock (1991). *Comprehensive Glossary of Psychiatry and Psychology.* Baltimore, Williams and Wilkins.

Kardiner, A. (1941). *The traumatic neuroses of war.* New York, Paul B. Hoeber.

Kaslow, F. W. (1982). Portrait of the healthy couple. *Psychiatric Clinics of North America* **5**: 519–527.

Kaufman, R., and F. Kaufman (1980). The face-schema in 3- and 4-month old infants: The role of dynamic properties of the face. *Infant Behavior and Development* **3**: 331–339.

Kavey, N. B. (1992). Psychological aspects of narcolepsy in children and adolescents. *Loss, Grief, and Care* **5**: 91–101.

Kelly, D. D., Ed. (1986). Stress-induced analgesia. *Annals of the New York Academy of Sciences* **467**.

Kempe, C. H., F. N. Silverman, B. F. Steele, W. Droegemueller, and H. K. Silver (1962). The battered-child syndrome. *Journal of the American Medical Association* **181**: 17–24.

Kessler, R. C., A. Sonnega, E. Bromet, M. Hughes, and C. B. Nelson (1995). Posttraumatic stress disorder in the national comorbidity survey. *Archives of General Psychiatry* **52**: 1048–1060.

Kilgus, M., A. Pumariega, and S. Cuffe (1995). Influence of race on diagnosis in adolescent psychiatric inpatients. *Journal of the American Academy of Child and Adolescent Psychiatry* **34**: 67–72.

Kinzie, J., R. Sack, and C. Riley (1994). The polysomnographic effects of clonidine on sleep disorders in posttraumatic stress disorder: A pilot study with Cambodian patients. *Journal of Nervous and Mental Disease* **182**: 585–587.

Kinzie, J. D., and P. Leung (1989). Clonidine in Cambodian patients with posttraumatic stress disorder. *Journal of Nervous and Mental Disease* **177**: 546–550.

Kirby, J. S., J. A. Chu, and D. L. Dill (1993). Correlates of dissociative symptomatology in patients with physical and sexual abuse histories. *Comprehensive Psychiatry* **34**(4): 258–263.

Kirsch, I., G. Montgomery, and G. Sapirstein (1995). Hypnosis as an adjunct to cognitive-behavioral psychotherapy: A meta-analysis. *Journal of Consulting and Clinical Psychology* **63**: 214–220.

Kirsten, M. (1990). Multiple personality disorder and borderline personality disorder [letter; comment]. *American Journal of Psychiatry* **147**(10): 1386–1387.

Kluft, R. P. (1984a). Multiple personality in childhood. *Psychiatric Clinics of North America* **7**(1): 121–134.

Kluft, R. P. (1984b). Treatment of multiple personality disorder: A study of 33 cases. *Psychiatric Clinics of North America* **7**(1): 9–29.

Kluft, R. P. (Ed.). (1985a). Childhood multiple personality disorder: Predictors, clinical findings, and treatment results. In *Childhood antecedents of multiple personality*. Washington, DC, American Psychiatric Press. 167–196.

Kluft, R. P. (1985b). Hypnotherapy of childhood multiple personality disorder. *American Journal of Clinical Hypnosis* **27**: 201–210.

Kluft, R. P. (1985c). The natural history of multiple personality disorder. In R. P. Kluft (Ed.), *Childhood antecedants of multiple personality*. Washington, DC, American Psychiatric Press. 197–238.

Kluft, R. P. (1986). Treating children who have multiple personality disorder. *Treatment of multiple personality disorder*. Washington, DC, American Psychiatric Press. 81–105.

Kluft, R. P. (1987a). First-rank symptoms as a diagnostic clue to multiple personality disorder. *American Journal of Psychiatry* **144**: 293–298.

Kluft, R. P. (1987b). The parental fitness of mothers with multiple personality disorder: A preliminary study. *Child Abuse and Neglect* **11**: 273–280.

Kluft, R. P. (1988). The postunification treatment of multiple personality disorder: First findings. *American Journal of Psychotherapy* **42**(2): 212–228.

Kluft, R. P. (1991). Multiple personality disorder. In A. Tasman and S. Goldfinger (Eds.), *American Psychiatric Press review of psychiatry: Vol. 10*. Washington, DC, American Psychiatric Press. 161–181.

Kluft, R. P. (1994). Basic principles in conducting the psychotherapy of multiple personality disorder. *Clinical perspectives on multiple personality disorder.* Washington, DC, American Psychiatric Press. 19–50.

Kluft, R. P., B. G. Braun, and R. G. Sachs (1984). Multiple personality, intrafamilial abuse, and family psychiatry. *International Journal of Family Psychiatry* 5: 283–301.

Kluft, R. P., and R. Schultz (1993). Multiple personality disorder in adolescence. *Adolescent Psychiatry* 19: 259–279.

Knutson, J. (1995). Psychological characteristics of maltreated children: Putative risk factors and consequences. *Annual Review of Psychology* 46: 401–431.

Koepp, W., S. Schildbach, C. Schmager, and R. Rohner (1993). Borderline diagnosis and substance abuse in female patients with eating disorders. *International Journal of Eating Disorders* 14(1): 107–110.

Kolb, L. C., B. C. Burris, and S. Griffiths (1984). Propranolol and clonidine in the treatment of post-traumatic stress disorders of war. In B. A. van der Kolk (Ed.), *Post-traumatic stress disorder: Psychological and biological sequelae.* Washington, DC, American Psychiatric Press. 97–108.

Kolko, J. D., J. T. Moses, and S. R. Weldy (1988). Behavioral/emotional indications of sexual abuse in child psychiatric inpatients: A controlled comparison with physical abuse. *Child Abuse and Neglect* 12: 529–541.

Koopman, C., C. Classen, and D. Spiegel (1994). Predictors of posttraumatic stress symptoms among survivors of the Oakland/Berkeley, Calif., firestorm. *American Journal of Psychiatry* 151(6): 888–894.

Kopelman, M. D., H. Christensen, A. Puffett, and N. Stanhope (1994a). The great escape: A neuropsychological study of psychogenic amnesia. *Neuropsychologia* 32(6): 675–691.

Kopelman, M. D., R. E. Green, E. M. Guinan, P. D. Lewis, and N. Stanhope (1994b). The case of the amnesic intelligence officer. *Psychological Medicine* 24(4): 1037–1045.

Kopelman, M. D., C. P. Panayiotopoulos, and P. Lewis (1994c). Transient epileptic amnesia differentiated from psychogenic fugue: Neuropsychological, EEG, and PET findings. *Journal of Neurology, Neurosurgery and Psychiatry* 57(8): 1002–1004.

Kopp, C., and N. Wyer (1994). Self-regulation in normal and atypical development. In D. Cicchetti and S. L. Toth (Eds.), *Disorders and dysfunctions of the self.* Rochester, NY, University of Rochester Press. 31–56.

Kosten, T. R., J. B. Frank, E. Dan, C. J. McDougle, and E. L. Giller (1991). Pharmacotherapy for posttraumatic stress disorder using phenelzine or imipramine. *Journal of Nervous and Mental Disease* 179: 366–370.

Kovacs, M. (1991). *Children's Depression Inventory manual.* North Tonawanda, NY, Multi-Health Systems.

Krell, R. (1985). Therapeutic value of documenting child survivors. *Journal of the American Academy of Child and Adolescent Psychiatry* 24: 397–400.

Krystal, J. H., A. L. Bennett, D. J. Bremner, S. M. Southwick, and D. S. Charney (1995). Towards a cognitive neuroscience of dissociation and altered memory function in post-traumatic stress disorder. In M. J. Friedman, D. S. Charney, and A. Y. Deutch (Eds.), *Neurobiological and clinical conse-*

quences of stress: From normal adaptation to post-traumatic stress disorder. Philadelphia, Lippincott–Raven. 239–269.

Krystal, J. H., L. P. Karper, J. P. Seibyl, G. K. Freeman, R. Delaney, J. D. Bremner, G. R. Heninger, M. B. Bowers, and D. S. Charney (1994). Subanesthetic effects of the noncompetitive NMDA antagonist, ketamine, in humans. *Archives of General Psychiatry* 51: 199–214.

Kuyken, W., and C. R. Brewin (1995). Autobiographical memory functioning in depression and reports of early abuse. *Journal of Abnormal Psychology* 104: 585–591.

Lacey, J. H. (1990). Incest, incestuous fantasy and indecency: A clinical catchment study of normal-weight bulimic women. *British Journal of Psychiatry* 157: 399–403.

Lacey, J. H. (1993). Self-damaging and addictive behaviour in bulimia nervosa. A catchment area study. *British Journal of Psychiatry* 163: 190–194.

Ladwig, G. B., and M. D. Andersen (1989). Substance abuse in women: Relationship between chemical dependency and past reports of physical and/or sexual abuse. *International Journal of the Addictions* 24: 739–745.

Lamb, M. E., K. J. Sternberg, and P. W. Esplin (1994). Factors influencing the reliability and validity of statements made by young victims of sexual maltreatment. *Journal of Applied Developmental Psychology* 15: 225–280.

Lancet (1991). Neurological conversion disorders in childhood. *Lancet* 337: 889–890.

Langmeier, J., and Z. Matejcek (1973). *Psychological deprivation in childhood*. New York, Halsted Press.

Lanktree, C., and J. Briere (1995). Outcome of therapy for sexually-abused children: A repeated measures study. *Child Abuse and Neglect* 19: 1145–1155.

Laor, N., L. Wolmer, L. Mayes, A. Golomb, D. Silverberg, R. Weizman, and D. Cohen (1996). Israeli preschoolers under Scud missile attacks: A developmental perspective on risk-modifying factors. *Archives of General Psychiatry* 53: 416–423.

Lapedes, A. (1994). A complex systems approach to computational molecular biology. In G. Cowan, D. Pines, and D. Meltzer (Eds.), *Santa Fe Institute studies in the sciences of complexity, Proceedings: Vol. 19*. Reading, MA, Addison-Wesley. 287–308.

LaPorta, L. (1992). Childhood trauma and multiple personality disorder: The case of a 9-year-old girl. *Child Abuse and Neglect* 16: 615–620.

Laquatra, T. A., and J. R. Clopton (1994). Characteristics of alexithymia and eating disorders in college women. *Addictive Behaviors* 19(4): 373–380.

Larmore, K., A. Ludwig, and R. Cain (1977). Multiple personality: An objective case study. *British Journal of Psychiatry* 131: 35–40.

Latz, T., S. Kramer, and D. Hughes (1995). Multiple personality disorder among female inpatients in a state hospital. *American Journal of Psychiatry* 152: 1343–1348.

Law, J., and J. Conway (1992). Effect of abuse and neglect on the development of children's speech and language. *Developmental Medicine and Child Neurology* 34: 943–948.

Lechner, M. E., M. E. Vogel, L. M. Garcia-Shelton, J. L. Leichter, and K. R.

Steibel (1993). Self-reported medical problems of adult female survivors of childhood sexual abuse. *Journal of Family Practice* **36**: 633–638.

Leitenberg, H., and K. Henning (1995). Sexual fantasy. *Psychological Bulletin* **117**: 469–496.

LePage, K. E., D. W. Schafer, and A. Miller (1992). Alternating unilateral lachrymation. *American Journal of Clinical Hypnosis* **34**(4): 255–260.

Lesieur, H. R., and S. B. Blume (1993). Pathological gambling, eating disorders, and the psychoactive substance use disorders. *Journal of Addictive Disorders* **12**(3): 89–102.

Leslie, A. M. (1988). Some implications of pretense for mechanisms underlying the child's theory of mind. In J. W. Astington, P. L. Harris, and D. R. Olson (Eds.), *Developing theories of mind*. Cambridge, UK, Cambridge University Press. 19–46.

Levenson, J., and S. L. Berry (1983). Family intervention in a case of multiple personality. *Journal of Marital and Family Therapy* **9**: 73–80.

Lewis, D. O. (1996). Diagnostic evaluation of the child with dissociative identity disorder/multiple personality disorder. *Child and Adolescent Psychiatric Clinics of North America* **5**: 303–332.

Lewis, M. (1991). Psychiatric assessment of infants, children and adolescents. In M. Lewis (Ed.), *Child and adolescent psychiatry*. Baltimore, Williams and Wilkins. 447–463.

Li, D., and D. Spiegel (1992). A neural network model of dissociative disorders. *Psychiatric Annals* **22**: 144–147.

Liebert, R. M., and J. Sprafkin (1988). *The early window*. Elmsford, NY, Pergamon Press.

Lifton, R. (1980). The concept of the survivor. In J. E. Dimsdale (Ed.), *Survivors, victims, and perpetrators: Essays on the Nazi Holocaust*. New York, Hemisphere. 113–126.

Lindsay, D. S., and M. K. Johnson (1987). Reality monitoring and suggestibility. In S. J. Ceci, M. P. Toglai, and D. F. Ross (Eds.), *Children's eyewitness testimony*. New York, Springer-Verlag. 79–91.

Lindy, J., B. Green, and M. Grace (1992). Somatic reenactment in the treatment of posttraumatic stress disorder. *Psychotherapy and Psychosomatics* **57**: 180–186.

Liotti, G. (1992). Disorganized/disoriented attachment in the etiology of dissociative disorders. *Dissociation* **5**: 196–204.

Lipper, S. (1990). Carbamazepine in the treatment of posttraumatic stress disorder: Implications for the kindling hypothesis. In M. E. Wolf and A. D. Mosnaim (Eds.), *Posttraumatic stress disorder: Etiology, phenomenology, and treatment*. Washington, DC, American Psychiatric Press. 184–203.

Lipper, S., J. R. Davidson, T. A. Grady, J. Edinger, and J. O. Cavenar (1986). Preliminary study of carbamazepine in post-traumatic stress disorder. *Psychosomatics* **27**: 849–854.

Lisak, D. (1994). The psychological impact of sexual abuse: Content analysis of interviews with male survivors. *Journal of Traumatic Stress* **7**: 525–548.

Litz, B., F. Weathers, V. Monaco, D. Herman, M. Wulfsohn, B. Marx, and T. Keane (1996). Attention, arousal, and memory in posttraumatic stress disorder. *Journal of Traumatic Stress* **9**: 497–519.

Livington, R., A. Witt, and G. R. Smith (1995). Families who somatize. *Journal of Developmental and Behavioral Pediatrics* 16: 42–46.

Loeber, R., M. Stouthamer-Loeber, W. Van Kammen, and D. P. Farrington (1991). Initiation, escalation and desistance in juvenile offending and their correlates. *Journal of Criminal Law and Criminology* 82: 36–82.

Loewenstein, R. J. (1991a). An office mental status examination for complex chronic dissociative symptoms and multiple personality disorder. *Psychiatric Clinics of North America* 14(3): 567–604.

Loewenstein, R. J. (1991b). Psychogenic amnesia and psychogenic fugue: A comprehensive review. In A. Tasman and S. M. Goldfinger (Eds.), *American Psychiatric Press review of psychiatry: Vol. 10*. Washington, DC, American Psychiatric Press. 189–221.

Loewenstein, R. J. (1991c). Rational psychopharmacology in the treatment of multiple personality disorder. *Psychiatric Clinics of North America* 14(3): 721–740.

Loewenstein, R. J. (1993). Posttraumatic and dissociative aspects of transference and countertransference in the treatment of multiple personality disorder. In R. Kluft and C. Fine (Eds.), *Clinical perspectives on multiple personality disorder*. Washington, DC, American Psychiatric Press. 51–85.

Loewenstein, R. J., N. L. Hornstein, and B. Farber (1988). Open trial of clonazepam in the treatment of posttraumatic stress symptoms in MPD. *Dissociation* 1: 3–13.

Loewenstein, R. J., and F. W. Putnam (1988). A comparison study of dissociative symptoms in patients with partial complex seizures, MPD, and posttraumatic stress disorder. *Dissociation* 1: 17–32.

Loewenstein, R. J., and F. W. Putnam (1990). The clinical phenomenology of males with multiple personality disorder: A report of 21 cases. *Dissociation* 3: 135–143.

Loftus, E. F. (1979). *Eyewitness testimony*. Cambridge, MA, Harvard University Press.

Loftus, E. G., M. Garry, and J. Feldman (1994). Forgetting sexual trauma: What does it mean when 38% forget? *Journal of Consulting and Clinical Psychology* 62: 1177–1181.

Long, J. V., and G. E. Vaillant (1989). Escape from the underclass. In T. F. Dugan and R. Coles (Eds.), *The child in our times*. New York, Brunner/Mazel. 200–214.

Looff, D., P. Grimley, and F. Kuller (1995a, February). Carbamazepine found efficacious for some children, adolescents with PTSD. *Psychiatric Times* 23–24.

Looff, D., P. Grimley, F. Kuller, A. Martin, and L. Shonfield (1995b). Carbamazepine for PTSD [Letter]. *Journal of the American Academy of Child and Adolescent Psychiatry* 34: 703.

Lovinger, S. L. (1983). Multiple personality: A theoretical view. *Psychotherapy: Theory, Research and Practice* 20: 425–434.

Ludwig, A. M. (1983). The psychobiological functions of dissociation. *American Journal of Clinical Hypnosis* 26: 93–99.

Ludwig, A. M., J. M. Brandsma, C. B. Wilbur, F. Bendfeldt, and D. H. Jameson

(1972). The objective study of a multiple personality. *Archives of General Psychiatry* **26**: 298–310.

Lydic, R. (1987). State-dependent aspects of regulatory physiology. *Journal of Federated American Society for Experimental Biology* **1**: 6–15.

Lynn, S. J., J. W. Rhue, and J. P. Green (1988). Multiple personality and fantasy proneness: Is there an association or dissociation. *British Journal of Experimental and Clinical Hypnosis* **5**: 138–142.

Lyons, J. A. (1991). Self-mutilation by a man with posttraumatic stress disorder. *Journal of Nervous and Mental Disease* **179**: 505–507.

Maier, S. F. (1986). Stressor controllability and stress-induced analgesia. *Annals of the New York Academy of Sciences* **467**: 55–72.

Main, M., and E. Hesse (1996). Disorganization and disorientation in infant Strange Situation behavior: Phenotypic resemblance to dissociative states. In L. Michelson and W. Ray (Eds.), *Handbook of dissociation: Theoretical, empirical, and clinical perspectives*. New York, Plenum Press. 107–138.

Main, M., and J. Solomon (1986). Discovery of a new, insecure–disorganized/disoriented attachment pattern. In T. B. Brazelton and M. Yogman (Eds.), *Affective development in infancy*. Norwood, NJ, Ablex. 95–124.

Malenbaum, R., and A. T. Russell (1987). Multiple personality disorder in an 11 year old boy and his mother. *Journal of the American Academy of Child and Adolescent Psychiatry* **24**: 495–501.

Malinosky-Rummell, R., and T. S. Hoier (1991). Validating measures of dissociation in sexually abused and nonabused children. *Behavioral Assessment* **13**: 341–357.

Mancini, C., M. Van Ameringen, and H. MacMillan (1995). Relationship of childhood sexual and physical abuse to anxiety disorders. *Journal of Nervous and Mental Disease* **183**: 309–314.

Mann, B. J., and S. Sanders (1994). Child dissociation and the family context. *Journal of Abnormal Child Psychology* **22**: 373–388.

Mannarino, A., J. Cohen, J. Smith, and S. Moore-Motily (1991). Six and twelve month follow-up of sexually abused girls. *Journal of Interpersonal Violence* **6**: 494–511.

Manosevitz, M., S. Fling, and N. M. Prentice (1977). Imaginary companions in young children: Relationships with intelligence, creativity and writing ability. *Journal of Child Psychology and Psychiatry* **18**: 73–78.

Marans, S., and D. Cohen (1993). Children and inner-city violence: Strategies for intervention. *Psychological effects of war and violence on children*. Hillsdale, NJ, Erlbaum. 281–302.

Marmar, C. R., D. S. Weiss, W. E. Schlenger, J. A. Fairbank, B. K. Jordan, R. A. Kulka, and R. L. Hough (1994). Peritraumatic dissociation and posttraumatic stress in male Vietnam theater veterans. *American Journal of Psychiatry* **151**(6): 902–907.

Marmer, S. S., and D. Fink (1994). Rethinking the comparison of borderline personality disorder and multiple personality disorder. *Psychiatric Clinics of North America* **17**(4): 743–771.

Martin, B. (1994). The schema. In G. Cowan, D. Pines, and D. Meltzer (Eds.),

Santa Fe Institute studies in the sciences of complexity, Proceedings: Vol 19. Reading, MA, Addison-Wesley. 263–285.

Martinez, P., and J. E. Richters (1993). The NIMH community violence project: II. Children's distress symptoms assocated with violence exposure. *Psychiatry* 56: 22–36.

Martinez-Taboas, A. (1989). Preliminary observations on MPD in Puerto Rico. *Dissociation* 2: 128–131.

Marx, J. (1995). How the glucorticoids suppress immunity. *Science* 270: 232–233.

Marzurek, A. J. (1994). Epidemiology of pediatric injury. *Journal of Accidents and Emergency Medicine* 11: 9–16.

Mathew, R. J., R. A. Jack, and W. S. West (1985). Regional cerebral blood flow in a patient with multiple personality. *American Journal of Psychiatry* 142: 504–505.

Mausert-Mooney, R. (1992). *Appeal and vulnerability patterns in girl victims of incest.* Unpublished doctoral dissertation, Western Michigan University, Kalamazoo.

McAdams, H. H., and L. Shapiro (1995). Circuit simulation of genetic networks. *Science* 269: 650–656.

McBride, P. A., R. P. Brown, M. DeMeo, J. Keilp, T. Mieczkowski, and J. J. Mann (1994). The relationship of platelet $5-HT_2$ receptor indices to major depressive disorder, personality traits, and suicidal behavior. *Biological Psychiatry* 35(5): 295–308.

McCann, J., J. Voris, and M. Simon (1992). Genital injuries resulting from sexual abuse: A longitudinal study. *Pediatrics* 79: 307–317.

McElroy, L. P. (1992). Early indicators of pathological dissociation in sexually abused children. *Child Abuse and Neglect* 16: 833–846.

McElroy, S. L., P. E. Keck, Jr., and K. A. Phillips (1995). Kleptomania, compulsive buying, and binge-eating disorder. *Journal of Clinical Psychiatry* 56(Suppl. 4): 14–26 (discussion, 27).

McHugh, P., and F. W. Putnam (1995). Resolved: Multiple personality disorder is an individually and socially created artifact. *Journal of the American Academy of Child and Adolescent Psychiatry* 34: 957–963.

McNally, R. J. (1991). Assessment of posttraumatic stress disorder in children. *Psychological Assessment* 3: 531–537.

McNally, R. J. (1995). Cognitive processing of trauma-relevant information in PTSD. *PTSD Research Quarterly* 6: 1–3.

Meiselman, K. (1978). *Incest.* San Francisco, Jossey-Bass.

Melges, F., and M. Swartz (1989). Oscillations of attachment in borderline personality disorder. *American Journal of Psychiatry* 146: 1115–1120.

Mennen, F. (1995). The relationship of race/ethnicity to symptoms in childhood sexual abuse. *Child Abuse and Neglect* 19: 115–124.

Merry, S., and L. Andrews (1994). Psychiatric status of sexually abused children 12 months after disclosure of abuse. *Journal of the American Academy of Child and Adolescent Psychiatry* 33: 939–944.

Merskey, H. (1992). The manufacture of personalities: The production of multiple personality disorder. *British Journal of Psychiatry* 160: 327–340.

Merskey, H. (1993). Professional and lay opinions on multiple personality disorder [Letter]. *British Journal of Psychiatry* **162**: 271.

Messerschmidt, R. (1927–1928). A quantitative investigation of the alleged independent operation of conscious and unconscious processes. *Journal of Abnormal and Social Psychology* **22**: 325–340.

Mesulam, M. M. (1981). Dissociative states with abnormal temporal lobe EEG: Multiple personality and the illusion of possession. *Archives of Neurology* **38**(3): 176–181.

Miller, B. A., W. R. Downs, D. M. Gondoli, and A. Keil (1987). The role of childhood sexual abuse in the development of alcoholism in women. *Violence and Victims* **2**: 157–172.

Miller, F. T., T. Abrams, R. Dulit, and M. Fyer (1993). Substance abuse in borderline personality disorder. *American Journal of Drug and Alcohol Abuse* **19**(4): 491–497.

Miller, N. S., M. S. Gold, and K. Stennie (1995). Benzodiazepines: The dissociation of addiction from pharmacological dependence/withdrawal. *Psychiatric Annals* **25**: 149–157.

Miller, P. P., T. A. Brown, P. A. DiNardo, and D. H. Barlow (1994). The experimental induction of depersonalization and derealization in panic disorder and nonanxious subjects. *Behaviour Research and Therapy* **32**(5): 511–519.

Miller, S. D. (1989). Optical differences in cases of multiple personality disorder. *Journal of Nervous and Mental Disease* **177**(8): 480–486.

Miller, S. D., T. Blackburn, G. Scholes, G. L. White, and N. Mamalis (1991). Optical differences in multiple personality disorder: A second look. *Journal of Nervous and Mental Disease* **179**: 132–135.

Modestin, J., G. Ebner, M. Junghan, and T. Erni (1996). Dissociative experiences and dissociative disorders in acute psychiatric patients. *Comprehensive Psychiatry* **37**: 355–361.

Moore, H. G., and J. L. Galloway (1992). *We were soldiers once . . . and young.* New York, Random House.

Morselli, G. W. (1953). Personalita alternate e patologia affectiva. *Archivo de Psicologia Neurologia e Psichiatria* **14**: 579–589.

Murphy, J. M., M. Jellinek, D. Quinn, G. Smith, F. G. Poitrast, and M. Goshko (1991). Substance abuse and serious child mistreatment: Prevalence, risk, and outcome in a court sample. *Child Abuse and Neglect* **15**: 197–211.

Murray, J. B. (1993). Relationship of childhood sexual abuse to borderline personality disorder, posttraumatic stress disorder, and multiple personality disorder. *Journal of Psychology* **127**(6): 657–676.

Myers, N. A., and M. Perlmutter (1979). Memory in the years from two to five. In P. A. Ornstein (Ed.), *Memory development in children.* Hillsdale, NJ, Erlbaum. 191–218.

Nash, M. R., T. L. Hulsey, M. C. Sexton, T. L. Harralson, and W. Lambert (1993). Long-term sequelae of childhood sexual abuse: Perceived family environment, psychopathology, and dissociation. *Journal of Consulting and Clinical Psychology* **61**(2): 276–283.

National Advisory Mental Health Council (1990). *National plan for research on child and adolescent mental disorders.* Rockville, MD, National Institute of Mental Health.

National Center on Child Abuse and Neglect (1988). *Study findings: Study of national incidence and prevalence of child abuse and neglect: 1988.* Washington, DC, U.S. Government Printing Office.

Newton, J. R., C. P. Freeman, and J. Munro (1993). Impulsivity and dyscontrol in bulimia nervosa: Is impulsivity an independent phenomenon or a marker of severity? *Acta Psychiatrica Scandinavica* 87(6): 389–394.

Nissen, M. J., J. L. Ross, D. B. Willingham, T. B. Mackenzie, and D. L. Schacter (1988). Memory and awareness in a patient with multiple personality disorder. *Brain and Cognition* 8: 117–134.

Oates, K., and S. Shrimpton (1991). Children's memories for stressful and nonstressful events. *Medical Science and Law* 31: 4–10.

Oates, R., B. O'Toole, D. Lynch, A. Stern, and G. Cooney (1994). Stability and change in outcomes for sexually abused children. *Journal of the American Academy of Child and Adolescent Psychiatry* 33: 945–953.

Oates, R., and A. Peacock (1984). Intellectual development of battered children. *Australian and New Zealand Journal of Developmental Disabilities* 10: 27–29.

Ogata, S. N., K. R. Silk, S. Goodrich, N. E. Lohr, D. Westen, and E. M. Hill (1990). Childhood sexual and physical abuse in adult patients with borderline personality disorder. *American Journal of Psychiatry* 147: 1008–1013.

Ornstein, P. A. (1995). Children's long-term retention of salient personal experiences. *Journal of Traumatic Stress* 8: 581–605.

Osofsky, J. D. (1995). The effects of exposure to violence on young children. *American Psychologist* 50: 782–788.

Paolo, A. M., J. J. Ryan, G. E. Dunn, and J. V. Fleet (1993). Reading level of the Dissociative Experiences Scale. *Journal of Clinical Psychology* 49(2): 209–211.

Paradise, J., L. Rose, L. Sleeper, and M. Nathanson (1994). Behavior, family function, school performance, and predictors of persistent disturbance in sexually abused children. *Pediatrics* 93: 452–459.

Paris, J., and H. Zweig-Frank (1992). A critical review of the role of childhood sexual abuse in the etiology of borderline personality disorder. *Canadian Journal of Psychiatry* 37: 125–128.

Park, J., B. Choe, M. Kim, H. Hnan, S. Yoo, S. Kim, and Y. Joo (1995). Standardization of the Dissociative Experiences Scale—Korean Version (I). *Korean Journal of Psychopathology* 4: 105–125.

Pashler, H. (1994). Dual-task interference in simple tasks: Data and theory. *Psychological Bulletin* 116(2): 220–244.

Paxton, J. W., and M. Dragunow (1993). Pharmacology. In J. S. Werry and M. G. Aman (Eds.), *Practitioner's guide to psychoactive drugs for children and adolescents.* New York, Plenum. 23–55.

Pelletier, G., J. Legendre-Roberge, B. Boileau, G. Geoffroy, and J. Leveille (1995). Case study: Dreamy state and temporal lobe dysfunction in a migrainous adolescent. *Journal of the American Academy of Child and Adolescent Psychiatry* 34: 297–301.

Perrine, K. R. (1991). Psychopathology in epilepsy. *Seminars in Neurology* **11**(2): 175–181.

Perry, B. D., R. Pollard, T. Blakely, W. Baker, and D. Vigilante (1995). Childhood trauma, the neurobiology of adaptation and "use-dependent" development of the brain: How "states" become "traits." *Infant Mental Health Journal* **16**: 271–291.

Persinger, M. A. (1993). Vectorial cerebral hemisphericity as differential sources for the sensed presence, mystical experiences and religious conversions. *Perceptual and Motor Skills* **76**(3, Pt 1): 915–930.

Peters, S., G. Wyatt, and D. Finkelhor (1986). Prevalence. In D. Finkelhor (Ed.), *A sourcebook on child sexual abuse*. Beverly Hills, CA, Sage. 15–59.

Peterson, G. (1990). Diagnosis of childhood multiple personality. *Dissociation* **3**: 3–9.

Peterson, G. (1991). Children coping with trauma: Diagnosis of "dissociation identity disorder." *Dissociation* **4**: 152–164.

Peterson, G. (in press). Dissociative disorders. *Psicologia Contemporanea*.

Peterson, G., and F. W. Putnam (1994). Preliminary results of the field trial of proposed criteria for dissociative disorder of childhood. *Dissociation* **7**: 212–220.

Pinegar, C. (1995). Screening for dissociative disorders in children and adolescents. *Journal of Child and Adolescent Psychiatric Nursing* **8**: 5–16.

Piper, A., Jr. (1994). Multiple personality disorder. *British Journal of Psychiatry* **164**(5): 600–612.

Pipp, S., and R. J. Harmon (1987). Attachment as regulation: A commentary. *Child Development* **58**: 548–562.

Pitman, R. (1987). Pierre Janet on obsessive–compulsive disorder (1903). *Archives of General Psychiatry* **44**: 226–232.

Pitman, R., S. Orr, B. van der Kolk, M. Greenberg, J. Meyerhoff, and E. Mougey (1990). Analgesia: A new dependent variable for the biological study of posttraumatic stress disorder. In M. Wolf and A. Mosnaim (Eds.), *Posttraumatic stress disorder: Etiology, phenomenology, and treatment*. Washington, DC, American Psychiatric Press. 141–147.

Plomin, R., and R. Rende (1991). Human behavioral genetics. *Annual Review of Psychology* **58**: 161–190.

Plotnick, A. B., P. A. Payne, and D. J. O'Grady (1991). Correlates of hypnotizability in children: Absorption, vividness of imagery, fantasy play, and social desirability. *American Journal of Clinical Hypnosis* **34**: 51–58.

Polusny, M. A., and V. M. Follette (1995). Long term correlates of child sexual abuse: Theory and review of the empirical literature. *Applied and Preventive Psychology* **4**: 143–166.

Pope, H. G., and J. L. Hudson (1992). Is childhood sexual abuse a risk factor for bulimia nervosa? *American Journal of Psychiatry* **149**: 455–463.

Pope, H. G., J. L. Hudson, and J. Mialet (1985). Bulimia in the late nineteenth century: The observations of Pierre Janet. *Psychological Medicine* **15**: 739–743.

Post, R. M., S. R. Weiss, and M. A. Smith (1995). Sensitization and kindling. In M. J. Friedman, D. S. Charney, and A. Y. Deutch (Eds.), *Neurobiological and clinical consequences of stress: From normal adaptation to post-traumatic stress disorder*. Philadelphia, Lippincott–Raven. 203–224.

Prentky, R. A., A. N. Burgess, F. Rokous, A. Lee, C. Hartman, R. Ressler, and J. Douglas (1989). The presumptive role of fantasy in serial sexual homicide. *American Journal of Psychiatry* **146**: 887–891.

Pribor, E. F., and S. H. Dinwiddie (1992). Psychiatric correlates of incest in childhood. *American Journal of Psychiatry* **149**: 52–56.

Pribor, E. F., S. Yutzy, J. Dean, and R. Wetzel (1993). Briquet's syndrome, dissociation and abuse. *American Journal of Psychiatry* **150**: 1507–1511.

Pribram, K., Ed. (1994). *Origins: Brain and self organization*. Hillsdale, NJ, Erlbaum.

Price, M. (1993). The impact of incest on identity formation in women. *Journal of the American Academy of Psychoanalysis* **21**: 213–228.

Prince, M. (1927). Suggestive repersonalization. *Archives of Neurology and Psychiatry* **18**: 159–189.

Prince, M., and F. Peterson (1908). Experiments in psychogalvanic reactions from co-conscious ideal in a case of multiple personality. *Journal of Abnormal Psychology* **3**: 114–131.

Putnam, F. W. (1984). The psychophysiologic investigation of multiple personality disorder. *Psychiatric Clinics of North America* **7**: 31–40.

Putnam, F. W. (1985a). Dissociation as a response to extreme trauma. In R. P. Kluft (Ed.), *Childhood antecedents of multiple personality*. Washington, DC, American Psychiatric Press. 66–97.

Putnam, F. W. (1985b). Pieces of the mind: Recognizing the psychological effects of abuse. *Justice for Children* **1**: 6–7.

Putnam, F. W. (1986a). The scientific investigation of multiple personality. In J. M. Quen (Ed.), *Split minds/split brains*. New York, New York University Press. 109–126.

Putnam, F. W. (1986b). The treatment of multiple personality: State of the art. In B. G. Braun (Ed.), *Treatment of multiple personality disorder*. Washington, DC, American Psychiatric Press. 175–198.

Putnam, F. W. (1988). The switch process in multiple personality disorder and other state-change disorders. *Dissociation* **1**: 24–32.

Putnam, F. W. (1989a). *Diagnosis and treatment of multiple personality disorder*. New York, Guilford Press.

Putnam, F. W. (1989b). Pierre Janet and modern views of dissociation. *Journal of Traumatic Stress* **2**(4): 413–429.

Putnam, F. W. (1990). Disturbances of "self" in victims of childhood sexual abuse. In R. P. Kluft (Ed.), *Incest-related syndromes of adult psychopathology*. Washington, DC, American Psychiatric Press. 113–133.

Putnam, F. W. (1991a). Dissociative phenomena. In A. Tasman and S. M. Goldfinger (Eds.), *American Psychiatric Press review of psychiatry: Vol. 10*. Washington, DC, American Psychiatric Press. 145–160.

Putnam, F. W. (1991b). Recent research on multiple personality disorder. *Psychiatric Clinics of North America* **14**: 489–502.

Putnam, F. W. (1991c). The satanic ritual abuse controversy. *Child Abuse and Neglect* **15**: 175–179.

Putnam, F. W. (1992). Using hypnosis for therapeutic abreactions. *Psychiatric Medicine* 10: 51–56.

Putnam, F. W. (1993a). Dissociation in the inner city. In R. P. Kluft and C. G. Fine (Eds.), *Clinical perspectives on multiple personality disorder*. Washington, DC, American Psychiatric Press. 179–200.

Putnam, F. W. (1993b). Dissociation: A North American perspective. *Dissociation* 6: 80–86.

Putnam, F. W. (1993c). Dissociative disorders in children: Behavioral profiles and problems. *Child Abuse and Neglect* 17: 39–45.

Putnam, F. W. (1994). Dissociative disorders in children and adolescents. In S. J. Lynn and J. W. Rhue (Eds.), *Dissociation: Clinical and theoretical perspectives*. New York, Guilford Press. 175–189.

Putnam, F. W. (1995). Development of dissociative disorders. In D. Cicchetti and D. Cohen (Eds.), *Developmental psychopathology: Vol. 2*. New York, Wiley–Interscience. 581–608.

Putnam, F. W. (1996a). Child development and dissociation. *Child and Adolescent Psychiatric Clinics of North America* 5: 285–302.

Putnam, F. W. (1996b). Special methods for trauma research with children. In E. Carlson (Ed.), *Trauma research methodology*. Lutherville, MD, Sidran Press. 153–173.

Putnam, F. W. (1996c). Posttraumatic stress disorder in children and adolescents. In L. Dickstein, M. Riba, and J. Oldham (Eds.), *Review of Psychiatry: Vol. 15*. Washington, DC, American Psychiatric Press. 447–468.

Putnam, F. W. (1996d). Child development and dissociation. *Child and Adolescent Psychiatric Clinics of North America* 5: 285–302.

Putnam, F. W., M. S. Buchsbaum, F. Howland, and R. M. Post (1982, May). *Evoked potentials in multiple personality disorder: New Research Abstract #137*. Presented at the annual meeting of the American Psychiatric Association, New Orleans.

Putnam, F. W., M. S. Buchsbaum, and R. M. Post (1993a). Differential brain electrical activity in multiple personality disorder. Unpublished manuscript.

Putnam, F. W., and E. B. Carlson (in press). Dissociation, hypnosis and trauma: Myths, metaphors and mechanisms. *Dissociation, memory and trauma*. Washington, DC, American Psychiatric Press.

Putnam, F. W., E. B. Carlson, C. A. Ross, G. Anderson, P. Clark, M. Torem, E. Bowman, P. Coons, J. Chu, D. Dill, R. J. Loewenstein, and B. G. Braun (1996a). Patterns of dissociation in clinical and non-clinical samples. *Journal of Nervous and Mental Disease* 184: 673–679.

Putnam, F. W., J. J. Guroff, E. K. Silberman, L. Barban, and R. M. Post (1986). The clinical phenomenology of multiple personality disorder: Review of 100 recent cases. *Journal of Clinical Psychiatry* 47(6): 285–293.

Putnam, F. W., K. Helmers, L. A. Horowitz, and P. K. Trickett (1994). Hypnotizability and dissociativity in sexually abused girls. *Child Abuse and Neglect* 19: 645–655.

Putnam, F. W., K. Helmers, and P. K. Trickett (1993b). Development, reliability and validity of a child dissociation scale. *Child Abuse and Neglect* 17: 731–741.

Putnam, F. W., N. L. Hornstein, and G. Peterson (1996b). Clinical phenomenology of child and adolescent dissociative disorders: Gender and age effects. *Child and Adolescent Psychiatric Clinics of North America* 5: 351–360.

Putnam, F. W., and R. J. Loewenstein (1993). Treatment of multiple personality disorder: A survey of current practices. *American Journal of Psychiatry* 150: 1048–1052.

Putnam, F. W., and G. Peterson (1994). Further validation of the Child Dissociative Checklist. *Dissociation* 7: 204–211.

Putnam, F. W., and P. Trickett (1997). The psychobiological effects of sexual abuse: A longitudinal study. *Annals of the New York Academy of Sciences* 821: 150–159.

Putnam, F. W., P. K. Trickett, L. Burke, and M. D. De Bellis (1995). *Somatic symptoms in sexually abused and matched comparison girls.* Unpublished manuscript.

Putnam, F. W., T. P. Zahn, and R. M. Post (1990). Differential autonomic nervous system activity in multiple personality disorder. *Psychiatry Research* 31: 251–260.

Putnam, N., and M. Stein (1984). Self-inflicted injuries in childhood. *Clinical Pediatrics* 24: 514–518.

Pynchon, T. (1973). *Gravity's rainbow.* New York, Viking.

Pynoos, R. S., and S. Eth (1984). The child as witness to homicide. *Journal of Social Issues* 40: 87–108.

Pynoos, R. S., and S. Eth (1985). Children traumatized by witnessing acts of personal violence: Homicide, rape or suicidal behavior. In S. Eth and R. S. Pynoos (Eds.), *Post-traumatic stress disorder in children.* Washington, DC, American Psychiatric Press. 17–44.

Pynoos, R. S., C. Frederick, K. Nader, W. Arroyo, A. Steinberg, S. Eth, F. Nunez, and L. Fairbanks (1987). Life threat and posttraumatic stress in school-age children. *Archives of General Psychiatry* 44: 1057–1063.

Pynoos, R. S., and K. Nader (1988). Children who witness the sexual assaults of their mothers. *Journal of the American Academy of Child and Adolescent Psychiatry* 28: 236–241.

Quen, J. M., Ed. (1986). *Split minds/split brains.* New York, New York University Press.

Rauch, S., B. van der Kolk, R. Fisler, N. Alpert, S. Orr, C. Savage, A. Fischman, M. Jenike, and R. Pitman (1996). A symptom provocation study of posttraumatic stress disorder using positron emission tomography and script-driven imagery. *Archives of General Psychiatry* 53: 380–387.

Reagor, P. A., J. D. Kasten, and N. Morelli (1992). A checklist for screening dissociative disorders in children and adolescents. *Dissociation* 5: 4–19.

Reddy L. A., and S. I. Pfeiffer (1997). Effectiveness of treatment foster care with children and adolescents: A review of outcome studies. *Journal of the American Academy of Child and Adolescent Psychiatry* 36: 581–588.

Reiter, R. C., L. R. Shakerin, J. C. Gambone, and A. K. Milburn (1990). Correlation between sexual abuse and somatization in women with somatic and nonsomatic pelvic pain. *American Journal of Obstetrics and Gynecology* 165: 104–109.

Renz, B. M., and R. Sherman (1992). Child abuse by scalding. *Journal of the Medical Association of Georgia* **81**: 574–578.

Resnick, H., D. G. Kilpatrick, B. S. Dansky, B. G. Saunders, and C. L. Best (1993). Prevalence of civilian trauma and posttraumatic stress disorder in a representative national sample of women. *Journal of Consulting and Clinical Psychology* **61**: 984–991.

Resnick, H. S., R. Yehuda, R. Pitman, and D. W. Foy (1995). Effect of previous trauma on acute plasma cortisol level following rape. *American Journal of Psychiatry* **152**: 1675–1677.

Richters, J. E., and P. Martinez (1993). The NIMH community violence project: I. Children as victims of and witness to violence. *Psychiatry* **56**: 7–21.

Riddle, M. A. (1991). Pharmacokinetics with children and adolescents. In M. Lewis (Ed.), *Child and adolescent psychiatry*. Baltimore, Williams and Wilkins. 767–769.

Riggs, S., A. J. Alario, and C. McHorney (1990). Health risk behaviors and attempted suicide in adolescents who report prior maltreatment. *Journal of Pediatrics* **116**: 815–821.

Riley, R. L., and J. Mead (1988). The development of symptoms of multiple personality disorder in a child of three. *Dissociation* **1**: 41–46.

Robins, E., and S. B. Guze (1970). Establishment of diagnostic validity in psychiatric illness: Its application to schizophrenia. *American Journal of Psychiatry* **126**: 983–987.

Robins, L., and J. Barrett, Eds. (1989). *The validity of psychiatric diagnoses*. New York, Raven Press.

Romans, S. E., J. L. Martin, J. C. Anderson, G. P. Herbison, and P. E. Mullen (1995). Sexual abuse in childhood and deliberate self-harm. *American Journal of Psychiatry* **152**: 1336–1342.

Root, M. P. (1989). Treatment failures: The role of sexual victimization in women's addictive behavior. *American Journal of Orthopsychiatry* **59**: 542–549.

Rosenbaum, M. (1980). The role of the term schizophrenia in the decline of multiple personality. *Archives of General Psychiatry* **37**: 1383–1385.

Rosenberg, R. (1994). Borderline states: Pharmacotherapy and psychobiology of personality. A discussion of Soloff's article. *Acta Psychiatrica Scandinavica* (Suppl. 379): 56–60.

Rosenfeld, A. A., D. J. Pilowsky, P. Fine, M. Thorpe, E. Fein, M. D. Simms, N. Halfon, M. Irwin, J. Alfaro, R. Saletsky, and S. Nickman (1997). Foster care: An update. *Journal of the American Academy of Child and Adolescent Psychiatry* **36**: 448–457.

Rosenheck, R., and J. Thomson (1986). "Detoxification" of Vietnam War trauma: A combined family–individual approach. *Journal of Family Process* **25**: 559–570.

Rosenthal, P. A., and S. Rosenthal (1984). Suicidal behavior by preschool children. *American Journal of Psychiatry* **141**: 520–525.

Ross, C. A. (1989). *Multiple personality disorder: Diagnosis, clinical features and treatment*. New York, Wiley.

Ross, C. A. (1990). Twelve cognitive errors about multiple personality disorder. *American Journal of Psychotherapy* **44**(3): 348–356.

Ross, C. A. (1991). Epidemiology of multiple personality disorder. *Psychiatric Clinics of North America* 14(3): 503–518.

Ross, C. A., S. Heber, and G. R. Norton (1989a). Differentiating multiple personality disorder and complex seizures. *General Hospital Psychiatry* 11: 54–58.

Ross, C., S. Heber, G. Norton, D. Anderson, G. Anderson, and P. Barchet (1989b). The Dissociative Disorders Interview Schedule: A structured interview. *Dissociation* 2: 169–189.

Ross, C. A., S. Heber, G. R. Norton, and G. Anderson (1989c). Somatic symptoms in multiple personality disorder. *Psychosomatics* 30: 154–160.

Ross, C. A., S. Heber, G. R. Norton, and G. Anderson (1989d). Differences between multiple personality disorder and other diagnostic groups on structured interview. *Journal of Nervous and Mental Diease* 177(8): 487–491.

Ross, C. A., S. Joshi, and R. Currie (1989e). Dissociative experiences in the general population. *American Journal of Psychiatry* 147: 1547–1552.

Ross, C. A., S. D. Miller, L. Bjornson, P. Reagor, G. Fraser, and G. Anderson (1990). Structured interview data on 102 cases of multiple personality disorder from four centers. *American Journal of Psychiatry* 147: 596–601.

Ross, C. A., S. D. Miller, L. Bjornson, P. Reagor, G. A. Fraser, and G. Anderson (1991). Abuse histories in 102 cases of multiple personality disorder. *Canadian Journal of Psychiatry* 36: 97–101.

Ross, C. A., G. R. Norton and K. Wozney (1989f). Multiple personality disorder: An analysis of 239 cases. *Canadian Journal of Psychiatry* 34: 413–418.

Ross, C. A., L. Ryan, H. Voigt, and L. Eide (1989g). Dissociative experiences in adolescents and college students. *Dissociation* 2: 239–242.

Rossini, E., D. Schwartz, and B. Braun (1996). Intellectual functioning of inpatients with dissociative identity disorder and dissociative disorder not otherwise specified. *Journal of Nervous and Mental Disease* 184: 289–294.

Rossiter, E. M., W. S. Agras, C. F. Telch, and J. A. Schneider (1993). Cluster B personality disorder characteristics predict outcome in the treatment of bulimia nervosa. *International Journal of Eating Disorders* 13(4): 349–357.

Rovee, C. K., L. W. Kaufman, G. H. Collier, and G. C. Kent (1976). Periodicity of death feigning by domestic fowl in response to simulated predation. *Physiology and Behavior* 17: 891–895.

Rubin, D. C., Ed. (1986). *Autobiographical memory.* Cambridge, UK, Cambridge University Press.

Rubin, K. H., R. J. Coplan, N. A. Fox, and S. D. Calkins (1995). Emotionality, emotion regulation, and preschoolers' social adaptation. *Development and Psychopathology* 7: 49–62.

Rubinow, D., and F. W. Putnam (1981). Sleep-induced mood state switches in a rapid cycling bipolar patient. Unpublished manuscript.

Rubonis, A. V., and L. Blickman (1991). Psychological impairment in the wake of disaster: The disaster–psychopathology relationship. *Psychological Bulletin* 109: 384–399.

Russell, D. E. H. (1986). *The secret trauma: Incest in the lives of girls and women.* New York, Basic Books.

Russell, W. D., and D. L. Weeks (1994). Attentional style in ratings of perceived exertion during physical exercise. *Perceptual and Motor Skills* **78**(3, Pt. 1): 779–783.

Ryan, R., E. Deci, and W. Grolnick (1995). Autonomy, relatedness, and the self: Their relation to development and psychopathology. *Developmental Psychopathology, Vol 1*. New York, Wiley–Interscience. 618–658.

Salzinger, S., S. Kaplan, D. Pelcovitz, C. Samit, and R. Krieger (1984). Parent and teacher assessment of children's behavior in child maltreating families. *Journal of the American Academy of Child Psychiatry* **23**: 458–464.

Sandberg, D. A., and S. J. Lynn (1992). Dissociative experiences, psychopathology and adjustment, and child and adolescent maltreatment in female college students. *Journal of Abnormal Psychology* **101**(4): 717–723.

Sanders, B. (1992). The imaginary companion experience in multiple personality disorder. *Dissociation* **5**: 159–162.

Sapolsky, R. (1996). Social subordinance as a marker of hypercortisolism: Some unexpected subtleties. *Annals of the New York Academy of Sciences* **771**: 626–639.

Saporta, J. A., and J. Case (1993). The role of medications in treating adult survivors of childhood trauma. In P. Paddison (Ed.), *Treating adult survivors of incest*. Washington, DC, American Psychiatric Press. 101–134.

Sar, V., L. Yargic, and H. Tutkun (1996). Structured interview data on 35 cases of dissociative identity disorder in Turkey. *American Journal of Psychiatry* **153**: 1329–1333.

Sarbin, T. R. (1995). On the belief that one body may be host to two or more personalities. *International Journal of Experimental Hypnosis* **43**(2): 163–183.

Saunders, B. E., L. A. Villeponteaux, J. A. Lipovsky, D. G. Kilpatrick, and L. J. Veronen (1992). Child sexual assault as a risk factor for mental health disorders among women: A community sample. *Journal of Interpersonal Violence* **7**: 189–204.

Saxe, G. N., G. Chinman, R. Berkowitz, K. Hall, G. Lieberg, J. Schwartz, and B. A. van der Kolk (1994). Somatization in patients with dissociative disorders. *American Journal of Psychiatry* **151**(9): 1329–1334.

Saxe, G. N., B. A. van der Kolk, R. Berkowitz, G. Chinman, K. Hall, G. Lieberg, and J. Schwartz (1993). Dissociative disorders in psychiatric inpatients. *American Journal of Psychiatry* **150**(7): 1037–1042.

Saxe, G. N., R. G. Vasile, T. C. Hill, K. Bloomingdale, and B. A. van der Kolk (1992). SPECT imaging and multiple personality disorder. *Journal of Nervous and Mental Disease* **180**: 662–663.

Schacter, D. L., J. F. Kihlstrom, L. C. Kihlstrom, and M. B. Berren (1989). Autobiographical memory in a case of multiple personality disorder. *Journal of Abrnormal Psychology* **98**(4): 1–7.

Scheeringa, M. S., C. H. Zeanah, M. J. Drell, and J. A. Larrieu (1995). Two approaches to the diagnosis of posttraumatic stress disorder in infancy and early childhood. *Journal of the American Academy of Child and Adolescent Psychiatry* **34**: 191–200.

Scheflin, A. W., and D. Brown (1996). Repressed memory or dissociative amnesia: What the science says. *Journal of Psychiatry and Law* **Summer**: 143–188

Schenk, L., and D. Bear (1981). Multiple personality and related dissociative phenomena in patients with temporal lobe epilepsy. *American Journal of Psychiatry* **138**(10): 1311–1316.

Schmidt, U., A. Jiwany, and J. Treasure (1993). A controlled study of alexithymia in eating disorders. *Comprehensive Psychiatry* **34**(1): 54–58.

Schneider-Rosen, K., and D. Cicchetti (1991). Early self-knowledge and emotional development: Visual self-recognition and affective reactions to mirror self-image in maltreated and non-maltreated toddlers. *Developmental Psychology* **27**: 471–478.

Schultz, R., B. G. Braun, and R. P. Kluft (1989). Multiple personality disorder: Phenomenology of selected variables in comparison to major depression. *Dissociation* **2**(1): 45–51.

Schwab-Stone, M. E., T. S. Ayers, W. Kasprow, C. Voyce, C. Barone, T. Shriver, and R. P. Weissberg (1995). No safe haven: A study of violence exposure in an urban community. *Journal of the American Academy of Child and Adolescent Psychiatry* **34**: 1343–1352.

Schwartz, I., J. Rendon, and C. Hsieh (1994). Is child maltreatment a leading cause of delinquency? *Child Welfare* **73**: 639–655.

Schwarz, E. D., and J. M. Lowalski (1991). Posttraumatic stress disorder after a school shooting: Effects of symptom threshold selection and diagnosis by DSM-III, DSM-III-R, or proposed DSM-IV. *American Journal of Psychiatry* **148**: 592–597.

Scialli, J. V. (1982). Multiple identity processes and the development of the observing ego. *Journal of the American Academy of Psychoanalysis* **10**(3): 387–405.

Seghorn, T., R. Prentky, and R. Boucher (1987). Childhood sexual abuse in the lives of sexually aggressive offenders. *Journal of the American Academy of Child and Adolescent Psychiatry* **26**: 262–267.

Seine, S., D. F. Becker, T. H. McGlashan, D. Vojvoda, S. Hartman, and J. P. Robbins (1995). Adolescent survivors of "ethnic cleansing": Observations on the first year in America. *Journal of the American Academy of Child and Adolescent Psychiatry* **34**: 1153–1159.

Shanks, D., and M. St. John (1994). Characteristics of dissociable human learning systems. *Behavioral and Brain Sciences* **17**: 367–447.

Shatan, C. (1973). The grief of soldiers: Vietnam combat veterans' self-help movement. *American Journal of Orthopsychiatry* **43**: 640–653.

Shaw, J., A. Campo-Bowen, B. Applegate, D. Perez, L. Antoine, E. Hart, B. Lahey, R. Testa, and A. Devaney (1993). Young boys who commit serious sexual offenses: Demographics, psychometrics, and phenomenology. *Bulletin of the American Academy of Psychiatry and the Law* **21**: 399–408.

Shaw, M. (1992). A teenager who firebombed his parents while in a dissociative state. *European Child and Adolescent Psychiatry* **1**: 196–199.

Shay, J. (1994). *Achilles in Vietnam: Combat trauma and the undoing of character.* New York, Atheneum/Macmillan.

Shearer, S. L. (1994). Dissociative phenomena in women with borderline personality disorder. *American Journal of Psychiatry* **151**(9): 1324–1328.

Shearer, S. L., C. P. Peters, M. S. Quayman, and R. L. Ogden (1990). Frequency and correlates of childhood sexual and physical abuse histories in adult female borderline patients. *American Journal of Psychiatry* **147**: 214–216.

Sidis, J. J. (1986). Can neurological disconnection account for psychiatric dissociation? In J. M. Quen (Ed.), *Split minds/split brains*. New York, New York University Press. 127–148.

Silberg, J. (1996). Psychological testing with dissociative children and adolescents. In J. Silberg (Ed.), *The dissociative child*. Lutherville, MD, Sidran Press. 85–102.

Silberman, E. K., F. W. Putnam, H. Weingartner, B. G. Braun, and R. M. Post (1985). Dissociative states in multiple personality disorder: A quantitative study. *Psychiatry Research* **15**: 253–260.

Singer, M. I., and M. K. Petchers (1989). The relationship between sexual abuse and substance abuse among psychiatrically hospitalized adolescents. *Child Abuse and Neglect* **13**: 319–325.

Siraganian, P., and F. W. Putnam (1997). *Diagnostic confirmation and clinical phenomenology of dissociative disorder outpatients*. Manuscript in preparation.

Skodol, A. E., J. M. Oldham, S. E. Hyler, H. D. Kellman, N. Dodge, and M. Davies (1993). Comorbidity of DSM-III-R eating disorders and personality disorders. *International Journal of Eating Disorders* **14**(4): 403–416.

Skuse, D., A. Albanese, R. Stanhope, J. Gilmour, and L. Voss (1996). A new stress-related syndrome of growth failure and hyperphagia in children, associated with reversibility of growth-hormone insufficiency. *The Lancet* **348**: 353–348.

Smith, S., and J. Howard (1994). The impact of previous sexual abuse on childrens adjustment in adoptive placement. *Social Work* **39**: 491–501.

Sohlberg, S., and C. Norring (1995). Co-occurrence of ego function change and symptomatic change in bulimia nervosa: A six-year interview-based study. *International Journal of Eating Disorders* **18**(1): 13–26.

Solomon, J. (1942). Reactions of children to blackouts. *American Journal of Neuropsychiatry* **12**: 361–362.

Solomon, S. D., E. T. Gerrity, and A. M. Muff (1992). Efficacy of treatments for posttraumatic stress disorder: An empircal review. *Journal of the American Medical Association* **261**(8): 633–638.

Southwick, S. M., R. Yehuda, and E. L. Giller (1993). Personality disorders in treatment-seeking combat veterans with posttraumatic stress disorder. *American Journal of Psychiatry* **150**: 1020–1023.

Spaccarelli, S. (1994). Stress, appraisal, and coping in child sexual abuse: A theoretical and empirical review. *Psychological Bulletin* **116**: 340–362.

Spanos, N. P. (1986). Hypnosis, nonvolutional responding, and multiple personality: A social psychological perspective. *Progress in Experimental Personality Research* **14**: 1–62.

Spiegel, D. (1986). Dissociation, double binds, and posttraumatic stress in multiple personality disorder. In B. G. Braun (Ed.), *Treatment of multiple personality disorder*. Washington, DC, American Psychiatric Press. 61–78.

Spielberger, C. D. (1973). *State–Trait Anxiety Inventory for Children*. Palo Alto, CA, Consulting Psychologists Press.

Spitz, R. A. (1945). Hospitalism: An inquiry into the genesis of psychiatric conditions in early childhood. *Psychoanalytic Study of the Child* 1: 53–74.

Spitz, R. A. (1946). Hospitalism: A follow-up report. *Psychoanalytic Study of the Child* 2: 113–117.

Sprick, R. S. (1985). *Discipline in the secondary classroom*. West Nyack, NJ, Center for Applied Research in Education.

Squire, L. R. (1986). Mechanisms of memory. *Science* 232: 1612–1619.

Sroufe, L. A., and M. Rutter (1984). The domain of developmental psychopathology. *Child Development* 55: 17–29.

Steiger, H., F. Leung, J. Thibaudeau, L. Houle, and A. M. Ghadirian (1993). Comorbid features in bulimics before and after therapy: Are they explained by axis II diagnoses, secondary effects of bulimia, or both? *Comprehensive Psychiatry* 34(1): 45–53.

Steiger, H., S. Stotland, and L. Houle (1994). Prognostic implications of stable versus transient borderline features in bulimic patients. *Journal of Clinical Psychiatry* 55(5): 206–214.

Stein, M. B., C. Koverola, C. Hanna, M. Torchia, and B. McClarty (in press). Hippocampal volume in women victimized by childhood sexual abuse. *Psychological Medicine* 27.

Stein, M. B., and T. W. Uhde (1989). Depersonalization disorder: Effects of caffeine and response to pharmacotherapy. *Biological Psychiatry* 26: 315–320.

Steinberg, A., and M. Steinberg (1994). Systematic assessment of multiple personality disorder in an adolescent who is blind. *Dissociation* 7: 117–128.

Steinberg, M. (1991). The spectrum of depersonalization: Assessment and treatment. In A. Tasman and S. M. Goldfinger (Eds.), *American Psychiatric Press review of psychiatry: Vol. 10*. Washington, DC, American Psychiatric Press. 223–247.

Steinberg, M. (1994). *Structured Clinical Interview for DSM-IV Dissociative Disorders—Revised (SCID-D-R)*. Washington, DC, American Psychiatric Press.

Steinberg, M. (1996). Diagnosis and assessment of dissociation in children and adolescents. *Psychiatric Clinics of North America* 5: 333–350.

Steinberg, M., B. Rounsaville, and D. Cicchetti (1991). Detection of dissociative disorders in psychiatric patients by a screening instrument and a structured diagnostic interview. *American Journal of Psychiatry* 148: 1050–1054.

Steinberg, M., and A. Steinberg (1995). Systematic assessment of MPD in adolescents using the SCID-D: Three case studies. *Bulletin of the Menninger Clinic* 59: 221–251.

Stevens-Simon, C., and E. McAnarney (1994). Childhood victimization: Relationship to adolescent pregnancy. *Child Abuse and Neglect* 18: 569–575.

Stone, M. H. (1981). Borderline syndromes: A consideration of subtypes and an overview of directions for research. *Psychiatric Clinics of North America* 4: 3–13.

Sutherland, S. M., and J. R. Davidson (1994). Pharmacotherapy for post-traumatic stress disorder. *Psychiatric Clinics of North America* 17: 409–423.

Svendson, M. (1934). Children's imaginary companions. *Archives of Neurology and Psychiatry* 32: 985–999.

Swica, Y., D. Lewis, and M. Lewis (1996). Child abuse and multiple personality: The objective documentation of childhood maltreatment. *Child and Adolescent Psychiatric Clinics of North America* 5: 431–448.

Szostak, C., R. Lister, M. Eckardt, and H. Weingartner (1994). Dissociative effects of mood on memory. In R. M. Klein and B. K. Doane (Eds.), *Psychological concepts and dissociative disorders*. Hillsdale, NJ, Erlbaum. 187–206.

Szostak, C., R. Lister, F. W. Putnam, and H. Weingartner (1997). *Characterization of implicit and explicit retrieval functions in multiple personality disorder: Three case studies*. Manuscript in preparation.

Tariot, P. N., and H. Weingartner (1986). A psychobiologic analysis of cognitive failures: Structures and mechanisms. *Archives of General Psychiatry* 43: 1183–1188.

Tart, C. T. (1972). States of consciousness and state-specific sciences. *Science* 176: 1203–1210.

Tart, C. T. (1975). *States of consciousness*. New York, E. P. Dutton.

Tart, C. T. (1990). Multiple personality, altered states and virtual reality: The world simulation process approach. *Dissociation* 3: 222–233.

Tarter, R. E., A. M. Hegedus, N. E. Winsten, and A. I. Alterman (1984). Neuropsycholgical, personality, and familial characteristics of physically abused delinquents. *Journal of the American Academy of Child Psychiatry* 23: 668–674.

Taylor, M., B. S. Cartwright, and S. M. Carlson (1991). *Fantasy and theory of mind: A developmental investigation of children's imaginary companions*. Paper presented at the biennial meeting of the Society for Research in Child Development, Seattle, WA.

Teicher, M., C. Glod, J. Surrey, and C. Swett (1993). Early childhood abuse and limbic system ratings in adult psychiatric outpatients. *Journal of Neuropsychiatry and Clinical Neuroscience* 5: 301–306.

Terr, L. (1979). Children of Chowchilla: A study of psychic trauma. *Psychoanalytic Study of the Child* 34: 547–623.

Terr, L. (1981). "Forbidden games": Post-traumatic child's play. *Journal of the American Academy of Child and Adolescent Psychiatry* 20: 741–760.

Terr, L. (1983). Chowchilla revisited: The effects of psychic trauma after a school-bus kidnapping. *American Journal of Psychiatry* 140: 1543–1550.

Thackwray, D. E., M. C. Smith, and J. Bodfish (1991). Unsolicted reports of sexual abuse in a comparative study of treatments of bulimia [Letter]. *American Journal of Psychiatry* 148: 1754.

Thelen, E., and L. B. Smith (1994). *A dynamic systems approach to the development of cognition and action*. Cambridge, MA, Bradford.

Thigpen, C. H., and H. Cleckley (1954). A case of multiple personality. *Journal of Abnormal and Social Psychology* 49: 135–151.

Thompson, R., and B. Wilcox (1995). Child maltreatment research. *American Psychologist* 50: 789–793.

Thompson, R. A. (1991). Attachment theory and research. In M. Lewis (Ed.), *Child and adolescent psychiatry*. Baltimore, Williams and Wilkins. 100–108.

Thormaehlen, D. J., and E. R. Bass-Feld (1994). Children: The secondary victims of domestic violence. *Maryland Medical Journal* **43**: 355–359.

Thygesen, P., K. Hermann, and R. Willanger (1970). Concentration camp survivors in Denmark: Persecution, disease, disability, compensation. *Danish Medical Bulletin* **17**: 65–108.

Tiller, J., U. Schmidt, S. Ali, and J. Treasure (1995). Patterns of punitiveness in women with eating disorders. *International Journal of Eating Disorders* **17**(4): 365–371.

Trickett, P., C. McBride-Chang, and F. W. Putnam (1994). The classroom performance and behavior of sexually abused females. *Development and Psychopathology* **6**: 183–194.

Trickett, P., A. Reiffman, L. Horowitz, and F. W. Putnam (in press). Characteristics of sexual abuse trauma and the prediction of developmental outcomes. In D. Cicchetti and S. Toth (Eds.), *Rochester Symposium on Developmental Psychopathology: Vol 8: The effects of trauma on the developmental process*. Rochester, NY, University of Rochester Press.

Tromp, S., M. P. Koss, A. J. Figueredo, and M. Tharan (1995). Are rape memories different? A comparison of rape, other unpleasant, and pleasant memories among employed women. *Journal of Traumatic Stress* **8**: 607–627.

Trujillo, K., D. O. Lewis, C. A. Yeager, and B. Gidlow (1996). Imaginary companions of school boys and boys with dissociative identity disorder: A normal to pathological continuum. *Child and Adolescent Psychiatric Clinics of North America* **5**: 375–392.

Tulving, E., and D. L. Schacter (1990). Priming and human memory. *Science* **247**: 301–306.

Tyson, G. M. (1992). Childhood MPD/dissociation identity disorder: Applying and extending current diagnostic checklists. *Dissociation* **5**: 20–27.

Uddo, M., J. T. Vasterling, K. Brailey, and P. B. Sutker (1993). Memory and attention in posttraumatic stress disorder. *Journal of Psychopathology and Behavioral Assessment* **15**: 43–52.

U.S. Department of Health and Human Services (1996). *The Third National Incidence Study of Child Abuse and Neglect*. Washington, DC, U.S. Government Printing Office.

U.S. Department of Health and Human Services, and National Center on Child Abuse and Neglect (1996). *Child maltreatment 1994: Reports from the States to the National Center on Child Abuse and Neglect*. Washington, DC, U.S. Government Printing Office.

van der Hart, O., and B. Friedman (1989). A reader's guide to Pierre Janet on dissociation: A neglected intellectual heritage. *Dissociation* **2**: 3–16.

van der Kolk, B. A. (1996). The complexity of adaptation to trauma: Self-regulation, stimulus discrimination, and characterological development. In B. A. van der Kolk, A. C. McFarlane, and L. Weisaeth (Eds.), *Traumatic stress: The effects of overwhelming experience on mind, body, and society*. New York, Guilford Press. 182–213.

van der Kolk, B. A., D. Dreyfuss, M. Michaels, D. Shera, R. Berkowitz, R. Fisler and G. Saxe (1994). Fluoxetine in posttraumatic stress disorder. *Journal of Clinical Psychology* **155**: 517–522.

van der Kolk, B. A., and C. Ducey (1989). The psychological processing of traumatic experience: Rorschach patterns in PTSD. *Journal of Traumatic Stress* 2: 259–263.

van der Kolk, B. A., and R. Fisler (1995). Dissociation and the fragmentary nature of traumatic memories: Overview and exploratory study. *Journal of Traumatic Stress* 8: 505–525.

van der Kolk, B. A., M. Greenberg, H. Boyd, and J. H. Krystal (1985). Inescapable shock, neurotransmitters and addiction to trauma: Towards a psychobiology of post traumatic stress disorder. *Biological Psychiatry* 22: 314–325.

van der Kolk, B. A., and W. Kadish (1987). Amnesia, dissociation and the return of the repressed. *Psychological Trauma*. Washington, DC, American Psychiatric Press. 173–190.

van der Kolk, B., D. Pelcovitz, S. Roth, F. Mandel, A. McFarlane, and J. Herman (1996). Dissociation, somatization, and affect dysregulation: The complexity of adaptation to trauma. *American Journal of Psychiatry* 153: 83–93.

van der Kolk, B. A., J. C. Perry, and J. L. Herman (1991). Childhood origins of self-destructive behavior. *American Journal of Psychiatry* 148: 1665–1671.

van IJzendoorn, M., and C. Schuengel (1996). The measurement of dissociation in normal and clinical populations: Meta-analytic validation of the Dissociative Experiences Scale (DES). *Clinical Psychology Review* 16: 365–382.

Vincent, M., and M. R. Pickering (1988). Multiple personality disorder in childhood. *Canadian Journal of Psychiatry* 33: 524–529.

Walker, E. A., A. N. Gelfand, M. D. Gelfand, M. P. Koss, and W. J. Katon (1995). Medical and psychiatric histories in female gastroenterology clinic patients with histories of sexual victimization. *General Hospital Psychiatry* 17: 85–92.

Walker, E., W. J. Katon, J. Harrop-Griffiths, L. Holm, J. Russo, and L. R. Hickok (1988). Relationship of chronic pelvic pain to psychiatric diagnoses and childhood sexual abuse. *American Journal of Psychiatry* 145: 75–80.

Walker, E. A., W. J. Katon, K. Neraas, R. P. Jemelka, and D. Massoth (1992). Dissociation in women with chronic pelvic pain. *American Journal of Psychiatry* 149: 534–537.

Waller, G. (1991). Sexual abuse as a factor in eating disorders. *British Journal of Psychiatry* 159: 664–671.

Waller, G. (1993a). Association of sexual abuse and borderline personality disorder in eating disordered women. *International Journal of Eating Disorders* 13(3): 259–263.

Waller, G. (1993b). Sexual abuse and eating disorders: Borderline personality disorder as a mediating factor? *British Journal of Psychiatry* 162: 771–775.

Waller, N. G. (1995). The Dissociative Experiences Scale. In J. C. Conoley and J. C. Impara (Eds.), *Twelfth mental measurements yearbook*. Lincoln, NE, Buros Institute of Mental Measurement. 122.

Waller, N. G., F. W. Putnam, and E. B. Carlson (1996). Types of dissociation and dissociative types. *Psychological Methods* 1: 300–321.

Waller, N. G., and C. Ross (in press). The prevalence of pathological dissociation in the general population. *Journal of Abnormal Psychology*.

Watkins, B., and A. Bentovim (1992). The sexual abuse of male children and
adolescents: A review of current research. *Journal of Child Psychology and
Psychiatry* **33**: 197–248.

Weingartner, H. J. (1978). Human state dependent learning. In B. T. Ho, D. W.
Richards, and D. C. Chute (Eds.), *Drug discrimination and state dependent
learning*. New York, Academic Press. 361–382.

Weingartner, H. J., F. W. Putnam, D. T. George, and P. L. Ragan (1995). Drug
state-dependent autobiographical knowledge. *Experimental and Clinical
Psychopharmacology* **3**: 304–307.

Weiss, D. S., C. R. Marmar, T. J. Metzler, and H. M. Ronfeldt (1995). Predicting
symptomatic distress in emergency services personnel. *Journal of Consulting and Clinical Psychology* **63**(3): 361–368.

Weiss, M., P. J. Sutton, and A. J. Utecht (1985). Multiple personality in a 10-
year-old girl. *Journal of the American Academy of Child Psychiatry* **24**:
495–501.

Weller, E., and R. Weller (1991). Grief. In M. Lewis (Ed.), *Child and adolescent
psychiatry*. Baltimore, Williams and Wilkins. 389–393.

Werry, J. S., and M. G. Aman, Eds. (1993). *Practitioner's guide to psychoactive
drugs for children and adolescents*. New York, Plenum Press.

West, L. J. (1967). Dissociative reaction. In A. M. Freedman and H. I. Kaplan
(Eds.), *Comprehensive textbook of psychiatry, second edition*. Baltimore,
Williams and Wilkins. 885–899.

Westen, D., P. Ludoplh, B. Misle, S. Ruffins, and J. Block (1990). Physical and
sexual abuse in adolescent girls with borderline personality disorder. *American Journal of Orthopsychiatry* **60**: 55–66.

Wetzler, S. E., and J. A. Sweeney (1986). Childhood amnesia: An empirical
demonstration. In D. C. Rubin (Ed.), *Autobiographical memory*. Cambridge, UK, Cambridge University Press. 191–201.

Wherry, J. N., J. B. Jolly, J. Feldman, B. Adam, and S. Manjanatha (1994). The
Child Dissociative Checklist: Preliminary findings of a screening instrument. *Child Sexual Abuse* **3**: 51–66.

White, R., and B. Shevach (1942). Hypnosis and the concept of dissociation.
Journal of Abnormal and Social Psychology **37**: 309–328.

Widom, C., and M. Ames (1994). Criminal consequences of childhood sexual
victimization. *Child Abuse and Neglect* **18**: 303–318.

Wiggins, M. E., E. Akeman, and A. P. Weiss (1994). The management of dog
bites and dog bite infections to the hand. *Orthopedics* **17**: 617–623.

Wilens, T., J. Biederman, and T. Spencer (1994). Clonidine for sleep disturbances associated with attention-deficit hyperactivity disorder. *Journal
of the American Academy of Child and Adolescent Psychiatry* **33**: 424–
426.

Williams, L. M. (1994). Amnesia for childhood trauma: A prospective study of
women's memories of child sexual abuse. *Journal of Consulting and Clinical Psychology* **62**: 1167–1176.

Williams, L. M. (1995). Recovered memories of abuse in women with documented child sexual victimization histories. *Journal of Traumatic Stress* 8: 649–673.

Williams, M. B. (1991). Clinical work with families of MPD patients: Assessment and issues for practice. *Dissociation* 4: 92–98.

Williams, T. H., Ed. (1986). *The impact of television: A natural experiment in three communities.* Orlando, FL, Academic Press.

Wilson, S. C., and T. X. Barber (1983). The fantasy-prone personality: Implications for understanding imagery, hypnosis, and parapsychological phenomena. *Imagery: Current theory, research, and application.* New York, Wiley. 340–387.

Wind, T., and L. Silvern (1994). Parenting and family stress as mediators of the long-term effects of child abuse. *Child Abuse and Neglect* 18: 439–453.

Windle, M. (1994). Substance use, risky behaviors, and victimization among a US national adolescent sample. *Addiction* 89: 175–182.

Wissow, L. S. (1995). Child abuse and neglect. *New England Journal of Medicine* 332: 1425–1431.

Wolf, D. P. (1990). Being of several minds: Voices and versions of the self in early childhood. In D. Cicchetti and M. Beeghly (Eds.), *The self in transition: Infancy to childhood.* Chicago, University of Chicago Press. 183–212.

Wolf, M. E., A. Alavi, and A. D. Mosnam (1988). Posttraumatic stress disorder in Vietnam veterans: Clinical and EEG findings. Possible therapeutic effects of carbamazepine. *Biological Psychiatry* 23: 642–644.

Wolfe, B. E., D. C. Jimerson, and J. M. Levine (1994). Impulsivity ratings in bulimia nervosa: Relationship to binge eating behaviors. *International Journal of Eating Disorders* 15(3): 289–292.

Wolfe, V. V., C. Gentile, and D. A. Wolfe (1989). The impact of sexual abuse on children: A PTSD formulation. *Behavior Therapy* 20: 215–228.

Wolff, P. H. (1987). *The development of behavioral states and the expression of emotions in early infancy.* Chicago, University of Chicago Press.

Wolff, P. H. (1993). Behavioral and emotional states in infancy: A dynamic perspective. In L. Smith and E. Thelen (Eds.), *A dynamic systems approach to development: Applications.* Cambridge, MA, MIT Press. 189–208.

Wolpaw, J., J. Schmidt, and T. Vaughan, Eds. (1991). Activity-driven CNS changes in learning and development. *Annals of the New York Academy of Sciences* 627.

Wurtele, S. K., G. M. Kaplan, and M. Keairnes (1990). Childhood sexual abuse among chronic pain patients. *Clinical Journal of Pain* 6: 110–113.

Yarrow, M., J. Campbell, and R. Burton (1970). Recollections of childhood: A study of the retrospective method. *Monographs of the Society for Research in Child Development* 35: 1–83.

Yates, A. (1982). Children eroticized by incest. *American Journal of Psychiatry* 139: 482–485.

Yeager, C. A., and D. O. Lewis (1996). The intergenerational transmission of violence and dissociation. *Child and Adolescent Psychiatric Clinics of North America* 5: 393–430.

Yehuda, R., B. Kahana, K. Binder-Byrnes, S. M. Southwick, J. W. Mason, and E.

L. Giller (1995). Low urinary cortisol excretion in Holocaust survivors with posttraumatic stress disorder. *American Journal of Psychiatry* **152**: 982–986.

Yehuda, R., and A. C. McFarlane (1995). Conflict between current knowledge about posttraumatic stress disorder and its original conceptual basis. *American Journal of Psychiatry* **152**: 1705–1713.

Yule, W. (1993). Technology-related disasters. In C. F. Saylor (Ed.), *Children and disaster*. New York, Plenum Press. 104–121.

Zahn, T. P., R. Moraga, and W. J. Ray (1996). Psychophysiological assessment of dissociative disorders. In L. Michelson and W. Ray (Eds.), *Handbook of dissociation: Theoretical, empirical, and clinical perspectives*. New York, Plenum Press. 269–287.

Zanarini, M. C., J. G. Gunderson, M. F. Marino, E. O. Schwartz, and F. R. Frankenburg (1989). Childhood experiences of borderline patients. *Comprehensive Psychiatry* **30**: 18–25.

Zatzick, D. F., C. R. Marmar, D. S. Weiss, and T. Metzler (1994). Does trauma-linked dissociation vary across ethnic groups. *Journal of Nervous and Mental Disease* **182**: 576–582.

Zetlin, S. B., and R. J. McNally (1991). Implicit and explicit memory bias for threat in posttraumatic stress disorder. *Behaviour Research and Therapy* **29**: 451–457.

Zinberg, N. E. (Ed.). (1977). The study of consciousness states: Problems and progress. In *Alternate states of consciousness*. New York, Free Press. 1–36.

Zlotnick, C., C. Ryan, I. Miller, and G. Keitner (1995). Childhood abuse and recovery from depression. *Child Abuse and Neglect* **19**: 1513–1516.

Zweig-Frank, H., J. Paris, and J. Guzder (1994). Psychological risk factors for dissociation and self-mutilation in female patients with borderline personality disorder. *Canadian Journal of Psychiatry* **39**(5): 259–264.

Index